The
Unprocessed
Plate

RHIANNON LAMBERT

DK
[RED]

The Unprocessed Plate

**Simple, flavorful UPF-free
recipes to transform your life**

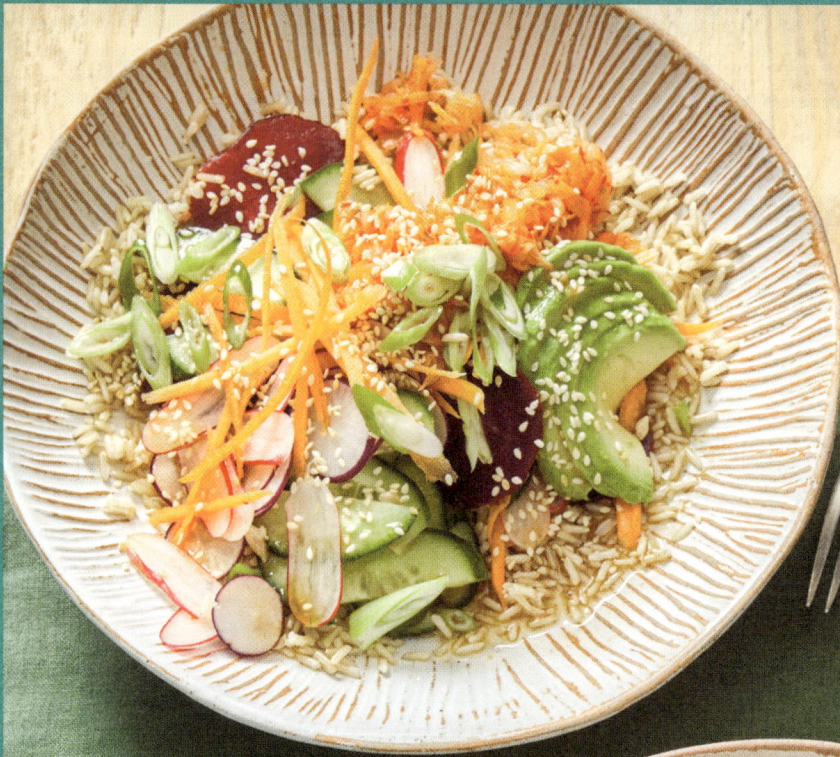

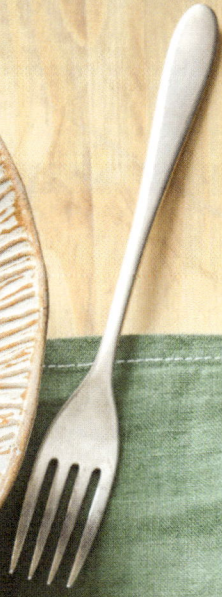

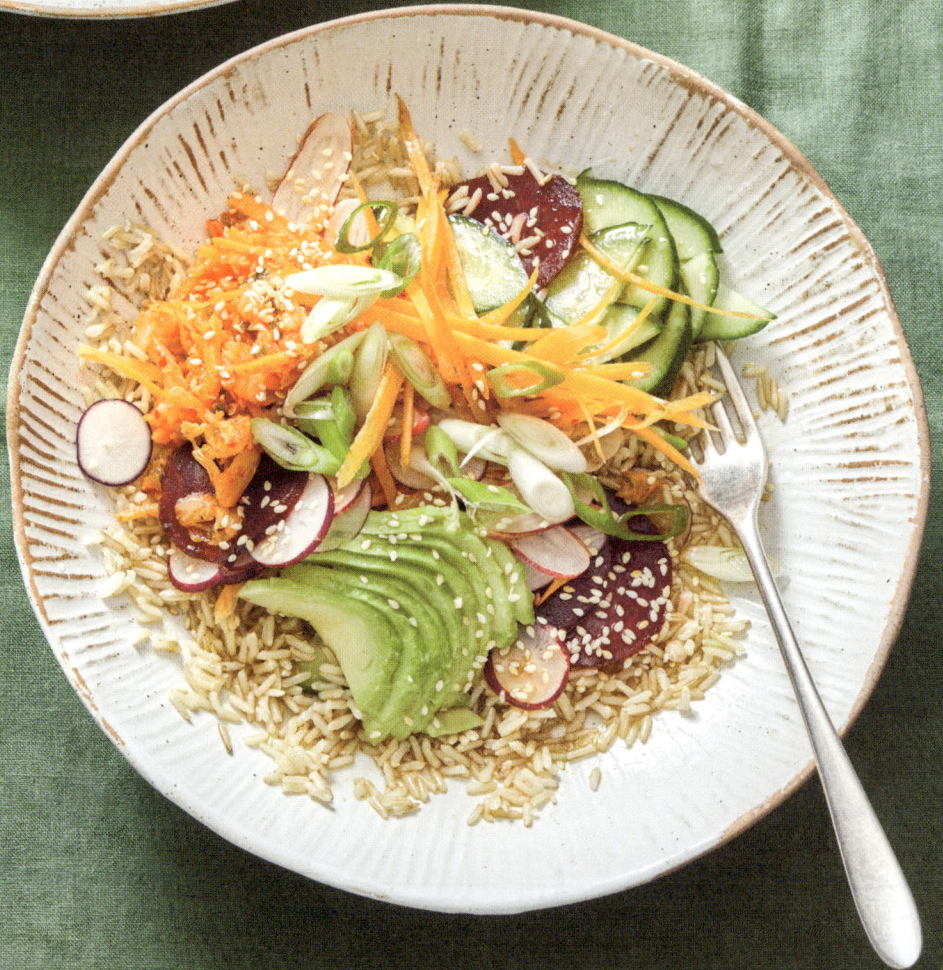

Contents

Foreword   006

Know your nutrition   008

What are ultra-processed foods?   010

How to build a UPF-free life   060

Recipes to unprocess your plate   088

Recipe notes   216

References   217

Index   218

About the author   222

Acknowledgments   223

Foreword

A few decades ago, fat was in the firing line. We were told to avoid it at all costs if we wanted to stay healthy. "Fat makes you fat," was the mantra. In reality, unsaturated fats are an important component of a healthy diet. Then, it was carbs' turn to be reviled—people made millions promoting low-carb diets rich in animal fats. Again, the reality is that low-carb, high-fat, or high-protein diets were never the secret to long-term good health.

Rarely out of the news, ultra-processed foods (UPFs) have become the latest nutritional pariah; a status that—given the broad range of products and added chemicals—is only partially deserved. In this timely book, Rhiannon helps cut through the almost deafening noise that currently surrounds these products.

While there certainly is good evidence that a diet rich in UPFs is linked to poorer health outcomes, it's not as simple as "cut out all UPFs." The latest science shows that not all UPFs have the same negative impact on health measures. In fact, some might be linked to a reduced risk of chronic disease, so simply throwing them all in the naughty corner is both unhelpful and impractical. UPFs are accessible and cheap and, if you avoid the worst of the worst, can form part of a healthy diet. With so much nonsense written about nutrition in the media at large, this book is a breath of fresh air.

In *The Unprocessed Plate*, Rhiannon outlines the often-ignored nuances in the UPF debate bringing some much-needed clarity. She tackles thorny issues that are often overlooked, like inequality and accessibility and their pivotal role in diet and health. Alongside solid evidence-based advice, Rhiannon shares delicious recipes that are not reliant on ingredients that are out of reach.

She also provides advice on how meal planning can be healthy, thrifty, and, importantly, slotted into a busy schedule—an essential for any modern cookbook to be genuinely useful.

Unsurprisingly, the mixed messages about UPFs have caused widespread confusion, which the food industry thrives on. This is why ZOE—the science and nutrition company I cofounded—has designed a new tool called the ZOE Processed Food Risk Scale, which allows people to understand the different health risks associated with processed foods.

We all want to eat well for a longer life, but as we are constantly buffeted by a conflicting maelstrom of messaging, many of us don't know where to turn. This book offers shelter from the storm.

The Unprocessed Plate takes the reader on a journey through the essentials of nutrition science and metabolism, the current evidence regarding UPFs' links to health, and provides simple, sensible advice to keep you and your family well-fed and healthy. Rhiannon's writing brings you a sense of calm, helping the reader take back control of their diet, while allowing them to spot and avoid nutrition misinformation, navigate our baffling food environment, and build a healthy, well-rounded diet for you and your family.

Tim Spector MD OBE

Professor of epidemiology Kings College London
Co-founder of ZOE Ltd and author of *Food for Life*

Know your nutrition

What exactly are UPFs, and how do they affect our health? Should we avoid them completely, or is there room for nuance? Enter *The Unprocessed Plate*—this book tackles one of the most contentious topics in modern nutrition: **ultra-processed foods (UPFs)**. Rarely has a term sparked such debate, fear, and misunderstanding, but within these pages I aim to answer everyone's most common concerns in a way that is clear, compassionate, and firmly rooted in science.

In a world saturated with conflicting messages about food and health, navigating nutrition has become a daunting challenge for many. Buzzwords, pseudoscience, and diet fads dominate headlines, leaving people confused, overwhelmed, and disconnected from the joy of eating. This book was born out of a desire to change that—to provide clarity, empower individuals with evidence-based knowledge, and help them embrace a healthy relationship with food that supports both their bodies and minds.

This is not just a book about what to avoid—it's a book about what to embrace. It's about finding balance, equipping yourself with the knowledge to make informed choices, and letting go of perfection in favor of progress. Throughout these pages, you'll find not only the latest scientific insights, but also practical strategies to navigate the modern food environment, no matter your circumstances.

The conversation around UPFs is nuanced and often deeply emotional. Food isn't just sustenance: it's tied to culture, identity, and our unique psychological and emotional connections. We all eat for different reasons, and not everyone has the same access, choices, or opportunities. As you delve into this book, I urge you to be kind to yourself. Acknowledge that everyone is doing their best to navigate their circumstances and live a happy, fulfilling life. This interplay between food and psychology is one of the reasons I entered this field—to help others find balance without judgment or guilt.

As a mother of two young boys, I understand firsthand the challenges of balancing family life, work, and health in today's fast-paced world. My hope is that this book becomes a guide you can turn to, whether you're striving to improve your diet, better understand the science, or simply make peace with your plate.

Together, let's cut through the noise, embrace a healthier relationship with food, and pave the way for a brighter, healthier future for ourselves and the generations to come.

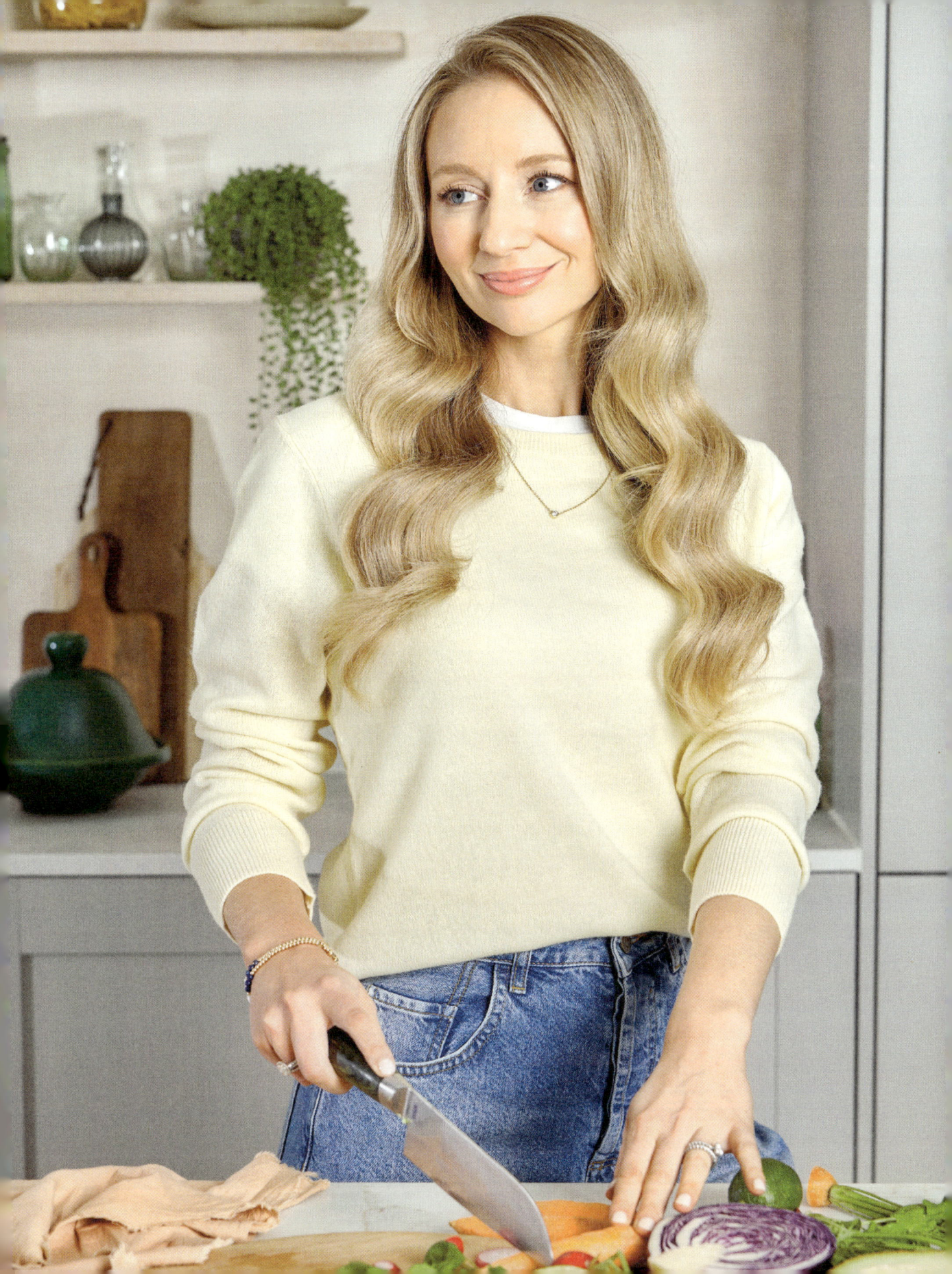

What are ultra-

Let's dive into the science, the facts, and the bigger picture! Without a deeper understanding of why UPFs exist in the first place, it's easy to feel overwhelmed or even confused by the debate surrounding them. Recognizing that these foods have a place in our modern diets, while also acknowledging that they're best consumed in moderation, is essential for maintaining both mental and physical well-being.

This chapter serves as your go-to guide to untangle the complex web of UPFs and their impact on our lives, arming you with the knowledge to make informed food choices. We'll explore the long-term effects of UPFs on health, including their connections to gut health, fertility, the environment, and social circumstances. You'll also gain clarity on the additives in your food: what they are, why they're used, and whether they're truly necessary.

processed foods?

How do we define processed and ultra-processed foods?

Currently, there are no universally agreed upon definitions of "processed" or "ultra-processed foods". The most commonly agreed upon framework that we have to date is the NOVA classification as defined by Carlos Monteiro. This is the framework we will use throughout this book when discussing, unprocessed, processed, and ultra-processed foods.

While the exact definitions are being agreed upon, what scientists do agree on is that regularly consuming excessive amounts of UPFs may have long-term health consequences. There might be situations when choosing UPFs is necessary, however, many people consume them without even realizing it. Without clear information, it can be challenging to make informed decisions about the place of UPFs in your diet.

The four NOVA food groups

Carlos Monteiro and a team of nutritional scientists developed the NOVA classification in response to their observations of changing dietary patterns in Brazil. The classification splits food products up into four different categories.

1. Unprocessed or minimally processed foods

Unprocessed or minimally processed food is food that has not been altered and/or has no added ingredients. Washed and bagged spinach, precut fresh fruit, or frozen vegetables are all minimally processed. They might have been made more convenient to consume, but their nutritional value hasn't been altered.

2. Processed culinary ingredients

Processed culinary ingredients are made from unprocessed foods through simple processing techniques. This group includes oil, butter, sugar, salt, dried herbs, and spices. Processed culinary ingredients are added to other foods, rather than eaten by themselves.

3. Processed foods

Processed foods are partially altered by adding sugar, oil, fat, salt, and other culinary ingredients to unprocessed or minimally processed foods, often to extend their shelf life. Foods like cheese, homemade or artisanal bread, and tofu have been processed, but not in a way that's necessarily negative for our health.

4. Ultra-processed foods

UPFs are foods that have been entirely altered and may have high levels of unhealthy fats, refined sugars, and/or salt. They also undergo industrial processes like hydrogenation and molding, and contain additives like dyes, stabilizers, flavor enhancers, emulsifiers, and defoaming agents. These foods are usually very calorie-dense and don't contain many, if any, valuable nutrients.

Processed food

Processing food involves changing its natural state; this is often done to prolong shelf life, make products safe to store and/or eat, enhance taste, or even increase nutritional value. This is not a bad thing—processing methods such as pasteurizing, canning, fermenting, freezing, and drying have enabled us to feed large and growing populations, particularly in difficult times when food is sparse. In fact, processed food is not just a thing of the present. Fermentation is as old as human civilization. The earliest form of fermentation was discovered by analyzing the stone mortars found at Natufian burial sites. The findings revealed that fermented cereals have been used for beer-brewing for over 13,000 years.

These days, most food products are processed to some degree. With the exception of freshly harvested, organic fruit and vegetables, it's almost impossible to avoid consuming processed food in today's modern society.

Ultra-processed food

UPFs are engineered to be convenient, extra tasty, and highly profitable for the companies that make them, and they have also helped to save lives. Ultra-processing food involves changing the natural state of foods using industrial-scale methods and ingredients that you may not recognize. A useful way of understanding the different types of food processing is by looking at the NOVA food classification. Through extensive research and analysis of nationwide food consumption, the Brazilian epidemiologist Carlos Monteiro and his team identified two distinct dietary patterns: one centered on traditional, minimally processed foods, and the other on ultra-processed foods. The NOVA classification was ultimately created to understand the relationship between food processing, nutrition, and health outcomes, helping to address the complexities of the modern food environment.

Your pantry at a glance

Here are how some familiar food items fit into the four NOVA food groups.

1. Unprocessed or minimally processed foods	2. Processed culinary ingredients	3. Processed foods	4. Ultra-processed foods
• Oranges	• Butter	• Cheese	• Soft drinks
• Carrots	• Olive oil/avocado oil	• Canned chickpeas	• Prepackaged meals
• Frozen spinach	• Flour	• Tofu	• Store-bought mayonnaise/ketchup/salad dressing
• Seeds	• Salt	• Kimchi	• Store-bought hummus
• Nuts	• Honey	• Canned or jarred fish	• Chips
• Packaged rice	• Vinegar	• Freshly made bread	• Breakfast cereals
• Oats	• Table sugar	• Salted or sugared nuts	• Jarred sauces
• Lentils/chickpeas/beans etc.		• Salted, dried, smoked, or cured meat or fish	• Packaged baked goods
• Dried fruit			• Flavored yogurts
• Dried herbs and spices			• Infant formula
			• Instant soups
			• Ice cream
			• Margarine

Why do we process food?

Processing food is important for numerous reasons. Often food is processed to extend shelf life and therefore increase its availability, or it can be processed to make it more convenient for us if we're on the go. Sometimes processing happens in order for food to meet food safety requirements, or to fortify and enrich products by adding ingredients that are good for our health. Some foods are processed to tailor them to certain dietary needs. Processing can also have the added benefits of reducing food waste, lowering price, and preserving nutritional quality.

Methods of food processing

Food processing is so ubiquitous in our society that there are some common methods that might be surprising.

Inclusion of additives

Additives such as flavorings, colorings, and emulsifiers manipulate aspects of food to make them more appealing (see pages 26–29 for more information).

Smoking

Smoking involves exposing food to smoke from burning materials, or other chemical methods, to preserve it. This technique is commonly used for meats, fish, and cheese, enhancing both flavor and shelf life.

Juicing

Fresh fruit and vegetables are juiced to create different products.

Packaging

The packaging of food is a form of processing and plays a key role in protecting food from contamination and extending its shelf life. This can range from simply washing and sealing items such as spinach leaves, to more advanced methods like vacuum packing, which removes air to slow spoilage and prevent oxidation.

Pasteurization

A heat treatment process used to kill harmful bacteria in foods like milk, juice, and eggs while maintaining quality and extending shelf life.

Heating

Heat processing methods such as boiling, roasting, and baking are used to cook or preserve food, often altering texture and flavor.

Freezing

This is a great way to preserve fresh foods, from meat and fish to fruit and vegetables.

Dried or dehydrated

Fruit, vegetables, and other food items can be dried or dehydrated to extend their shelf life. Dehydration is a more intensive process that removes even more moisture than drying.

Fermentation

This is a natural process in which bacteria, yeast, or other microorganisms break down sugars, often enhancing flavor and nutritional value.

Canning

Fruit, vegetables, and legumes, can be sealed in airtight containers after heat treatment to prevent spoilage.

The pros and cons of food processing

Processing food is a major part of how we access and consume it, and it's important to remember that while "processed food" might have negative connotations, processing food isn't all bad. Many everyday processes that place food in the processed category go largely unnoticed by consumers. However, it is important to be aware of and consider the positive and negative effects of food processing.

Positives

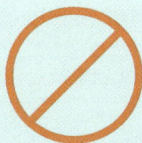

Catering to dietary needs: Food processing can help make foods more accessible for people with specific dietary needs. Examples include gluten-free products, fortified cereals (with added vitamins and minerals), or lactose-free and dairy alternatives.

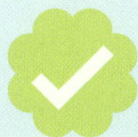

Convenience: Preprepared fruit, vegetables, canned soups, and ready-to-eat meals are all processed to make meals quicker and easier to prepare, while also helping to extend shelf life in the store and at home.

Food safety: Processing methods such as pasteurization, canning, and refrigeration help reduce the risk of foodborne illnesses by eliminating harmful bacteria and pathogens.

Reducing food waste: Food processing can help extend the shelf life of products that are perishable which may reduce the amount of food that is thrown away.

Negatives

Inclusion of added sugar, fat, and salt: Adding sugar, fat, and salt in controlled amounts can enhance flavor and texture in processed foods. However, our excessive consumption of these ingredients may increase our risk of some chronic diseases such as obesity, heart disease, and diabetes.

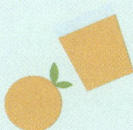

Overconsumption due to changes in food form: Processing can lead to overeating by altering the food's form and making it easier to consume large quantities.

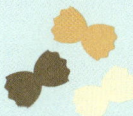

Reduction in nutrients: Many forms of processing, especially high-heat methods like boiling or frying, can reduce the nutrient content of foods. Water-soluble vitamins, like vitamin C and B vitamins, are particularly susceptible to degradation during cooking, leading to nutrient loss in processed foods.

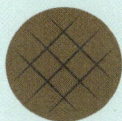

Introduction of contaminants: Some processing methods can introduce unwanted chemicals or contaminants, such as plastic from packaging, which may leaching into food, or adding preservatives or artificial additives, which may be linked to an increased risk of chronic illnesses.

How much UPF are we eating?

Ultra-processed foods now make up a huge portion of people's diets around the globe and there are many different reasons for this that vary across countries, cultures, and population demographics (see pages 18–19). However, the ubiquity of UPFs in people's diets is broadly due to the fact that they are created to be hyper-palatable and their long shelf life makes them convenient. As well as this, their formulation, presentation, marketing, and low price point often promote overconsumption.

In recent years, there has also been a global increase in both obesity and malnutrition. It's becoming apparent that it's not a coincidence that this is the case at the same time as our diets have become more heavily reliant on UPFs. Consumers are buying and eating less sugar, salt, and fat in its original state (NOVA group 2) but are in fact consuming more sugar, salt, and fat via UPFs (NOVA group 4). As our consumption of UPFs grows, more associations with serious illnesses (obesity, type 2 diabetes, and some cancers—page 56) come to light.

The most eaten UPFs
(percentage of calories in a typical diet)

This data is based on the UK, but is also reflective of diets in the US, Canada, and Australia, showing that UPF overconsumption is a global issue.

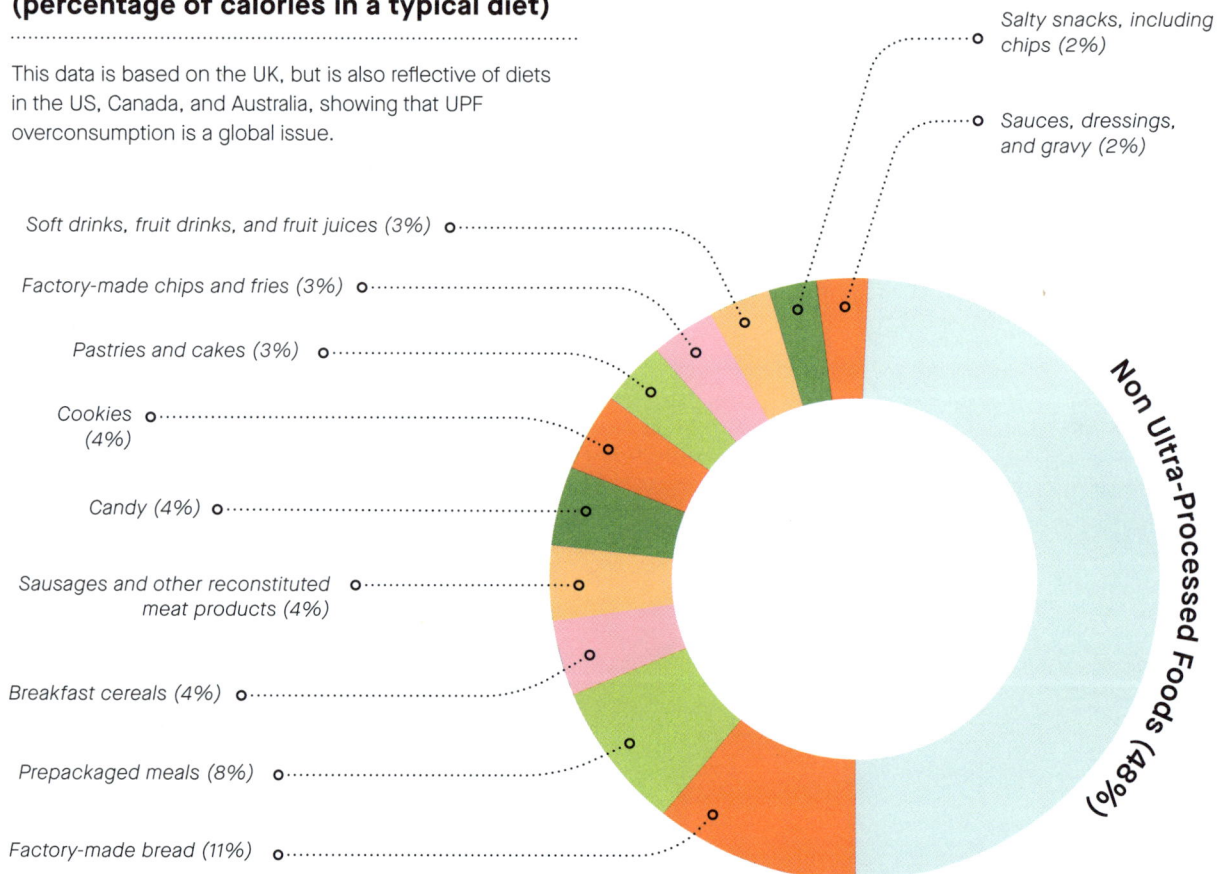

Salty snacks, including chips (2%)

Sauces, dressings, and gravy (2%)

Soft drinks, fruit drinks, and fruit juices (3%)

Factory-made chips and fries (3%)

Pastries and cakes (3%)

Cookies (4%)

Candy (4%)

Sausages and other reconstituted meat products (4%)

Breakfast cereals (4%)

Prepackaged meals (8%)

Factory-made bread (11%)

Non Ultra-Processed Foods (48%)

Here's a snapshot of the average percentage of energy of an adult's diet that is derived from UPFs around the world:

- US: 58%
- UK: 57%
- Australia: 40%
- South Africa: 39%
- Mexico: 30%
- Japan: 28%
- Chile: 28%
- Brazil: 22%
- South Korea: 21%
- Indonesia: 18%
- Italy: 18%

Are all UPFs equal?

How to categorize UPFs in more detail has long been debated by scientists. Using the original NOVA classifications as a basis (page 12), the ZOE science team, led by Tim Spector, is now researching the effects of UPFs on our health. The aim is to have a system that advises on which UPFs are healthy to consume, and which UPFs are best avoided or consumed minimally.

For example, sugar-sweetened beverages, processed meats, and prepackaged brown bread are all UPFs and therefore categorized as NOVA group 4; however, their effects on our health are all different. It is this nuance that scientists are hoping to resolve in the near future, and which will hopefully push the food industry to reformulate their products and inform consumers better.

As our consumption of UPFs grows, more associations with serious illnesses come to light.

What causes us to eat more UPFs?

When we eat any kind of food, whether it's processed or not, the food itself undergoes a degree of change and physical breakdown as we chew it. Foods that have been altered, or processed, to any degree to break down their complex structure of nutrients—what food scientists call "the food matrix"—are easier for us to absorb as a result. This means that foods in any processed form, whether minimally processed or ultra-processed, can be consumed more quickly and in larger amounts. For example, it's much easier to drink the juice of six oranges, where the fiber has been removed, than to eat six whole oranges intact. Similarly, a soft white roll is often easier to eat and can be consumed faster, than a more dense sourdough slice due to the different level of processing that these two breads have undergone.

Research suggests that UPFs may contribute to overeating because they are quickly digested, delaying the brain's ability to register fullness. This may disrupt the gut—brain communication and bypass hormones that signal satiety, leading to overeating. Additionally, the hyper-palatability of UPFs may further encourage excessive consumption (page 22). It's also worth noting that food manufacturers are aware that when they process food it's easier for you to digest, leaving you wanting more, and so offer products that will lead you to buy more, too.

How is privilege linked to UPFs?

Before diving any deeper into the role of UPFs in our diets, it's important to understand and appreciate the link between privilege and food.

Before 2018, a PubMed search using the term "ultra-processed" retrieved 137 papers. By November 2023, this search retrieved 1,558 papers, and this number is growing at a rapid rate. It is evident that the consumption of UPFs is growing globally. There are many driving factors behind this: environment, education, and culture changes across the world mean traditional diets are shifting to favor UPFs.

This rise in consumption of UPFs can, in part, be attributed to household income. Research shows that children from poorer households eat larger amounts of UPFs than others. This could be because these foods are highly palatable and more likely to be eaten (and less likely to end up in the trash); and it may also be because UPF products are often more affordable and require less time to prepare than lots of ingredients. Not all UPFs are necessarily negative for our health (page 44), but this disparity does potentially put us in a position where those less privileged are consuming higher amounts of salt, sugar, fat, and industrialized ingredients with little nutritional value. In combination with a lack of food education and cooking knowledge (trends on the rise among all income groups), this could have more serious health implications for those with low incomes.

Everyone deserves equal access to food education and a healthy diet and lifestyle, but we're often at the mercy of the food industry and food policies. When advocating for healthier food choices and changes in policy relating to

Who eats the most ultra-processed foods?

This map shows the UPF consumption from a selection of countries around the world, along with the privilege-linked factors that may impact these consumption levels.

Percentage figures

Share of the UPFs in adults' diets as a proportion of total calories consumed.

Demographics

Common sociodemographic groups of UPF eaters within each country.

♂ male gender

♀ female gender

⚥ younger age range

🏛 urban living

🎓 higher education level

🎓 lower education level

Ⓢ higher income level

Ⓢ lower income level

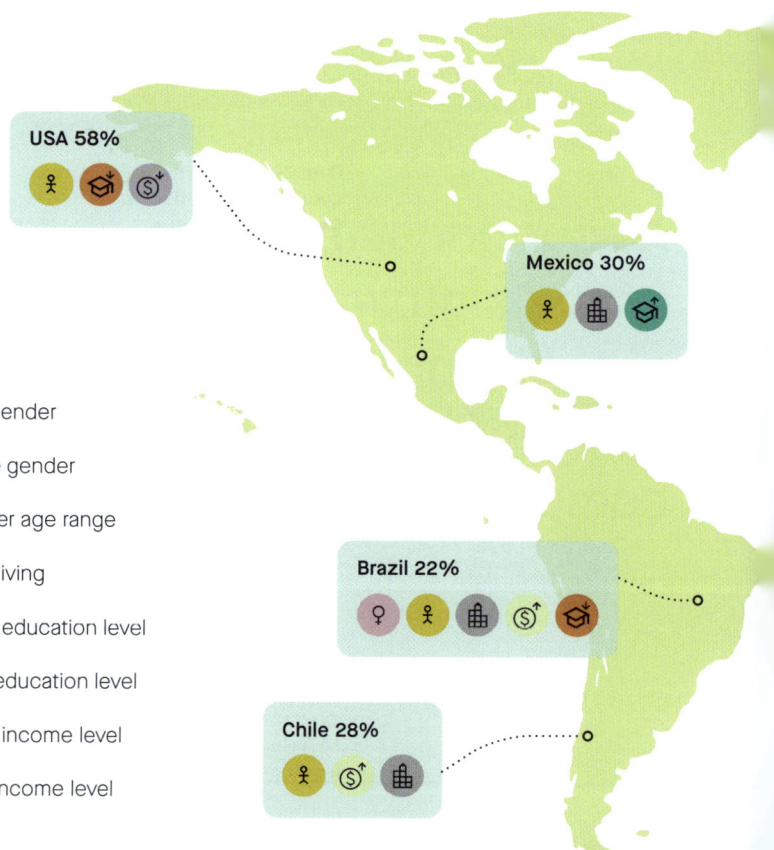

USA 58%

Mexico 30%

Brazil 22%

Chile 28%

UPFs, it's important to consider the effects this might have to those in less privileged sociodemographic groups and the access they have to food.

Culture matters

As you can see from the map below, average UPF intake varies greatly across countries, but within each country, a number of sociodemographic variables are independently associated with UPF intake. These are likely a reflection of social injustice. It's interesting to note that whereas in some countries those at a lower income level consume more UPFs, in others it is those who earn a higher income who consume the most UPFs, showing how privilege and the culture of what is considered a luxury food item changes depending on where you are in the world. The magnitude of the differences in UPF intake across sociodemographic levels are comparable to the magnitudes associated with increased risks of obesity and cardiometabolic disease, highlighting the importance of policy action and interventions to minimize the health inequalities relating to social injustice.

The growing cost of eating well is exacerbating health inequality

In 2025 the Food Foundation published a report that uses 13 key metrics to provide a snapshot of the current food environment. What it showed is that eating healthily has never been more expensive in the UK. Healthier food – based on its nutrient profile – is more than twice as expensive per calorie as "junk" food. Healthier options have increased in price at twice the rate of less healthy options in the past two years.

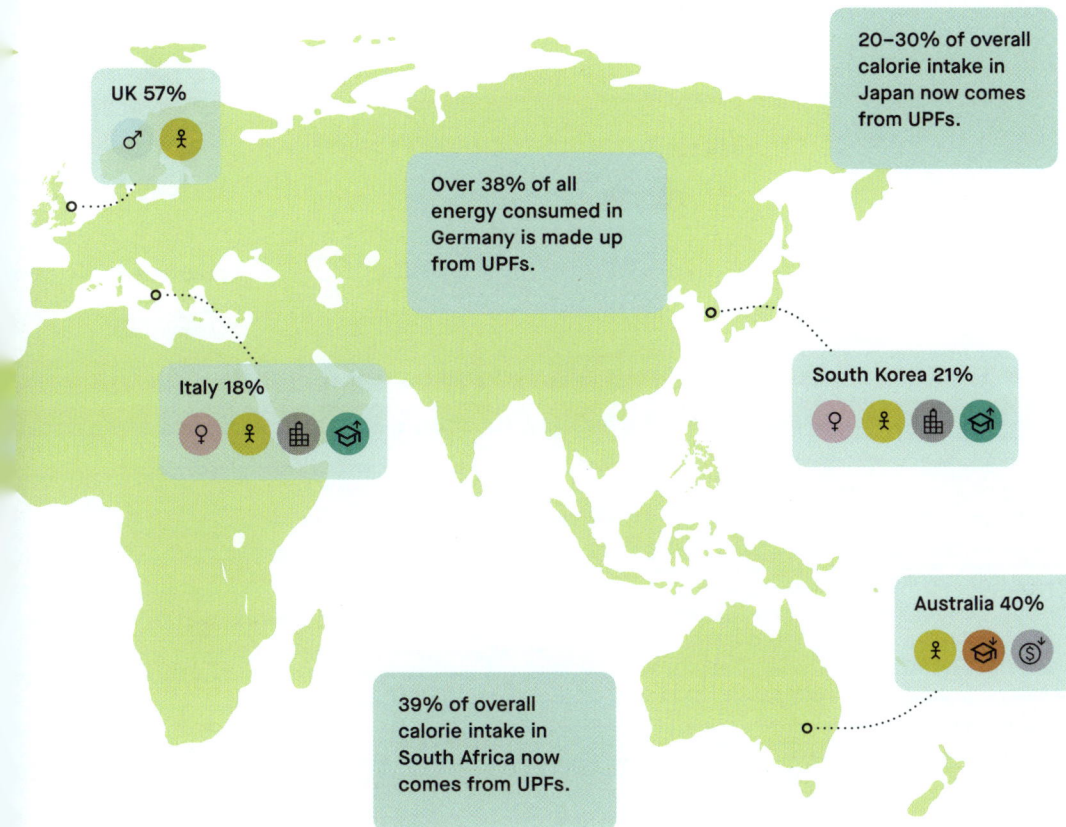

20–30% of overall calorie intake in Japan now comes from UPFs.

UK 57%

Over 38% of all energy consumed in Germany is made up from UPFs.

Italy 18%

South Korea 21%

Australia 40%

39% of overall calorie intake in South Africa now comes from UPFs.

How do we build a healthy relationship with food?

Before we dive into UPFs on a more scientific level, it's important to note that psychology and nutrition go hand in hand.

Everyone's nutritional goal should be to have a healthy relationship with food, but depending on birthplace, culture, and food education, relationships with food can vary. Understanding that we all have a unique relationship with food is essential though, and what seems healthy or acceptable to you might not be the same for others.

"Disordered Eating" (different from "Eating Disorders," which are classified using the *Diagnostic and Statistical Manual of Mental Disorders* and require professional medical help) has no official definition. Generally, it refers to disturbed and abnormal eating behaviors that might include skipping meals, restrictive dieting, or rigid rules around eating (for example, removing a major food group from your diet). It's important to note that a healthy relationship with food does not involve dieting and weight loss, despite this being the new normal for many.

Building a healthy relationship with food requires four key components

1. Regular eating

Eating at consistent intervals throughout the day helps regulate hunger and fullness cues, preventing extreme hunger that can lead to overeating. Skipping meals or going long periods without food can disrupt energy levels, mood, and overall well-being, making it harder to maintain a balanced diet.

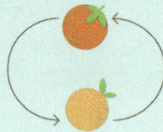

2. Being flexible with food choices

Avoiding certain foods or labeling them as "bad" can make them more desirable, often leading to cravings and overeating. By including all foods in moderation and listening to your body's natural cues, you remove the emotional charge around them, and normalizing them. Over time, this balanced approach can help reduce cravings and make eating feel more intuitive and enjoyable.

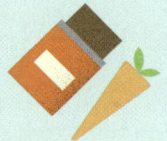

3. Eating with enjoyment

Food is more than just nutrition, it's part of social events, traditions, and everyday life. Being too rigid with food choices can lead to stress, guilt, and a strained relationship with eating. Allowing for spontaneity and making room for different foods, including those often labeled as 'treats,' supports a sustainable and healthy mindset around food.

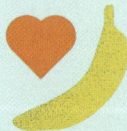

4. Diet variety (not cutting out food groups or particular foods unnecessarily)

Enjoying food is an important part of overall well-being, and feeling guilty about eating can take away from this experience. Rather than focusing solely on "good" or "bad" foods, shifting the focus to how food makes you feel, both physically and mentally, can help create a more positive relationship with eating.

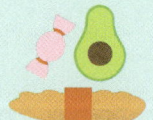

Common signs that you may not have a healthy relationship with food

- You feel guilty about eating.
- You avoid or restrict foods that are "bad" for you.
- You have developed a long list of rules surrounding the foods you can and cannot eat.
- You rely on calorie counters or apps to tell you when you're done eating for the day.
- You ignore your body's natural hunger cues.
- You have a history of yo-yo dieting or following the latest fad diets.
- You feel immense stress and anxiety when eating in social settings due to fear of what others may think of your food choices.

Working toward having a healthy relationship with food can be challenging, but it can also be a very rewarding journey. After a decade of working with clients on relationships with food, I assure you that it is entirely possible for everyone to improve their relationship with food and be happy and healthy.

It is important to note that a healthy relationship with food does not involve dieting and weight loss.

Tips for building a healthy relationship with food

- Don't discuss body shape and size around children.
- Never comment on somebody's shape or size.
- Create a relaxing, positive, and calm environment at mealtimes, especially if eating as a family.
- Don't allow technology at the dinner table. Play music instead and/or treat it as wind down time.
- Think, "what can I add in to my diet?" instead of dwelling on what to remove from it.
- Instead of counting calories, set yourself goals like "how many different colored vegetables can I eat this week?"
- If you need to reduce certain foods, aim to reduce them slowly rather than all at once.
- Identify if you are in a "binge-restrict cycle" and take steps to break it.
- Practice mindful eating where you engage all of the five senses as you eat—this can help build your trust with food and help you tune into hunger and satiety signals.
- Try intuitive eating—it's not for everyone, but this approach encourages listening to your body's hunger and fullness cues, rather than following external diets or restrictions. It focuses on making peace with food and developing a healthy relationship with eating.
- See a registered dietitian who specializes in eating disorders and/or relationship to food and body image.
- If you need support with your relationship with food, contact a therapist.

Are UPFs addictive?

Food addiction is frequently documented, but there is a very blurred line between what is "addiction" and what is simply a "poor relationship with food." Scientists are divided on this, with most stating that food addictions are not the same as an addiction to a substance like alcohol or nicotine.

Food addiction is typically characterized by a compulsion to consume excessive amounts of unhealthy "junk foods" such as high-calorie, sugary, salty, or fatty foods and drinks. When this compulsion evolves to the point where it becomes a requirement to function in daily life, the behavior develops into compulsive overeating. This is usually defined as eating far beyond the number of calories your body needs to function normally. Certain types of foods, such as high-sugar foods, react with the brain's dopamine receptors to create feelings of pleasure. Once you become used to a certain level of dopamine, you may start craving those items, which can manifest in what people refer to as becoming addicted to food.

How dopamine impacts our eating habits

Eating sugar- and fat-laden UPF foods may cause a dopamine response in the brain; however, with repeated consumption your dopamine receptors will become less receptive. Over time, this means you become reliant on these foods because, to get the same dopamine hit, you need to consume bigger quantities of these foods, placing you in a cycle of UPF overconsumption.

The dopamine cycle

UPFs may be considered addictive because after prolonged consumption our reward system becomes desensitized causing us to crave UPFs more and thereby exacerbate the problem.

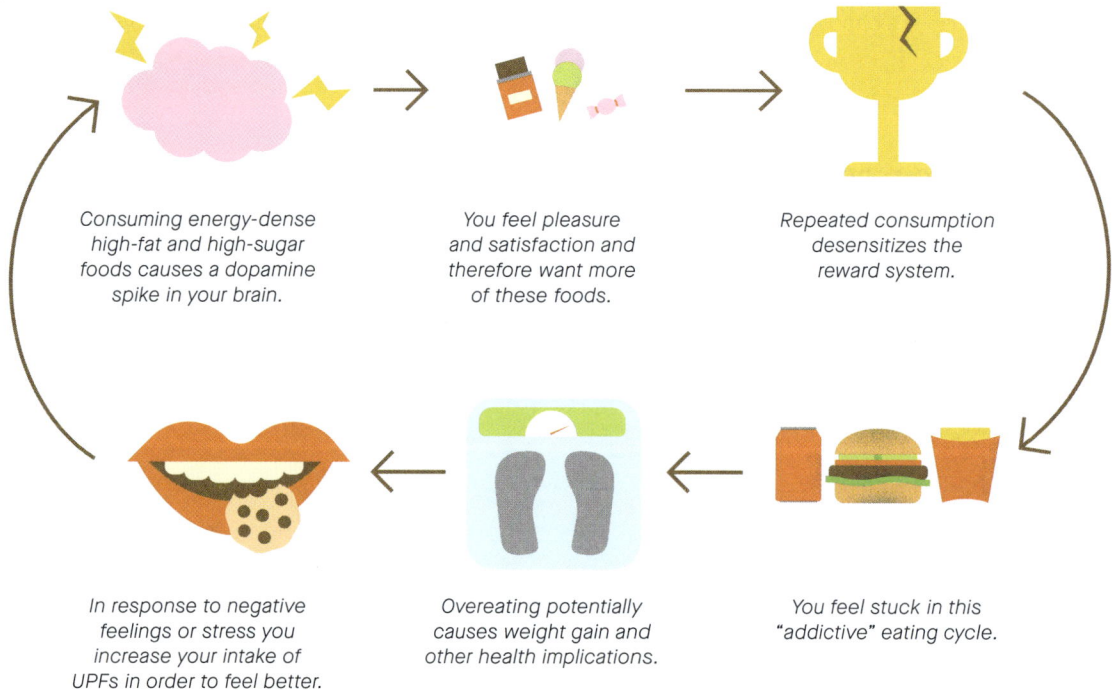

Consuming energy-dense high-fat and high-sugar foods causes a dopamine spike in your brain.

You feel pleasure and satisfaction and therefore want more of these foods.

Repeated consumption desensitizes the reward system.

In response to negative feelings or stress you increase your intake of UPFs in order to feel better.

Overeating potentially causes weight gain and other health implications.

You feel stuck in this "addictive" eating cycle.

Mind over matter

Food addiction is classified as a "behavioral addiction" or a "process addiction". The physical act of overeating is often a symptom of an underlying psychological issue, such as stress or low self-esteem. It's little wonder over the past decade in my clinic, that I have seen hundreds of cases of individuals who feel completely addicted to food. Behaviors include intense cravings, difficulty controlling intake, and continued consumption even when there are negative health consequences.

UPFs often contain high levels of both refined carbohydrates and fats, which make them extremely palatable. Unlike whole foods, which typically contain one dominant macronutrient, UPFs pack both refined carbs and fats into more equal proportions, amplifying their effects on the brain's reward systems.

It's also important to recognize that when food is processed to have a softer, smoother, less fibrous texture, it becomes easier to consume in larger quantities. Whole foods require more chewing and digestion, slowing down the eating process, whereas UPFs are absorbed more quickly. This can lead to overeating and may contribute to weight gain over time.

The rapid absorption of refined carbohydrates, combined with saturated fat, can lead to a quicker spike in dopamine, intensifying cravings and reinforcing addictive eating behaviors. This contrast highlights not only the balance of nutrients but also the quality of those nutrients as a factor in food addiction. So, the balance of nutrients in a chocolate bar mimics the way the brain responds to addictive substances, triggering more intense dopamine releases than either nutrient alone would. The simultaneous hit from carbs and fats creates a "supra-additive" effect, leading to greater stimulation of reward pathways and making that particular food more difficult to resist. This is similar to how addictive drugs work: substances like nicotine or alcohol that enter the bloodstream, and therefore reach the brain rapidly, have a higher potential for addiction.

Evidence shows that people exhibit addictive behaviors toward UPFs, including overconsumption, impulsivity, and difficulty in quitting. These behaviors are similar to those seen in substance use disorders, suggesting that UPFs can trigger addictive-like responses in vulnerable individuals. However, unlike known addictive substances like nicotine, there is no single chemical in UPFs identified as being directly responsible for addiction. While UPFs activate reward systems, critics argue that the absence of a specific addictive ingredient weakens the case for labeling them as addictive in the same way substances like alcohol or nicotine are classified.

The broad category of UPFs mapped out in NOVA (page 12), contains many different foods, some of which may not have strong addictive potential, such as certain meat alternatives. Additionally, homemade versions of foods containing sugar and fat could also seem addictive but are not classified as UPFs. This complicates the debate about which foods should be considered addictive, and much more research is needed in this area to understand this issue fully.

Which would you choose?

....

Combining fat and carbs in equal proportions activates reward systems (which is typical of UPFs). Salmon is higher in protein and fat, keeping you fuller for longer. Whereas chocolate is higher in combined carbs and fat, which is highly rewarding and provides a quick boost of energy, but provides less longer-lasting satiety. Type of fat also plays a role in the addictive potential of foods. In salmon, fat is primarily unsaturated, which has different effects on the body compared to the saturated fats in chocolate.

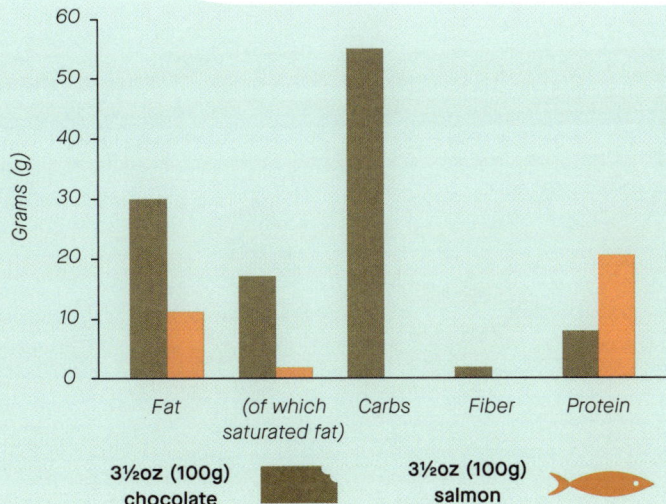

3½oz (100g) chocolate

3½oz (100g) salmon

How are calories linked to UPFs?

Calories were once hailed as the go-to dieter's tool to lose or gain body weight and are based on an equation that was devised by a man called Nicolas Clément in the early 19th century. Clément's definition was based on the amount of heat required to raise the temperature of one kilogram of water by one degree Celsius. The term "calorie" comes from the Latin word "calor," which means "heat," and it was originally used for fuel efficiency in steam engines. A world away from food at its conception, this unit of energy has now become the preferred unit of energy in the world of nutrition and dietetics.

In simple terms, if you consume more calories (energy) than your body requires to function, the more body fat you may gain and store. However, the concept of calories in relation to food is far more nuanced (see below). Throw into the mix the fact that agencies like the FDA allow a 20% wiggle room in calorie counts on packets, we can't really know for sure how much energy we are consuming.

1 calorie = 4184 joules of energy
1 calorie = 4.184 kilo joules (kj) of energy

Not all calories are equal

The way our bodies process the calories of different foods varies depending on their nutritional profile. For example, how can we compare 100 calories of steamed broccoli to 100 calories of chocolate and expect our body to react to that energy in the same way?

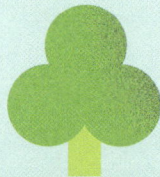

8¼oz (234g) steamed broccoli = 100 kcal

Protein	Fiber	Carbs	Fat
9.7g	8.9g	8.5g	1.2g
		of which sugars 4.7g	of which saturates 0.3g

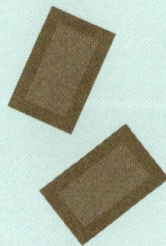

⅔oz (19.2g) milk chocolate = 100 kcal

Protein	Fiber	Carbs	Fat
1.4g	0.5g	10g	6g
		of which sugars 10g	of which saturates 3.6g

How do our bodies metabolize nutrition?

This diagram explains the thermic effect of food (TEF), which simply means the amount of energy it takes for your body to digest, absorb, and metabolize the food we eat. TEF is a component of our daily calorie expenditure, typically accounting for around 10% of total energy intake in healthy adults consuming a balanced diet. TEF varies depending on the type of food consumed. Protein and complex carbs have a higher thermic effect than fats or simple carbs because the body has to work harder to break them down, thus spending more energy and burning more calories to do so. Several factors influence TEF, including meal size, macronutrient composition, and individual characteristics, such as age.

Over 140 years ago, the varying energy absorption rates of different foods was noted by a scientist called Wilbur Olin Atwater. These days, his research has been built on to understand how the body metabolizes nutrients in our food and how this affects different people.

UPFs are often lower in protein and fiber, and higher in salt, fat, and sugar, which makes the calories (energy) they contain much easier for our bodies to access and absorb. However, food manufacturing has evolved far more rapidly than our bodies have. We originally evolved in a food environment where nutrients were harder to come by, and required more effort to digest. Diets based on whole foods that are rich in plants, fiber, and naturally occurring protein, demand more from our digestive systems, and help regulate appetite and energy balance more effectively. When energy becomes too easy to consume, as is often the case with ultra-processed options, the risk of overeating and weight gain rises.

This may sound alarming, but it's important to keep in mind that we eat food, not numbers. By focusing on the quality of your diet and consuming all food groups in a balanced manner, your body will be healthier. Counting calories does not help us build a healthy relationship with food (page 20) but noting the different ways in which foods impact us is key.

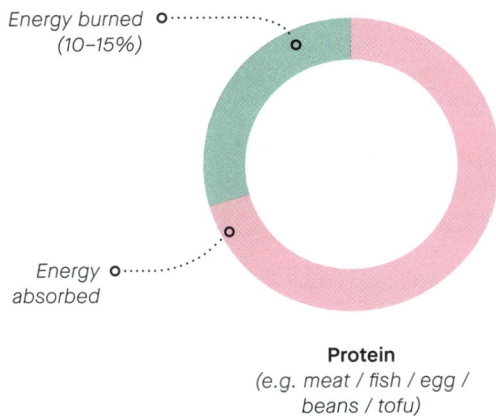

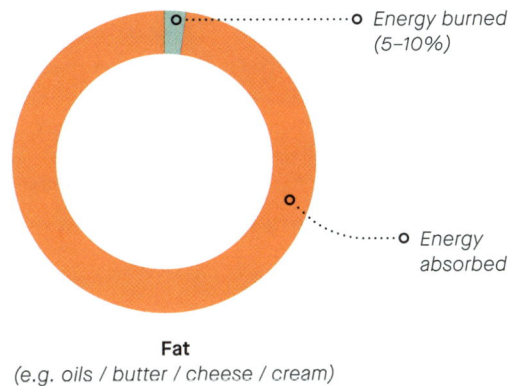

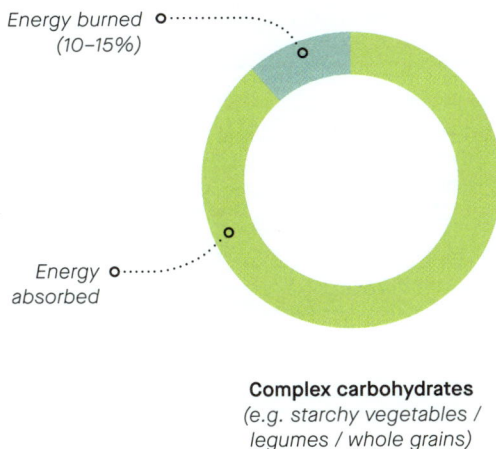

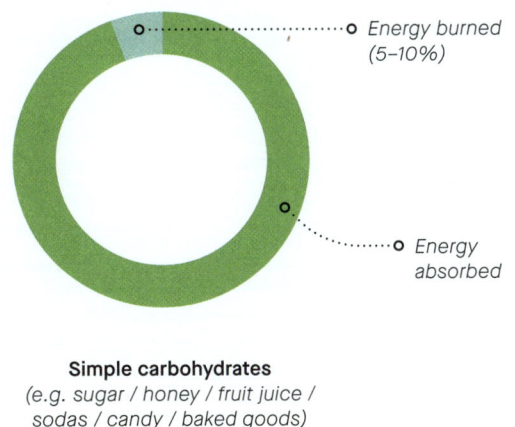

Energy burned (10–15%)
Energy absorbed

Protein
(e.g. meat / fish / egg / beans / tofu)

Energy burned (5–10%)
Energy absorbed

Fat
(e.g. oils / butter / cheese / cream)

Energy burned (10–15%)
Energy absorbed

Complex carbohydrates
(e.g. starchy vegetables / legumes / whole grains)

Energy burned (5–10%)
Energy absorbed

Simple carbohydrates
(e.g. sugar / honey / fruit juice / sodas / candy / baked goods)

Why do we use food additives?

Food has many qualities: texture, flavor, color, appearance and, of course, nutritional value. These are all elements that manufacturers of food want to preserve or manipulate to create an appealing product, make nutritional claims, and extend shelf life. To do this, they use additives. Food additives are substances that are added to processed foods—you won't find them in unprocessed or minimally processed foods. They are deemed safe by authorities for human consumption, and they have a variety of uses: to improve food safety, increase the amount of time a food can be stored, or to modify the sensory properties of food.

However, just because an additive is approved for use, that doesn't mean it can be added to any food and in any quantity. Legislation dictates when an additive may be used and how much can be added to a food item (this then varies across different food groups and additives).

Food additives tend to be made from either plants, animals or minerals and are sometimes chemically synthesized. There are thousands of food additives—too many to list here—but we can group them into three main categories (see below). To understand UPFs in more detail, and the nuance between them being simply "good" or "bad," it's necessary to understand this food language.

The main categories of food additives

While there are many different food additives, we can broadly categorize them into the three categories below in order to better understand why we use them.

1. Flavoring agents

These are added to foods to modify taste, smell, and aroma. Some common flavorings are:

- MSG (Monosodium Glutamate)
- Disodium Inosinate
- Disodium Guanylate
- Salt (Sodium Chloride)
- Vanillin
- Potassium Chloride
- Glycerol

2. Enzyme preparations

Enzymes are proteins that cause a reaction during food preparation (for example when making baked goods, wine, or cheese). They help move the process along and are used as alternatives to chemical-based technology. Enzyme preparations may or may not end up in the final food product. Some common enzymes are:

- Yeast
- Rennet
- Lysozyme
- Invertase
- Glucose Oxidase
- Transglutaminase

3. Other additives

There are many reasons additives are added to foods; they can alter flavor or color and aid with preservation. When food needs to be packaged and have shelf life, additives are added and become a part of the food. This category also includes artificial sweeteners (page 41). Some common additives are:

- Aspartame
- Sucralose
- Curcumin (coloring)
- Citric Acid
- Lecithins
- Xanthan Gum
- Guar Gum
- Sodium Nitrate

What do the authorities say?

It is important to note that the World Health Organization (WHO) suggests that international authorities monitor food additives closely. WHO encourages national authorities to monitor and ensure that food additives in food and drinks produced in their countries comply with permitted uses, conditions, and legislation. National authorities should oversee the food business, which carries the primary responsibility for ensuring that the use of a food additive is safe and complies with legislation.

While food additives are deemed safe, there have been many concerns over the years with regard to certain aspects of additives used in UPFs. For example, slushy drinks are not recommended for children under the age of four due to the levels of glycerol (sugar alternative) in them, which can cause severe headaches and nausea. Children have been hospitalized from excessive consumption of slushy drinks.

Underlying conditions can also dictate whether you need to steer clear of some (or all) additives in food, but this can be incredibly difficult to navigate and you'll need advice from a medical professional to manage this properly.

To put this knowledge of additives into practice, turn to page 62, which breaks down how to understand the ingredients lists and labeling on our most commonly purchased food items.

While food additives are deemed safe, there have been many concerns over the years with regard to certain aspects of UPFs.

What else is in our food?

Fortifiers

Fortifiers are added to food products to enhance nutrition and promote health, so you should not be put off by them. For example, in 1998, the UK government mandated that non-wholemeal wheat flour must be fortified with key nutrients to improve public health. That's why on packaged bread, the ingredients list will often begin with: Wheat Flour [Wheat Flour, **Calcium Carbonate**, **Iron**, **Niacin**, **Thiamine**], Water, Yeast, Salt. The additives highlighted here are simply fortifiers included to benefit health.

Interestingly, Switzerland fortifies on average 250 food products with folic acid (folic acid is a synthetic version of vitamin B9 [folate] that helps the body make healthy red blood cells). Since 2009, Australia has also fortified bread flour with folic acid, and in 2021 the UK government announced that folic acid will become a mandatory additive to non-wholemeal flour—coming into effect at the end of 2026, the aim of this initiative is to reduce neural tube defects by 20%. In Argentina, wheat flour must by law be fortified with iron, thiamine, riboflavin, niacin, and folic acid, while in Fiji studies have reported improved nutrient status due to wheat flour fortification.

What do common food additives do to our food?

Approved additives can be found in lots of different food products that we consume. Here are some common examples and the reasons why they include additives.

Foaming agents *maintain uniform aeration of gases in foods*

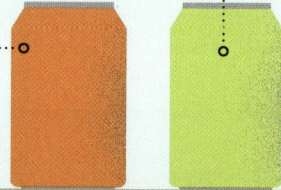

Soft drinks
- *Sulphite ammonia caramel is added to increase palatability and impart color.*
- *Phosphoric acid is added to impart tartness, reduce growth of bacteria and fungi, and improve shelf life.*
- *Caffeine is added for flavor.*

Flavor enhancers *increase the power of a flavor*

Glazing agents *improve appearance and can protect food*

Flour treatments *improve baking quality*

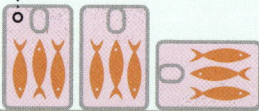

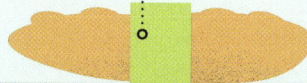

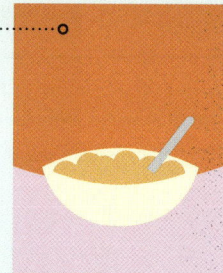

Mayonnaise
- *Lemon juice concentrate is added to provide acidity, which aids in emulsification, enhances flavor, and helps preserve freshness.*
- *Flavorings are added to enhance or modify the taste of mayonnaise, often to make it more palatable.*
- *The antioxidant calcium disodium EDTA is added to prevent the oxidation of fats and oils, helping to preserve the color, flavor, and texture.*
- *Paprika extract is likely added in a small amount to give mayonnaise a slightly deeper yellow color.*

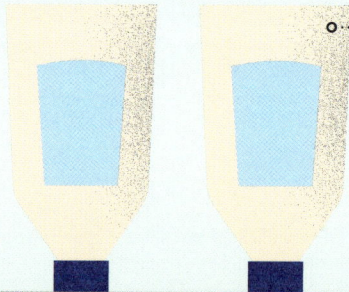

Food acids *maintain the right acid level*

Anticaking agents *stop ingredients from becoming lumpy*

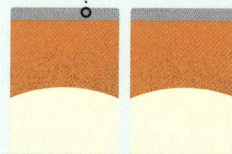

Baked beans
- *Modified corn starch is used as a thickening agent to give the sauce a smooth, consistent texture, and help it coat and stick to the beans.*
- *Spice and herb extracts are added to add depth of flavor without changing the texture of the sauce.*

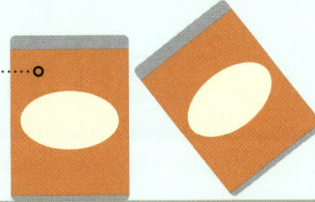

Colors *enhance or add color*

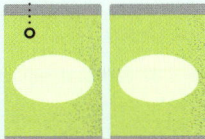

Emulsifiers *stop fats from clotting together*

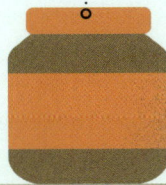

Antioxidants *prevent foods from oxidizing or going rancid*

Humectants *keep food moist*

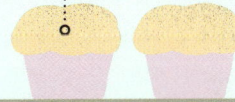

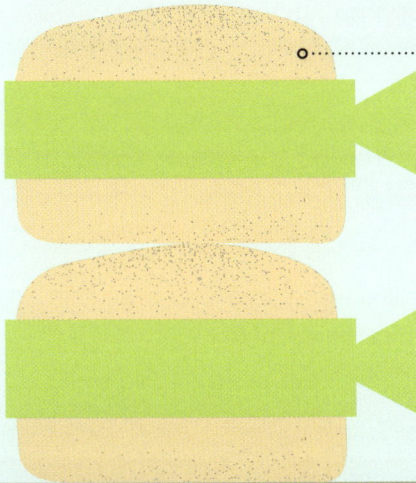

Store-bought bread
- *Soy flour is used to enhance the texture and moisture retention of bread, making it softer and longer-lasting.*
- *The preservative calcium propionate is added to extend the shelf life by preventing mold growth and bacterial contamination.*
- *Caramelized sugar is added to provide a mild sweetness and improve the bread's brown color and flavor.*
- *Emulsifiers are used to improve dough consistency, enhance the texture of the bread, and extend its freshness.*
- *Palm fat and oil contributes to the bread's softness and richness, improving the overall texture.*

Thickeners and vegetable gums *enhance texture and consistency*

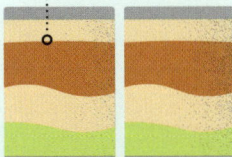

Preservatives *stop microbes from multiplying and spoiling food*

Gelling agents *alter the texture of foods through gel formation*

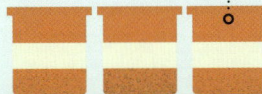

Does adding preservatives make something a UPF?

For as long as humans can remember, we have been trying to manipulate our food and make it last as long as possible. Food hasn't always been so readily available and sadly still isn't for some parts of the world. Dating back to the 14th century, humans used techniques such as salting and smoking with meat and fish to ensure it didn't go off. However, today, food safety is far more complex and requires vigorous testing and protocol, hence preservatives have become the norm in our food system, enhancing taste and shelf life. Preservatives are additives (page 26): additional items we add to food, working to prevent spoilage and deterioration of food. Getting poorly from food is to be avoided at all costs; food poisoning isn't only unpleasant, it can also be life threatening. Microorganisms (bacteria, molds, and yeasts) are always ready to get to work on the food we consume, therefore we must add preservatives to stop this antimicrobial activity.

Types of spoilage (and the reasons we need preservatives)

Preservatives are crucial to prevent microorganisms from growing and spoiling food products, and decreasing the risk of serious illness.

1. Water
Water is essential for all life. In order for microorganisms to grow, foods must contain a minimum of 18–20% water, which is why microorganisms do not grow in foods such as dried pasta, rice, and beans.

2. pH
Food acidity plays a role in spoilage. In foods with a pH of 5 or less, molds can form more easily. Citrus fruit, for example, has high acidity so mostly avoid bacterial spoilage but are susceptible to mold contamination.

3. Physical structure
Microorganisms cannot penetrate solid foods like meat in their original state, but a raw, ground version (such as ground meat or burger patties) can deteriorate rapidly because microorganisms exist both within the loosely packed ground meat as well as on the surface.

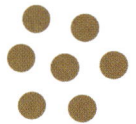

4. Chemical composition
Fruit supports organisms that metabolize sugars and carbohydrates, whereas meat supports protein decomposers. Starch-hydrolyzing bacterial cells and molds can be found on foods such as potatoes and rice.

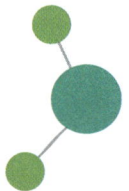

5. Oxidization
Oxidization is a type of chemical reaction that occurs when a substance reacts with oxygen, for example, the browning of an apple once it is cut and the flesh is exposed.

Preservatives used today are either natural or synthetic. Natural preservatives can be sourced from plants, animals, fungi, and algae, and also include using salt and sugar. For example, natamycin is commonly used to preserve cheese and is a bacteria present in our soil.

Our physical environment (temperature, light, and touch) impacts the preservation of food. For example, a fridge temperature is usually too cold for the growth of most spoilage organisms and a freezer temperature halts the growth of microbes completely. Whereas, in a warmer environment, these microbes tend to flourish. This is why food packaging often includes recommendations on how to store food, and why certain additives are added during processing. Some practical examples of protective storage to prevent spoilage include the canning of fish and tomato sauce, drying fresh fruit to make dried fruit, and adding salt to cabbage to make sauerkraut.

When food is properly vacuum sealed (for example, in cans or plastic packaging) oxygen is removed, creating an environment where harmful aerobic microbes (those that require oxygen to grow) cannot survive. However, if food is not prepared correctly and becomes contaminated with *C. botulinum*, a type of bacteria that can live without oxygen, it can thrive in vacuum-sealed foods. This can lead to the production of dangerous toxins, and the consumption of food contaminated with these toxins can result in botulism, a serious illness. This is why UPFs (for example, canned soups) have a place in our food system; by adding key preservatives, certain foods can be safely stored for longer on store shelves and in our kitchens without spoiling and causing food safety concerns.

Methods of food preservation

Humans have been using both physical and chemical methods of preservation for thousands of years. Physical preservation involves different techniques of alteration, whereas chemical preservation involves adding specific ingredients to food. The two methods are not mutually exclusive and one isn't better than the other.

Physical ○ ·········· Preservatives ·········· ○ Chemical

Drying *removes moisture from food, inhibiting microbial growth and enzymatic activity.*

Freezing *reduces microbial and enzymatic activity at low temperatures.*

Vacuum sealing *removes air from packaging to prevent oxidation and microbial contamination.*

Pasteurization *uses heat to kill harmful bacteria while preserving food quality.*

Canning *involves sealing food in airtight containers and heating to destroy pathogens and spoilage organisms.*

Irradiation *exposes food to controlled radiation to eliminate bacteria, parasites, and pests without affecting freshness.*

Salting *preserves food by drawing out moisture and creating a high-sodium environment that inhibits microbial growth.*

Pickling *uses acidic solutions to lower pH and prevent spoilage.*

Smoking *exposes food to antimicrobial and antioxidant compounds, extending shelf life.*

Sugaring *creates a high-sugar environment that dehydrates microbes and prevents fermentation.*

Antimicrobial *methods use sulphates, benzoates, sorbates, nitrates, sodium salts, and fruit extracts (e.g. grapes and pine).*

Antioxidant *methods use vitamins, polyphenols, thiols, phosphates, succinates, and lactates.*

What are emulsifiers?

Chemical emulsifiers are added to foods to bind ingredients that have different molecular polarities (like water and oil), making them more stable and preventing separation. This allows for food products to have longer shelf life and enhances texture; for this reason, emulsifiers are currently extensively used in the food industry in a variety of UPFs.

The European Food Safety Authority (EFSA) has concluded that there are no safety concerns regarding the use of common emulsifiers (see list, right). However, carboxymethyl cellulose, also called cellulose gum, (CMC), a type of cellulose, and polysorbate 80 (P80), have shown potential to disrupt the human gut microbiome. Research indicates that the ingestion of CMC and P80 can lead to a reduction in beneficial gut bacteria, changes that are also observed in those with IBS (see page 54 for more information on gut health.)

We currently need more research in humans on the impact of emulsifiers on our health, but there is growing debate around whether these emulsifiers contribute to inflammation and poor gut health alongside other UPF ingredients. More recently, a 2025 trial provided the first strong evidence linking emulsifiers to worsening symptoms and inflammation in people with Crohn's disease, however, more research is needed before firm recommendations can be made. Overall, being mindful of emulsifier intake may be beneficial, but there is not yet enough evidence to conclude they are a direct cause of poor health.

Common emulsifiers found in processed food items

- **Lecithins** – Derived from soybeans, sunflower seeds, canola, egg yolks, cheese, whey, or fish.
- **Monoglycerides and diglycerides** – Derived from coconut, palm, palm kernel, soy, canola, sunflower, cottonseed, corn, olive, tallow, or lard.
- **Guar gum** – The ground endosperm of seeds from strains of the guar plant, *Cyamopsis tetragonolobus.*
- **Xanthan gum** – Fermentation of a carbohydrate in a pure-culture of *Xanthomonas campestris,* recovered from the fermentation broth by precipitation.
- **Carrageenans** – Carbohydrate (polysaccharide) extracted from red seaweed.
- **Celluloses** – Microcrystalline cellulose, also known as cellulose gel or its abbreviation MCC. It is a naturally noncaloric indigestible dietary fiber that is widely used in food among other products.

How do emulsifiers work?

Emulsifier molecules have a water-loving (hydrophilic) end, which is attracted to water, and a water-hating (hydrophobic) end, which is attracted to oils.

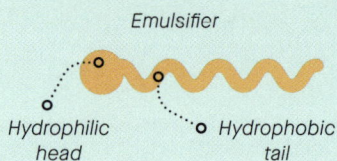

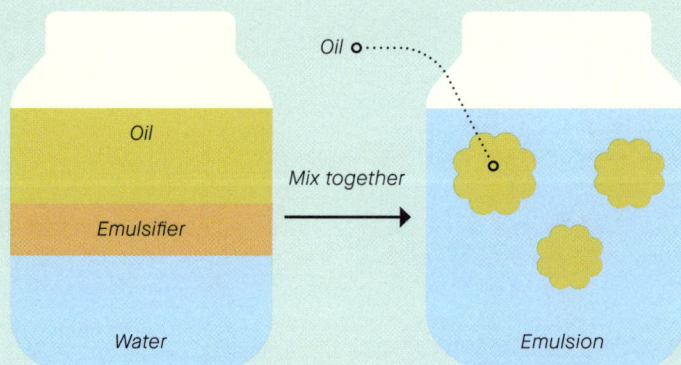

Emulsifier

Hydrophilic head

Hydrophobic tail

Oil

Emulsifier

Water

Mix together

Oil

Emulsion

Processed and ultra-processed foods found at your local supermarket that usually contain emulsifiers

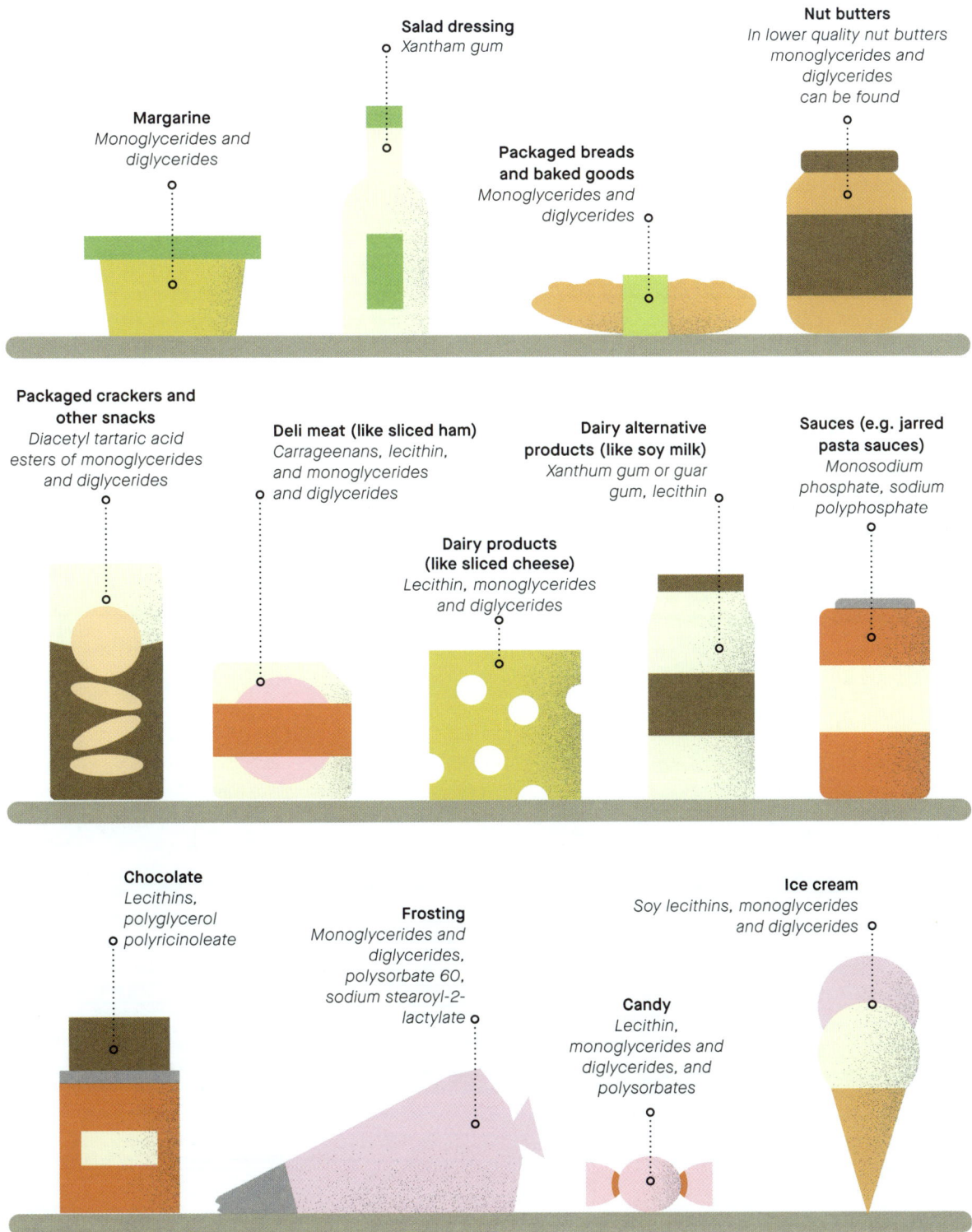

Salad dressing
Xantham gum

Nut butters
In lower quality nut butters monoglycerides and diglycerides can be found

Margarine
Monoglycerides and diglycerides

Packaged breads and baked goods
Monoglycerides and diglycerides

Packaged crackers and other snacks
Diacetyl tartaric acid esters of monoglycerides and diglycerides

Deli meat (like sliced ham)
Carrageenans, lecithin, and monoglycerides and diglycerides

Dairy alternative products (like soy milk)
Xanthum gum or guar gum, lecithin

Sauces (e.g. jarred pasta sauces)
Monosodium phosphate, sodium polyphosphate

Dairy products (like sliced cheese)
Lecithin, monoglycerides and diglycerides

Chocolate
Lecithins, polyglycerol polyricinoleate

Frosting
Monoglycerides and diglycerides, polysorbate 60, sodium stearoyl-2-lactylate

Ice cream
Soy lecithins, monoglycerides and diglycerides

Candy
Lecithin, monoglycerides and diglycerides, and polysorbates

What are the most common everyday UPFs?

It can be very confusing to navigate the world of UPFs. Items that appear to be fresh and labeled as "natural" can still contain a whole variety of additives, although this is not necessarily a bad thing (page 26). If you're able to recognize some of the most common UPFs, then you will be in a better position to make informed choices regarding your diet.

Occasionally enjoying the items listed here isn't a problem—it's when some become frequently consumed that it raises health concerns. However, in the case of some UPFs, like plant-based milk alternatives, research suggests that they can in fact have a positive impact on our health (see opposite).

Some brands are now choosing to make items (especially frozen products) without additives, where possible, but this is a tricky move for the food industry, where shelf life, profits, and food wastage all need to be considered and balanced.

What goes into your shopping basket?

In the US, more than half of the average food shop is now made up of UPFs. Here are some of the most common food products placed in shopping baskets.

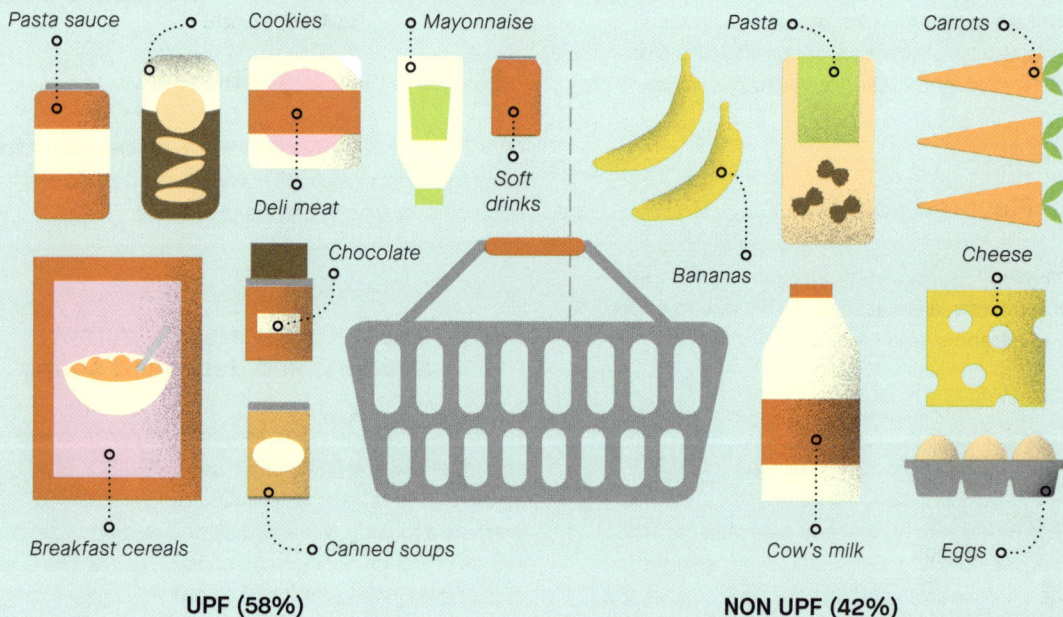

Pasta sauce

Cookies

Mayonnaise

Pasta

Carrots

Deli meat

Soft drinks

Chocolate

Bananas

Cheese

Breakfast cereals

Canned soups

Cow's milk

Eggs

UPF (58%)

NON UPF (42%)

1   Baked beans

Although considered a pantry staple for many, canned baked beans often contain added sugars, modified starches, and preservatives, which classify them as UPFs.

2   Breakfast cereals and granola

Many popular breakfast cereals contain refined sugars and artificial additives yet are marketed as a healthy way to start the day. These cereals cause rapid blood sugar spikes and crashes, which can lead to poor concentration and energy dips in both adults and children. We also now have evidence to suggest that those who consume a high-sugar breakfast will likely consume more sugar across the course of the day than those who consume a more balanced breakfast. Excess sugar also contributes to weight gain, dental cavities and increased risk of type 2 diabetes. Despite "wholegrain" or "fortified" labels, high sugar content could outweigh these benefits. Try making your own granola using the recipe on page 95.

3   Canned soups

Many canned or prepackaged soups branded as "healthy" are ultra-processed, containing additives, flavor enhancers, and preservatives to prolong shelf life.

4   Flavored yogurts

Many brands of flavored yogurts, including "low-fat" or "light" versions, are classed as UPFs due to added sugars, sweeteners, and flavorings.

5   Instant or "on-the-go" oats

On-the-go or flavored quick-cook oats often contain added sugars, flavorings, stabilizers, and anticaking agents to improve taste and texture. What's more, they might not always be vegetarian due to the glazing agent shellac, which is made from beetles.

6   Plant-based milk alternatives

Drinks like almond, oat, and soy milk are typically labeled as UPFs due to the inclusion of oils and additives like stabilizers and emulsifiers, while their dairy counterparts (like cow's milk and plain yogurt), are labeled as minimally processed. Recent research shows, however, that some fortified plant-based drinks can have similar or even better nutritional profiles than dairy products. For example, soy-based milks have fewer calories, less saturated fat, similar protein content, and a low glycaemic index, yet contain similar calcium content per cup, to dairy milk. They also contain beneficial components like polyphenols, folate, and trace minerals, which can offer potential health benefits.

7   Prepackaged cakes, muffins, and cookies

These items are high in saturated fat, refined sugars, and a range of artificial preservatives. Saturated fat is associated with increased levels of low-density lipoprotein (LDL) cholesterol, which can lead to heart disease. High consumption of these baked goods can also increase the risk of type 2 diabetes and obesity due to their calorie-dense yet nutritionally poor profile.

8   Store-bought hummus

While hummus is traditionally made with whole ingredients, many commercial versions contain preservatives and flavor enhancers, making them ultra-processed.

9   Ready-to-eat meals, instant noodles, and packaged soups

These convenience meals are often very high in sodium, preservatives, and flavor enhancers like MSG. High sodium intake is a known contributor to high blood pressure and heart disease. Just one serving of some brands of instant noodles can contain around one quarter of your daily intake of salt as an adult. While quick to prepare, convenience foods like this are nutritionally poor and often lack any real fiber, vitamins, or minerals.

10   Frozen fish sticks

Although made from fish, many frozen breaded fish stick brands contain emulsifiers, stabilizers, and artificial flavorings. Read more about them on page 39.

11   Soft drinks and energy drinks

These are some of the most heavily consumed UPFs, particularly among children and teenagers, and contain syrups or added sugars. Regular consumption of sugary beverages is directly linked to obesity, type 2 diabetes, and tooth decay. Research suggests that reducing soft drink intake should be a priority in tackling adolescent obesity. Interestingly, there is also research to suggest that consuming one or more soft drink servings daily can cause higher aggressive behaviour scores, attention problems, and withdrawn behaviour in children, with these effects increasing with higher soft drink consumption. Energy drinks are particularly harmful due to their high caffeine content, which can also lead to anxiety and sleep disturbances, all of which can be detrimental to both adults and children. Even bottled water with fruit flavors often contains sweeteners, flavorings, and preservatives, classifying it as a UPF despite the "natural" fruit label.

12   Margarine and spreadable butters

These products often contain emulsifiers, preservatives, and colorings, making them UPFs. They can be beneficial for lowering cholesterol as a butter alternative.

13   Processed meats (sausages, bacon, sliced ham, deli meats)

Processed meats are one of the most concerning UPFs due to their strong link to increased cancer risk (page 56), particularly bowel cancer. Studies have classified processed meats as "class 1 carcinogens." This classification is due to the use of preservatives like nitrates and nitrites, which, when digested, can form cancer-causing compounds. Regular consumption of processed meats is also linked to heart disease, diabetes, and obesity.

14   Ketchup and mayonnaise

Staples in our kitchen, and also when eating out, mayo and ketchup usually contain a long list of additives to improve taste and texture. There has recently been a rise in the availability of less processed alternatives, so check the ingredients lists; however, it's always best to make your own when possible (pages 206–207).

15   Jarred pasta sauces

While not inherently "bad" for us, jarred pasta sauces can contain sugar, modified starches, and preservatives to enhance flavor and extend shelf life, even if marketed as "healthy" or "natural".

16   Prepackaged bread

Of all the UPFs consumed in our diets, prepackaged bread is the most popular—globally, 78% of consumers purchased bread and bread products in 2024. Whether wholegrain or white, many supermarket breads contain preservatives, emulsifiers, and other additives. That doesn't necessarily mean that UPF bread is bad, but there is a sliding scale of options when it comes to the nutritional benefits of breads available. Cereal grain products can be a major source of iron, and in the UK, for example, a significant proportion of the population gets much of their iron intake from fortified cereals and breads. This is largely due to the mandatory fortification of flour with iron (along with other nutrients), which is essential for preventing deficiencies, especially in populations at risk like women of childbearing age and children (page 27). The key with buying prepackaged bread is to choose healthier options that prioritize whole grains, lower sugar content, and added micronutrients, thereby ensuring that the UPFs you are consuming still provide beneficial contributions to a balanced diet.

17   Fruit-based snacks

Fruit-based snacks, including some dried fruit, often have added sugars, oils, and preservatives, putting them in the UPF category despite the "fruit" label, which can be incredibly misleading.

18 Protein bars and snacks

These are often marketed as "healthy snacks," perfect for pre- or post-workout. But, in fact, they are usually highly processed and often contain sweeteners, emulsifiers, and other industrial ingredients.

19 Sweets and candy

While an occasional treat is fine, many children and adults consume high quantities of sweets, which are high in refined sugars, artificial colors, and preservatives. These foods contribute little to no nutritional value and are a leading cause of tooth decay, obesity, and behavioral issues in children due to blood sugar spikes and subsequent crashes. Regular and high sugar intake can negatively affect gut health by disrupting the balance of gut bacteria, increasing harmful bacteria that promote inflammation, and decreasing beneficial bacteria that support gut barrier function, leading to issues like low-grade inflammation and creating metabolic dysregulation.

20 Veggie burgers

Prepackaged veggie/plant-based burgers often contain additives like flavor enhancers, emulsifiers, and preservatives to maintain texture and shelf life, making them UPFs. Despite this, they can still be a better choice than a burger patty made of red meat (see right).

Items that appear to be fresh and labeled as "natural" can still contain a whole variety of additives.

Make the best choice for you

We shouldn't have to cut out all our favorite foods, but adapting or tweaking dishes is a great way to ensure our bodies are getting the right nutrition. Ensure meals contain good-quality protein and carbohydrates, healthy fats, and vegetables/fruit to remain on the right track (page 71). If one or more of these food groups is achieved via a UPF item, you may need to address your diet. For the biggest reduction in additives, salt, sugar, and saturated fat, a good trick is to try swapping out the UPF carbohydrate first, followed by swapping out the UPF protein, and so on. Let's use a burger as an example.

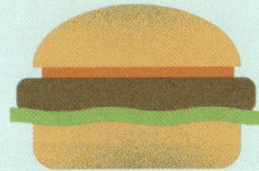

Worst

Red meat patty (class 1 carcinogen) in a low-quality UPF bun.

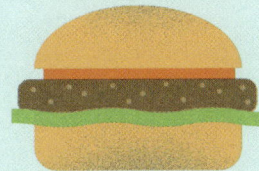

Better

UPF plant-based meat alternative patty in store-bought bun fortified with folic acid.

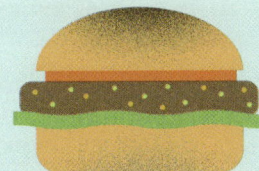

Best

Homemade bean burger in a homemade bun, both made with whole-food ingredients.

*Remember as a one off these items are fine, but frequent consumption may need to be addressed

Are processed meat and fish UPFs?

Traditionally our main sources of protein, meat and fish are now just two of many different protein sources readily available to us. In their original state they are, of course, whole foods, but consumerism and the demands of the food industry mean we have to delve a little deeper to understand what we're putting on our plates.

Meat

Fresh, raw meat loses nutrients over time, but by freezing it, or buying frozen meat in the first place, both nutrients and flavor are retained, meaning there is no need for most brands to add additives and preservatives. Fresh, raw red meats (like beef, pork, and venison) are not UPFs but there is evidence to suggest that they can lead to poor health. Read the label to check that the raw meat you buy contains no additives and is not a UPF.

However, there are many items that you wouldn't expect to be ultra-processed—and precooked meat is one of them. For example, precooked and prepackaged chicken often contains extra ingredients that go beyond just chicken. These added components, like rice flour, potato starch, corn starch and dextrose (a type of sugar), are used to improve texture, flavor, and shelf life. Additionally, stabilizers like triphosphates (pentasodium and pentapotassium triphosphate) are commonly added to retain moisture in cooked chicken, giving it a juicier texture and extending its freshness. Sugar and salt are frequently added to enhance taste and act as preservatives. While these additives aren't necessarily harmful in small amounts, consuming

processed products like prepackaged cooked chicken regularly may lead to higher intake of these unnecessary ingredients.

Heavily processed prepackaged meats, like sausages, sliced ham, and deli meats (commonly consumed by both adults and children on a daily basis), are more concerning as they are classified as "class 1 carcinogens" (page 56).

What about plant-based meat?

Although plant-based meat alternatives are usually classed as UPFs due to the inclusion of additives used to increase shelf life and mimic the texture and flavor of meat products, new research suggests that there are also positives to consuming these food items.

A Lancet study led by University College London found plant-based meat and milk were associated with a decreased risk of type 2 diabetes, while the animal products they are designed to replace were associated with a significantly increased risk. Researchers found that replacing conventional meat with plant-based meat for between one and eight weeks reduced LDL (or "bad" cholesterol) and helped with weight management. Plant-based meats have also scored highly in areas such as weight loss, gut health, and a reduced risk of cardiovascular disease, although there is always variation between products in nutritional value.

This shows that the role of UPFs in our diets is far more nuanced than simply labeling food products as "good" or "bad". In fact, the UK's Food Foundation recently found that, on average, plant-based meat products contained fewer calories, lower levels of saturated fat, and higher levels of fiber than the meat products analyzed. Plant-based meat products can be a stepping stone to encourage people to adopt healthier diets.

If you're aiming to reduce your meat consumption, then plant-based meat alternatives may be a good solution, especially if you're looking for products that mimic the taste and texture of meat. However, it's worth noting that these food items are still UPFs, so if you're already someone who doesn't eat meat, it's better to focus on eating whole foods when possible.

UPFs in our diets are far more nuanced than simply labeling food products "good" or "bad".

Fish

Fresh fish sold in supermarkets, whether raw or precooked, is rarely classified as a UPF as it tends to be minimally processed and retains much of its natural nutritional value. For example, a fresh precooked salmon fillet can be found to contain just "Salmon (Fish) (99%), Salt, Lemon Juice," which is a simple and nutritious whole food.

Things start to get a little more complicated with precooked fillets that include flavorings, like salmon packaged with sweet chili sauce. In this case, the ingredient list contains: "Salmon (fish) (86%), sweet chili sauce (6%) (water, sugar, distilled vinegar, corn starch, red chili purée, dried red pepper, salt, dried garlic, garlic purée, cayenne pepper)". All of these ingredients are minimally processed culinary ingredients, so the product is not technically a UPF, but they do mean the salmon is no longer a whole food.

Nonetheless, these types of products are good examples of how even flavored or precooked fish can be a healthy option, especially compared to some other precooked and packaged foods, like meat. However, it's always worth checking the label, because occasionally precooked products can include more additives or preservatives, which might shift them into the UPF category.

In contrast, processed fish products tell a different story (see below). Their ingredient lists often include a much smaller proportion of actual fish, heavily diluted with starches, sugars, flavorings, and additives to create a processed final product. Fish fingers, for example, are a highly processed food with ingredients far removed from their original form, making them a classic example of a UPF.

For a healthier choice, stick to fresh or simply prepared fish, and always check the label to understand exactly what you're buying.

What's actually in fish sticks?

Convenience wins out sometimes, and that's fine. When UPFs feel like the only option on busy days, know that fish products are usually a healthier choice than precooked and packaged meat products. Store-bought fish sticks are indeed UPFs; however, the research suggests that they can form part of a healthy diet. Cod (the most commonly used fish in fish sticks) is high in selenium (aids immune systems and thyroid function, as well as hair and nail growth) and is a decent source of phosphorus (essential for building strong bones and teeth). And the breadcrumbs aren't as bad as you think—their enhanced color comes from turmeric.

If you want to make a healthier swap, consider fish sticks made with pollock. This fish has nearly double the amount of omega-3 found in cod, and most big brands do a version made from it. Omega-3s are particularly important for heart health, brain health, and eye health. Deficiencies are linked to chronic disease, dementia, and heart attacks, and the US and the UK rank among the countries with the lowest levels of omega-3 in their diets.

If you have a little more time to spare, try making homemade fish sticks using the recipe on page 168.

Cod fish stick

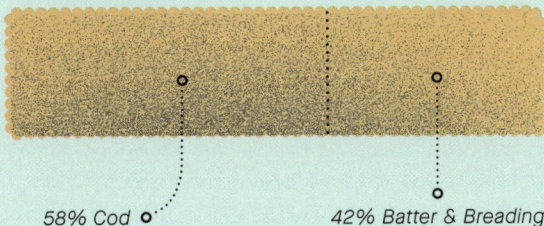

58% Cod   42% Batter & Breading

Pollock fish stick

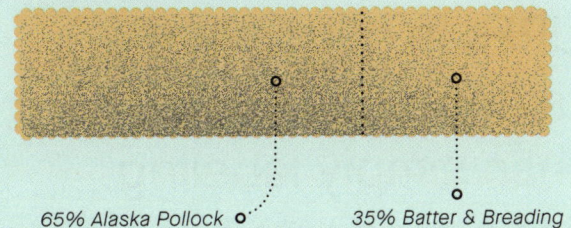

65% Alaska Pollock   35% Batter & Breading

Are sugar and artificial sweeteners UPFs?

Sugar is simply sucrose, which is made up of two molecules: fructose and glucose. It is a natural ingredient derived from sugar cane or sugar beet and humans have been using it for over two thousand years to sweeten and preserve food and enhance flavor, color, texture, aroma, and moisture levels. Sugar is minimally processed without any additives, so it is not a UPF.

What are glucose and fructose? Along with galactose, they are the three building blocks that make up all forms of carbohydrates. These three simple sugars are also known as monosaccharides. They bond with each other and themselves to make more complex carbohydrates. All carbohydrates are made up of one or more molecules of sugars. No matter how complex a carbohydrate is to start with, once in the body, all carbohydrates are broken down into these three simple sugars: glucose, fructose, and galactose.

Natural sugar is not necessarily "bad" for you and you don't need to fear it—you just need to be smart about it. Consuming high amounts of sugar is not advised since it can have negative effects on health, yet most people already consume more than the recommended daily amount. Issues arise because sugar is added in high levels to so many foods that are UPFs and, in combination with high levels of salt, saturated fats, and additives, this is not considered healthy. Sugar is best consumed in home-cooked items and avoided in convenience products when possible.

Added sugars

It is important to distinguish between added sugars and naturally occurring sugars. Added sugars are those added to foods and drinks such as baked goods, candy, cereals, flavored yogurts, and carbonated drinks. However, added sugars also include those found in honey, syrups (such as maple syrup and agave),

How is sucrose made?

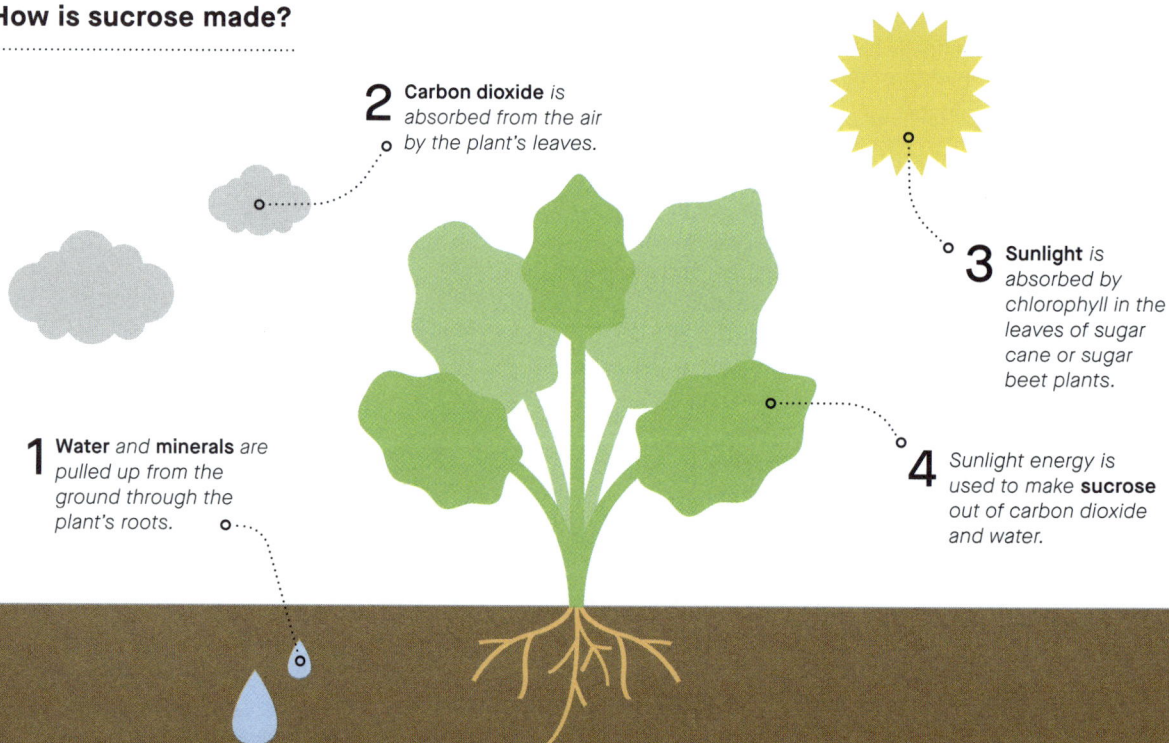

2 **Carbon dioxide** *is absorbed from the air by the plant's leaves.*

3 **Sunlight** *is absorbed by chlorophyll in the leaves of sugar cane or sugar beet plants.*

1 **Water** *and* **minerals** *are pulled up from the ground through the plant's roots.*

4 *Sunlight energy is used to make* **sucrose** *out of carbon dioxide and water.*

nectars, alternative sugars (such as coconut sugar) and unsweetened fruit juices, vegetable juices, and smoothies. The sugars in these foods occur naturally, and are often labeled as such, but still count as added sugars because to get them to a state in which they can be consumed they have to be heavily processed—something a lot of people are unaware of. Added sugars are linked to various health concerns, including weight gain and tooth decay. They can also impact our bodies in different ways. For example, agave syrup is approximately 80% fructose and 20% glucose (compared to refined sugar, which is made up of equal parts fructose and glucose). Unlike glucose, fructose is primarily processed by the liver. When consumed in large amounts, excessive fructose consumption can put strain on the liver and potentially lead to a host of negative effects. Therefore, "natural" alternative sugars may not actually be the best for our health.

Ultimately, when choosing alternatives to refined sugar, it's crucial to understand that many of these options still contribute to your "added sugar" intake and should be consumed with caution.

Artificial sweeteners

Artificial sweeteners were first created in the 20th century for the purpose of helping to reduce sugar levels and calorie intake in people's diets. You will find them in drinks, desserts, chewing gum, prepackaged meals, and even in toothpaste. They were initially hailed as a solution to a multitude of problems such as obesity and diabetes. Scientists at the time rightly had high hopes for them.

Artificial sweeteners work by mimicking the structure of sugar molecules so that they can fit into the sweetness receptors on your tongue. This triggers a signal to your brain that allows you to taste something sweet. However, there is a lot of confusion about whether artificial sweeteners are in fact "bad" for you. They are safe to consume and heavily tested, and some studies have even found that sugar substitutes can lead to modest weight loss for individuals. But in 2023, the WHO recommended against using non-sugar sweeteners to control body weight or reduce the risk of chronic diseases, suggesting that long-term consumption could increase the risk of diseases like type 2 diabetes and cardiovascular disease. They suggest that individuals should reduce artificial sugar intake by consuming more foods that contain naturally occurring sugars like fruit, or unsweetened foods and drinks.

Approved sweeteners in the UK

- Acesulfame
- Aspartame
- Erythritol
- Saccharin
- Sorbitol
- Steviol Glycosides
- Sucralose
- Xylitol

Approved sweeteners in the USA

- Saccharin (brand names include Sweet and Low, Sweet Twin, Sweet 'N Low, and Necta Sweet)
- Sucralose (brand name is Splenda)
- Neotame (brand name is Newtame)
- Advantame
- Acesulfame potassium (also known as Ace-K; brand names include Sweet One and Sunett)
- Aspartame (brand names include NutraSweet and Equal)
- Stevia
- Luo han guo (also known as monk fruit)
- Xylitol

Sweeteners and gut health

Natural sweeteners, such as stevia, may be a wiser choice compared to synthetic counterparts like aspartame and sucralose. However, sugar alcohols (polyols) such as xylitol and sorbitol, while naturally occurring, are not considered natural sweeteners as they are made from acid-treated fibers of birch wood using chemical processes in a laboratory. They should therefore be consumed in moderation, since they can cause gastrointestinal symptoms like diarrhea and bloating. It is important to note that this recommendation does not apply to certain products such as medications, facial products, or toothpastes. (Read more about gut health on page 54.)

Is fast food completely off-limits?

From a young age, many of us have been told that fast food is not the healthiest option. When we choose to eat at these places, often out of convenience, we do so knowing that it might not be the most nutritious choice. However, since scientists have been researching additives in more detail, there is now a lot more we can learn about our favorite fast-food chains in relation to UPFs.

You will notice that every single burger bun, chicken nugget, or fry from your favorite fast-food chain tastes the same wherever you are in the world. This uniformity is achieved by using a very limited supply chain as well as including a set range of UPF ingredients for each product, such as a specific type of wheat flour, or emulsifiers that stabilize texture and extend shelf life. While this consistency is great for quality control, it significantly reduces the diversity of nutrients we consume, especially in staple ingredients like wheat, impacting gut health and dietary variety. Over time, such uniformity, combined with a widespread consumption of these foods, can contribute to negative outcomes for both our microbiome and metabolic health, not to mention the landscape of the food system.

For children, the impact of fast food is particularly concerning; early exposure to these uniform and ultra-processed foods can shape lifelong dietary preferences, increase the risk of obesity, and limit the variety of whole foods in their diets.

Fast food in moderation

As you can see opposite, the amount of ingredients that go into a hamburger, box of chicken nuggets, or serving of fries is quite overwhelming. Even fast-food chain pickles are UPFs! While no one should feel that they must cut things from their diet completely, it's best to view fast food as an occasional treat rather than a regular go-to convenience food.

Even fast-food establishments that promote themselves as healthy should be met with caution. Fast food is more complex than its name suggests—it's not just about being made quickly. Marketing plays a significant role in influencing our choices, and brands often use nutritional claims to make certain options appear healthier. While products from some fast-food chains may indeed offer better nutrition, they still tend to contain a high number of additives.

According to the 2025 UK Broken Report, healthier foods cost, on average, more than twice as much per calorie as less healthy options, with prices rising at double the rate over the past two years. Given this financial barrier, it's no surprise that fast food remains a common choice for many.

Early exposure to uniform, ultra-processed foods can shape lifelong dietary preferences.

Will this meal really make you happy?

Common emulsifiers and preservatives—like potassium sorbate used in fast-food chain pickles—ensure a long shelf life and palatable texture, but could also be linked to gut microbiome disruption and inflammatory responses. Here's a breakdown of the ingredients that make up the items in your meal deal. (It's worth pointing out, though, that ingredients change depending on where you are in the world.)

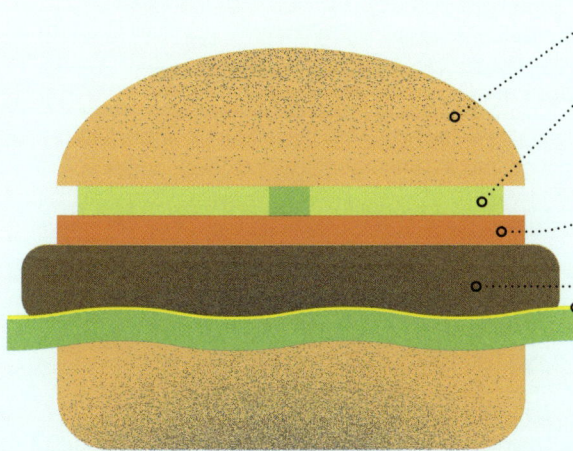

Bun: Wheat Flour (contains Calcium Carbonate, Iron, Niacin, Thiamin), Water, Sugar, Cream Yeast, Canola Oil, Salt, Wheat Fiber, Emulsifier (Mono- and Diacetyl Tartaric Acid Esters of Mono- and Diglycerides of Fatty Acids), Pea Protein, Wheat Starch, Wheat Maltodextrin, Dextrose, Maize Maltodextrin, Maize Starch.

Pickles: Cucumbers, Water, Distilled Vinegar, Salt, Firming Agent (Calcium Chloride), Natural Flavoring, Preservative (Potassium Sorbate).

Ketchup: 60% Tomato Purée, Glucose-Fructose Syrup, Distilled Vinegar, Salt, Spice Extracts.

Patty: 100% Pure Beef.

Mustard: Water, Distilled Vinegar, Mustard Seed (14%), Salt, Spices, Spice Extract.

Chicken nugget ingredients

Chicken Breast Meat 45%, Water, Vegetable Oils (Sunflower, Canola), Maize Flour, Wheat Flour (contains Calcium Carbonate, Iron, Niacin, Thiamin), Starches, Wheat Semolina, Breadcrumb (contains Wheat), Natural Flavorings (contains Celery), Potassium Chloride, Dried Glucose Syrup, Wheat Gluten, Salt, Raising Agents (Sodium Carbonates), Pepper, Celery, Dextrose.

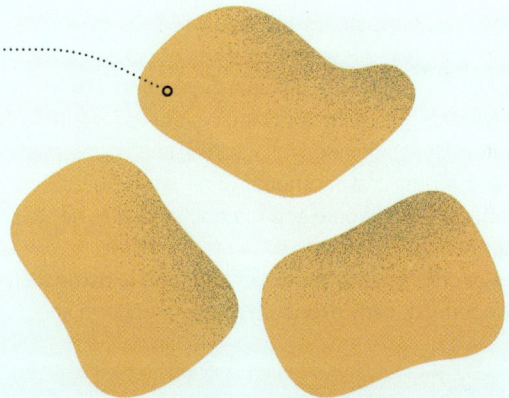

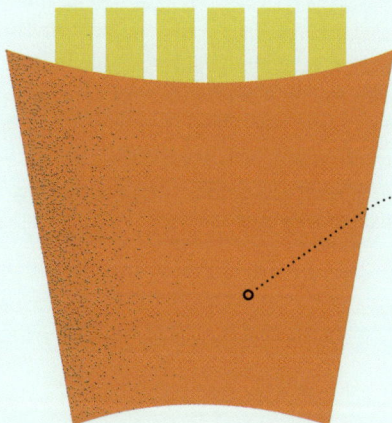

Fries ingredients

Potatoes, Non-Hydrogenated Vegetable Oils (Canola), Dextrose, Salt. (Prepared using a non-hydrogenated vegetable oil).

Are all UPFs unhealthy?

The simple answer is: no. It's important to remember that the purpose of UPFs is to help humans cope with adversity, illnesses, famine, cost of living, and to enhance taste and shelf life. UPFs have gained a bad reputation recently, but that's mainly due to the quantity and frequency of consumption of these products, as they are high in salt, sugars, fats and low in vitamins, minerals, and fiber.

Consuming a UPF item occasionally is not harmful. There is still a lot of research to be done on UPFs regarding weight gain, gut microbiome, and long-term health outcomes, but the variety of UPFs available to us means the issue is nuanced rather than black and white.

It is important to focus on our overall diet rather than isolating certain ingredients. Of course, if you can lower your consumption of UPFs, then that's great, but it's recommended to focus on other positive diet changes too.

Positive changes for your diet

- ☑ Aim to eat 30 different plants a week.
- ☑ Try one new fruit or vegetable each week.
- ☑ Swap your usual prepackaged meal for a home-cooked version.
- ☑ Add more legumes, such as beans, peas, and lentils, to your daily meals.
- ☑ Swap your white carbohydrates for whole grains where possible.
- ☑ Swap processed meats for other protein options.

It's important not to overlook the fact that there are many UPFs that have been created to provide options for those with illnesses or dietary requirements.

- **Plant-based drinks** – Fortified plant-based drinks like almond or soy milk can contain beneficial components like polyphenols, folate, and trace minerals, which can offer potential health benefits.
- **Cereal and bread products** – Cereal and bread products made primarily from whole grains with only a few additives are still classified as UPFs, but can also be fortified with essential nutrients like iron, folic acid, and B vitamins (page 27).
- **Canned legumes** – Although sometimes classified as UPFs, products like canned lentils and beans are much less processed compared to other UPF products and retain practically all their nutritional benefits.
- **Baby formula** – Baby formula ensures babies get all the nutrition they need when mothers are unable or choose not to breastfeed (page 49).
- **Popcorn** – Popcorn can be a much healthier snack alternative to chips and cookies. High-end brands usually contain minimal ingredients so often fall into the "processed" rather than UPF category.
- **Jarred sauces and pastes** – Although premade pasta sauces are usually UPFs, tomato-based products in particular can be packed with antioxidants. When it comes to products like this, it's usually better to look out for how much salt they contain, rather than the number of additives. There are all sorts of reasons for people to rely on convenience products like this—and this isn't a bad thing.

We can only wait and educate ourselves as scientists start to unravel the research and evidence surrounding UPFs in relation to our health. What is undeniable, is that home-cooked meals made with whole foods will have a better long-term effect on our body than consuming large proportions of UPFs.

What is a safe level of UPF consumption for adults?

In an ideal world, we would have enough research to concretely recommend how much of our daily energy could safely come from UPFs. Since there is no universally accepted guideline specifying an exact upper limit for UPF consumption, it is incredibly difficult to give an exact percentage.

The simple message is: try to reduce your intake of UPFs where possible but don't panic about it or let it interrupt a healthy relationship with food (page 20).

Factors of privilege (page 18), environment, culture, and background will all affect how much you are able to control your eating habits. Having the knowledge to make informed decisions about your diet and cooking from scratch, when possible, is key.

What we can do is look at the WHO recommendations for a healthy diet, particularly surrounding ingredients that are often contained within UPFs, like added sugars, fats, and salt.

The WHO recommendations for a healthy diet for adults

- [✓] Specific advice varies depending on country, so look up the guidelines based on where you are in the world; however, the WHO recommends a balanced diet for adults should include the following:

- [✓] Fruit, vegetables, legumes (e.g. lentils and beans), nuts and whole grains (e.g. unprocessed corn, millet, oats, wheat, and brown rice).

- [✓] Less than 10% of total energy intake from added sugar (page 40), which is equivalent to 50g (12 level teaspoons) for a person of healthy body weight consuming about 2,000 calories per day. Ideally, this would be less than 5% for a person with additional health benefits. Added sugars are all sugars added to foods or drinks by the manufacturer, cook, or consumer, as well as sugars naturally present in honey, syrups, fruit juices, and fruit juice concentrates.

- [✓] Less than 5g of salt (equivalent to about 1 teaspoon) per day.

- [✓] At least 14oz (400g) or five servings of fruit and vegetables per day, excluding potatoes, sweet potatoes, cassava, and other starchy vegetables.

- [✓] Less than 30% of total energy intake from fats. Unsaturated fats (found in fish, avocado, and nuts, and in sunflower, soybean, avocado, and olive oils) are preferable to saturated fats (found in fatty meat, butter, palm and coconut oil, cream, cheese, ghee, and lard) and trans fats of all kinds, including both industrially produced trans fats (found in baked and fried foods, and prepackaged foods, such as frozen pizza, pies, cookies, biscuits, wafers, and cooking oils and spreads) and ruminant trans fats (found in meat and dairy foods from ruminant animals, such as cows, sheep, goats, and camels). It is suggested that the intake of saturated fats be reduced to less than 10% of total energy intake and trans fats to less than 1% of total energy intake. In is important to note that industrially produced trans fats have been banned in the US. They are not part of a healthy diet and should be avoided.

What's the deal with supplements?

Health supplements have gained popularity in recent years and can be beneficial for many individuals. However, if the body doesn't require a supplement it is being supplied with, it can disrupt homeostasis (the body's tightly regulated balance), as the excess must be broken down and excreted, placing unnecessary strain on the body's regulatory systems.

In recent years, protein powders and dietary supplements have become sought-after staples in the fitness and wellness space. These products are marketed to help build muscle, support recovery, and enhance overall health, making them especially popular among athletes and bodybuilders. But are these products classified as UPFs? The answer in most cases is yes, yet they are still hailed as "natural" supplements by many.

Creatine

Creatine is one of the most widely researched and evidence-backed supplements in sports nutrition, often considered essential for active individuals and athletes looking to improve performance during high-intensity, short-duration activities like weightlifting or sprinting.

Creatine itself is naturally found in animal products like meat and fish, and our bodies can produce small amounts from amino acids. However, the supplement form, creatine monohydrate, is made through an industrial process that combines sarcosine, a compound found in many foods, with cyanamide, and this process technically classifies it as a UPF. However, unlike most ultra-processed products, creatine has no known risks to health and is recommended by sports nutritionists to support strength, power, and muscle recovery.

For non-athletes or those who don't engage in regular high-intensity exercise, creatine supplementation is likely unnecessary, as the body can produce sufficient amounts through a balanced diet. However, for active individuals, creatine is one of the few UPFs that may genuinely support health and performance.

Collagen

Collagen has gained popularity in recent years, particularly among individuals seeking to improve skin health and appearance. Products are often marketed as dietary supplements, promising benefits such as enhanced skin elasticity, reduced wrinkles, and improved joint health.

Many people may not realize that collagen is a UPF and is primarily derived from animal sources, including the skin, bones, and connective tissues of cows, pigs, and fish.

Despite claims by various collagen brands, scientific evidence supporting the effectiveness of collagen supplementation for skin health is limited. Current research suggests that while collagen supplementation may have a positive effect on several factors that relate to skin aging (such as skin hydration, elasticity, and wrinkles) the benefits may not be as significant as advertised. Interestingly, research has found that consuming a diet rich in whole foods and plants may offer comparable or even superior benefits for skin health due to their high vitamin E and antioxidant content.

Conversely, the research around the effect of collagen on joint health is stronger. Research has found that collagen supplementation may be a potential aid for joint health, particularly in individuals with degenerative conditions like osteoarthritis. Evidence suggests that collagen can enhance the structure and function of connective tissues, leading to improvements in joint functionality and reductions in pain.

For active individuals, creatine is one of the few UPFs that may genuinely support health and performance.

Protein powder

While the primary ingredient in protein powders is often a protein source—such as whey, soy, or pea protein—these products also typically contain many other ingredients designed to improve taste, texture and shelf life. While these ingredients make protein powders convenient and tasty, they also contribute to their classification as UPFs. The processing steps required to isolate the protein, combine it with other additives and create a shelf-stable product are far removed from original, whole-food sources of protein.

It's important to note that, although all protein powders and supplements are UPFs, they're not all created equally. Some products contain fewer additives or ingredients, focusing on natural ingredients and whole-food sources. It's always best practice to check the ingredients list (page 62).

Just because protein powders and supplements are classified as UPFs, it doesn't mean they are inherently "bad" for you. For many people, these products offer convenient and effective ways to meet their nutritional needs, especially when whole foods alone may not be enough. Current evidence shows that protein supplementation is effective for building muscle and increasing strength, especially when paired with regular, intense exercise. For most people, the recommended daily intake for protein is around 0.8g per kilogram of body weight per day and the average person is already consuming more protein than the recommended intake. Consuming protein above this level, particularly beyond 1.6g per kilogram is not understood to offer extra benefits, however, it's important to consider individual needs based on age, activity level, and training goals.

The key is to be informed about what you're consuming and to balance these products with a diet rich in whole, unprocessed foods.

Common ingredients in protein powders

Protein powders contain a multitude of ingredients to create a product that is convenient and easy to consume.

1. Protein isolates and concentrates

While these ingredients are derived from foods like milk, soy, or peas, they are heavily processed to strip away everything but the protein.

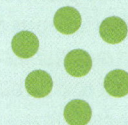

2. Artificial sweeteners and flavorings

Ingredients like sucralose, aspartame, and artificial flavorings, such as vanilla or chocolate, are commonly used to make the powders more palatable.

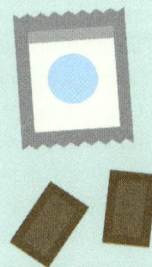

3. Thickeners and emulsifiers

Additives like xanthan gum, guar gum, and lecithin are used to improve the texture and mixability of the powders when blended with liquids.

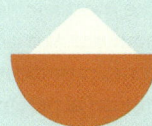

4. Preservatives and anticaking agents

These ingredients ensure that the powder remains stable over time and doesn't clump or degrade.

Am I giving my baby UPFs without realizing?

Simply put, children do not need store-bought snacks, but the need for convenience can be unavoidable as a parent. Children learn to eat via mouthfeel, texture, visuals, and smell, and eating whole foods is incredibly important to instill healthy eating patterns from an early age and grow a healthy child. Nutrition in particular plays a foundational role in a child's development. Poor nutrition in the first 1,000 days of a child's life can cause irreversible damage to growth and set the stage for chronic issues later in life.

Many common toddler snacks, including fruit pouches and flavored yogurts, fall into the UPF category due to their high levels of added sugars and artificial ingredients. The good news is that not all UPFs are bad—some vegetable pouches are packed with protein and fiber and are helpful when out and about or dealing with a phase of picky eating.

What should I look out for?

Where it's important to take note, is the high sugar content in many toddler snacks. Research shows that children in the highest quintile for UPF consumption exceed the recommended daily sugar intake, highlighting that many snacks marketed for toddlers are laden with added sugars that can lead to unhealthy dietary habits. Increased consumption of UPFs in toddlers is also linked to higher risks of obesity, diabetes, cardiovascular diseases, and other noncommunicable diseases (NCDs). These health issues are exacerbated by the low nutritional value of UPFs. It's also worth noting that many of these snack foods lack the fiber and protein required to help meet growing infants' nutritional needs.

These UPF products are heavily marketed toward families and children (how many faces of cartoon characters or bright colors have you seen in the baby and toddler snack aisle?), influencing parental choices and contributing to increased UPF consumption.

One study explored the impact of UPFs on the nutrient profiles of young children under the age of two. The analysis revealed that UPFs contributed significantly to the total energy intake of children, accounting for 47% of calories consumed. The most consumed UPFs were fruit drink concentrates, white bread, and low-fiber breakfast cereals. As UPF consumption increased, so did the intake of sugar and salt, with children in the highest UPF quintile consuming far more than the recommended daily amounts. These results suggest that UPFs substantially contribute to unhealthy dietary patterns in young children, raising concerns about their potential role in childhood obesity and nutrient deficiencies.

Public health guidelines emphasize the importance of minimizing UPF consumption among toddlers. Recommendations suggest prioritizing unprocessed or minimally processed foods, which are more beneficial for children's growth and development.

Artificial coloring in food

Here is a list of artificial colors that are commonly used in food and drinks, such as soft drinks, candy, cake, and ice cream:

- FD&C Yellow No. 5 (Tartrazine)

- FD&C Yellow No. 6 (Sunset Yellow FCF)

- FD&C Blue No. 1 (Brilliant Blue FCF)

- FD&C Blue No. 2 (Indigo Carmine)

- FD&C Green No. 3 (Fast Green FCF)

- FD&C Red 40 (Allura Red)

In January 2025 the United States banned the use of FD&C Red No. 3 (Erythrosine), joining Australia, New Zealand, Japan, and EU nations.

Is baby formula safe to use?

Baby formula is a good example of when a UPF has had a positive impact, helping women around the world raise healthy babies. For women who cannot breastfeed, or chose not to, baby formula is an essential UPF that is not harmful for babies or children.

Baby formula, whether in powdered or liquid form, is produced through specific industrial processes designed to ensure consistency, safety, and nutritional adequacy. The foundation of baby formulas consists of essential nutrients: proteins, fats, carbohydrates, vitamins, minerals, and trace elements. Each manufacturer develops their own unique formula, blending these nutrients from a variety of sources to create a product that meets their specific nutritional requirement goals. You will see that the ingredient composition can vary between brands, which is fine if they adhere to the legal nutritional standards, particularly for infant and follow-on formulas.

However, formulas intended for older children, particularly those marketed for use from one year of age, are subject to fewer regulatory requirements, leading to more variation in ingredients.

Additives in baby formula serve important functions and can contain a blend of natural and synthetic ingredients, stabilizers, emulsifiers, and nutrients added back in after processing. Some are included to prevent separation of ingredients, to regulate acidity, or to protect the formula from oxidation. In liquid formulas, emulsifiers are crucial to maintain a consistent mixture, preventing the separation of oils and water. Emulsifiers like soy lecithin help blend fats with water, ensuring the formula has a consistent texture and that nutrients are evenly distributed. These additives, while not essential for nutrition, are necessary to ensure that the formula remains stable and safe over time.

Children in the highest quintile for UPF consumption exceed the recommended daily sugar intake.

What is in baby formula?

In addition to essential nutrients for babies who are being raised with formula either as their only nutritional source, or as a supplementary source, there are also additives that are included to ensure consistency, safety, and to ensure that nutritional standards are met.

- Protein
- Fat
- Linoleic acid
- Vitamins A, D, E, K, C, B6, B12
- Niacin
- Thiamine
- Riboflavin
- Pantothenic acid
- Folic acid
- Calcium
- Phosphorus

- Magnesium
- Iron
- Zinc
- Manganese
- Copper
- Iodine
- Selenium
- Sodium
- Potassium
- Chloride
- Added DHA

Lactose is the main carbohydrate (sugar) in both breast milk and cow's milk. The lactose in some formulas may have been altered to make it easier to digest. Most baby formula contains added carbohydrates. These FDA-approved carbohydrates can include any or all of the following:

- Lactose
- Maltodextrin
- Corn syrup
- Corn syrup solids
- Sucrose

It's important to note that ingredients can vary slightly depending on the type of formula, especially those designed for specific allergy requirements.

How much UPF is being consumed by our children?

Alarmingly, studies have shown that children and adolescents are the leading consumers of UPF products. It is estimated that 65–70% of calories consumed by American children are derived from UPFs. This dietary pattern raises significant health concerns, since we know that excessive UPF consumption has been suggested to increase one's risk factor of developing chronic diseases, alongside a host of other negative health impacts.

One study found that, on average, children in the higher UPF consumption groups experienced a quicker increase in their BMI, weight, waist circumference, and body fat as they transitioned into adolescence and early adulthood. By the age of 24, individuals in the highest UPF consumption group had, on average, a higher BMI, were heavier, with a greater fat mass, and had a higher waist circumference than children who were not in this bracket.

School lunches are a prime example of the prevalence of UPFs in children's diets. A recent UK study revealed that British children have the highest levels of UPF consumption, with an alarming 73% of total lunch calories consumed by elementary school children and 78% for middle school children derived from UPFs. The analysis found that packed lunches contained higher UPF intakes compared to school-provided meals, particularly among middle school students and those from lower-income households. Fewer than two in every 100 packed lunches eaten by children in British elementary schools meet nutritional standards.

We've all been there—life is busy, and we want to make sure our children actually eat their meals. But this highlights why improving food policies and guidance is so essential. A better food environment, being one that supports accessible, nutritious options, makes it easier for parents and caregivers to provide lunches that truly fuel our children's growth, learning, and overall health. It is so important to have the right information about food, because every child should have access to nourishing meals both at home and at school.

The WHO recommendations for a healthy diet for children

Advice on a healthy diet for infants and children is similar to that for the WHO guidance for adults (page 45), but the following elements are also important:

- Infants should be breastfed* exclusively during the first 6 months of life.
- Infants should be breastfed continuously until 2 years of age and beyond.
- From 6 months of age, breast milk should be complemented with a variety of adequate, safe and nutrient-dense foods. Salt and sugars should not be added to complementary foods.
- In the first 2 years of a child's life, optimal nutrition fosters healthy growth and improves cognitive development. It also reduces the risk of becoming overweight or obese and developing NCDs later in life.

*It's important to note that breastfeeding is simply not possible for everyone.

What does a healthy plate look like for children?

A balanced plate for children is based on the four main food groups and nutritional benefits outlined below—if you include one or more of each of the foods suggested below, you'll be providing your children with a healthy diet.

Despite the evident risks associated with UPFs, current guidelines from health authorities do not provide specific recommendations for limiting UPF consumption in children. Although there is a lack of specific UPF guidelines, by adhering to the 5-4-3-2 rule and creating healthy plates, parents are likely to significantly lower their child's UPF consumption.

The 5-4-3-2 rule

A great way to consider whether your child is eating a balanced diet across the course of the day is to roughly follow the 5-4-3-2 rule. Although it can be hard to achieve this every day, it's a good aim of nutritional targets to strive for and bear in mind, although some children require more or less than others.

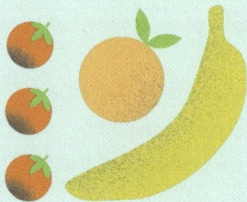

5 Fruit and vegetables

For **carotenes** (a form of vitamin A), **vitamin C**, **zinc**, **iron**, and **fiber**—including fresh, frozen, canned, and dried fruit, vegetables, and legumes.

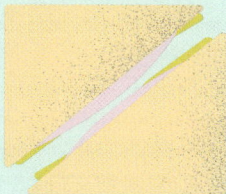

4 Starchy carbohydrates

For a range of nutrition such as, **fiber**, **energy**, **B vitamins**, and **iron**—including bread; potatoes, sweet potatoes, and other starchy root vegetables; pasta and noodles; rice and grains; and breakfast cereals.

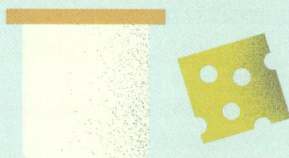

3 Dairy and plant-based alternatives

For a variety of nutrients, but especially **protein**, **calcium**, and **vitamin A**—including milk, cheese, and yogurt.

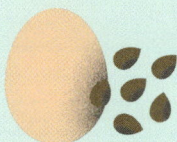

2 Proteins

For **protein**, and nutrients such as **iron**, **zinc**, **omega-3 fatty acids**, and **vitamins A** and **D**—including beans and legumes; nuts; meat and poultry; fish and shellfish; eggs; and meat alternatives.

Do UPFs affect fertility?

For some, fertility journeys are far from straightforward. If you take a moment to scour the internet, which isn't recommended, you will be bombarded with things to do (and not to do) when trying to conceive. When it comes to the relationship between fertility and UPFs, although research is being carried out, for the time being most scientists conclude that UPFs are not a driving factor in hindering chances of conception. Scientific concerns mainly focus on the broader issue of the impact of poor diet on fertility, but UPFs could exacerbate that issue.

A diet that is high in UPF consumption is associated with an increased risk of obesity and metabolic syndrome, which can include conditions like insulin resistance and high blood pressure, both well-known risk factors for fertility issues in both men and women. UPFs are often calorie-dense but nutritionally poor—in high-UPF diets, this excessive calorie intake combined with low nutritional intake isn't conducive for a healthy body, which is important for fertility success. Excess body weight can disrupt hormonal balance, impair ovulation in women, and reduce sperm quality in men, making conception more difficult. Additionally, in women, obesity is associated with conditions like polycystic ovary syndrome (PCOS), a leading cause of infertility.

What research is being done?

A study published in 2024 examined the relationship between the consumption of UPFs and male fertility. The researchers conducted a cross-sectional analysis involving more than 1,000 men who were attending fertility clinics in Spain. The findings revealed that higher consumption of UPFs was significantly associated with lower semen quality. The study concluded that reducing UPF intake might be a beneficial strategy for improving semen quality and, consequently, male fertility.

Another study published in 2022 explored the relationship between UPF consumption and the incidence of infertility among women. The researchers followed 3,685 women over an average of 8 years to assess dietary habits and fertility outcomes. They found that higher UPF consumption was associated with a significantly increased risk of infertility. The study suggested that diets high in UPFs, which are low in essential nutrients and high in harmful additives, could negatively impact hormonal balance and reproductive health, thereby increasing the likelihood of infertility.

In 2023, scientists looked at the association between UPF consumption and the diagnosis of endometriosis in a large cohort of French women. Endometriosis, a condition linked to infertility, was found to be more prevalent among women with higher UPF intake. The research indicated that women in the highest quartile of UPF consumption had a significantly higher risk of being diagnosed with endometriosis compared to those in the lowest quartile. The authors of the study suggested that the inflammatory properties of UPFs, along with their contribution to obesity and metabolic disorders, might explain the increased risk of endometriosis and its related fertility issues.

While more research needs to be done, one of the best things you can do when trying to conceive is to maintain a weight that's healthy for you, and eat a range of nutrient-dense whole foods. We are aware that both male and female fertility can be positively influenced by a healthy balanced diet, notably the Mediterranean diet, and certain nutrients and vitamins. That being said, the fertility journey can be a very vulnerable one and it's important to remember that no one single ingredient can have a bigger impact than overall diet quality.

Nutrients crucial for fertility

The essential nutrients for fertility vary between men and women.

♂ Men

Zinc
Found in: Meat (especially red meat), shellfish, beans, nuts, whole grains, dairy products, fortified cereals.

Selenium
Found in: Brazil nuts, seafood, meat, eggs, wholewheat bread, brown rice.

Omega-3 Fatty Acids
Found in: Oily fish (e.g. salmon, mackerel, trout, sardines), flaxseeds, chia seeds, walnuts, and hemp seeds.

Antioxidants
Found in: Berries (blueberries, strawberries, raspberries), dark chocolate, nuts, seeds, green leafy vegetables, and tea and coffee.

♀ Women

Folic Acid
Found in: Spinach, kale, Brussels sprouts, cabbage, broccoli, beans and legumes, nuts and seeds, fortified cereals (check the label), oranges and orange juice, eggs, poultry, pork, shellfish, and liver.

Calcium
Found in: Dairy products (milk, cheese, yogurt), fortified plant-based dairy alternatives (almond, soy, oat milks, and yogurts etc.), sardines with bones, leafy greens (spring greens, kale), calcium-fortified (calcium-set) tofu, fortified cereals, and wheat-flour products.

Iron
Found in: Red meat, legumes (beans, peas, lentils), dark green vegetables (spinach, kale, broccoli), nuts and seeds, fortified wheat-flour and cereal products.

Magnesium
Found in: Nuts and seeds, beans and legumes, leafy green vegetables (spinach, kale, arugula), grains, banana, avocado, dark chocolate with a high cocoa percentage, fish, and seafood.

Iodine
Found in: Fish and other seafood, seaweed, dairy products (milk, cheese, yogurt), and eggs.

Vitamin B6 (pyridoxine)
Found in: Poultry (chicken or turkey), pork, some fish, peanuts, oats, bananas, soy milk, fortified breakfast cereals (check the label).

Vitamin B12
Found in: Meat, fish, dairy products (milk, cheese, yogurt), eggs, and fortified cereals.

Vitamin D
Found in: Oily fish (salmon, sardines, herring, and mackerel), red meat, liver (avoid liver if you are pregnant), egg yolks, fortified foods such as some fat spreads and breakfast cereals.

One of the best things you can do when trying to conceive is to maintain a weight that's healthy for you.

What's the impact of UPFs on my gut?

Have you ever wondered if the food we eat directly impacts our gut bugs, known as the gut microbiota? The answer is yes. Gut health is still a fairly new field of research, but diet seems to have the most influence on the health of our gut. Recently, discussion has arisen around whether our gut bugs are able to recognize additives in our food.

Research suggests that food additives, commonly found in many UPFs, may have a negative impact on our gut health. There are some emulsifiers, sweeteners, and colorings that can influence various aspects of gut function, including the gut microbiome, permeability of the intestinal lining—a condition known as "leaky gut"—and intestinal inflammation. When gut function is influenced in this way it may potentially trigger systemic inflammation and diseases like diabetes and cardiovascular disease.

Why is gut health important?

- ☑ A healthier gut microbiome has been linked to improved mental health.

- ☑ 70–80% of the body's immune cells are located in the gut, highlighting the crucial role the digestive system plays in maintaining immune function.

- ☑ Up to 95% of serotonin is produced in the gut, highlighting the connection between our gut health and brain.

- ☑ The human gut contains about 10 times more microbial cells than the entire body, with an estimated 100 trillion microbes.

30 plants per week

We now have wonderful research that suggests the key to good gut health is to aim for diversity in our diets. People who eat 30 or more different plants per week are more likely to have certain "good" gut bugs than those who eat 10 different plants per week. By aiming to eat 30 different plants a week you can support a healthy gut microbiome, which is likely linked to a reduced risk of chronic diseases like obesity, type 2 diabetes, and inflammatory bowel disease.

Plants don't just mean fruit and vegetables; in fact, fruit and vegetables refer to only two out of the six groups of plants that are beneficial to our health (see opposite). We can use "plant points"—where eating a serving of a plant equates to one plant point (with the exception of dried herbs and spices which count as a quarter point each)—as an alternative metric to think about how to increase the diversity within our gut. To support a healthy gut microbiome, diversity is key here. For example, different colored vegetables such as red or green peppers, or red or white cabbage, contain different polyphenols, which all contribute to a diverse and healthy gut. As a result, incorporating different colors of the same plant counts as individual plant points. Plant points is a useful metric to use to measure the diversity within your diet.

The relationship between UPFs and gut health remains an area of active research. The evidence we have so far, particularly from observational studies, suggests a potential connection, but it is not yet definitive. Further research is needed to better understand how UPFs and the additives they contain directly impact gut health. However, what is known is that by balancing your diet with at least 30 plants over the course of a week you will be having a positive impact on your gut health, which can only be a good thing. Remember, 30 plants is just a suggestion, it's meant to inspire you to think about adding more variety to your diet, not to cause stress.

What do we mean by 30 plants per week?

Beneficial plants are generally split into the following six groups:

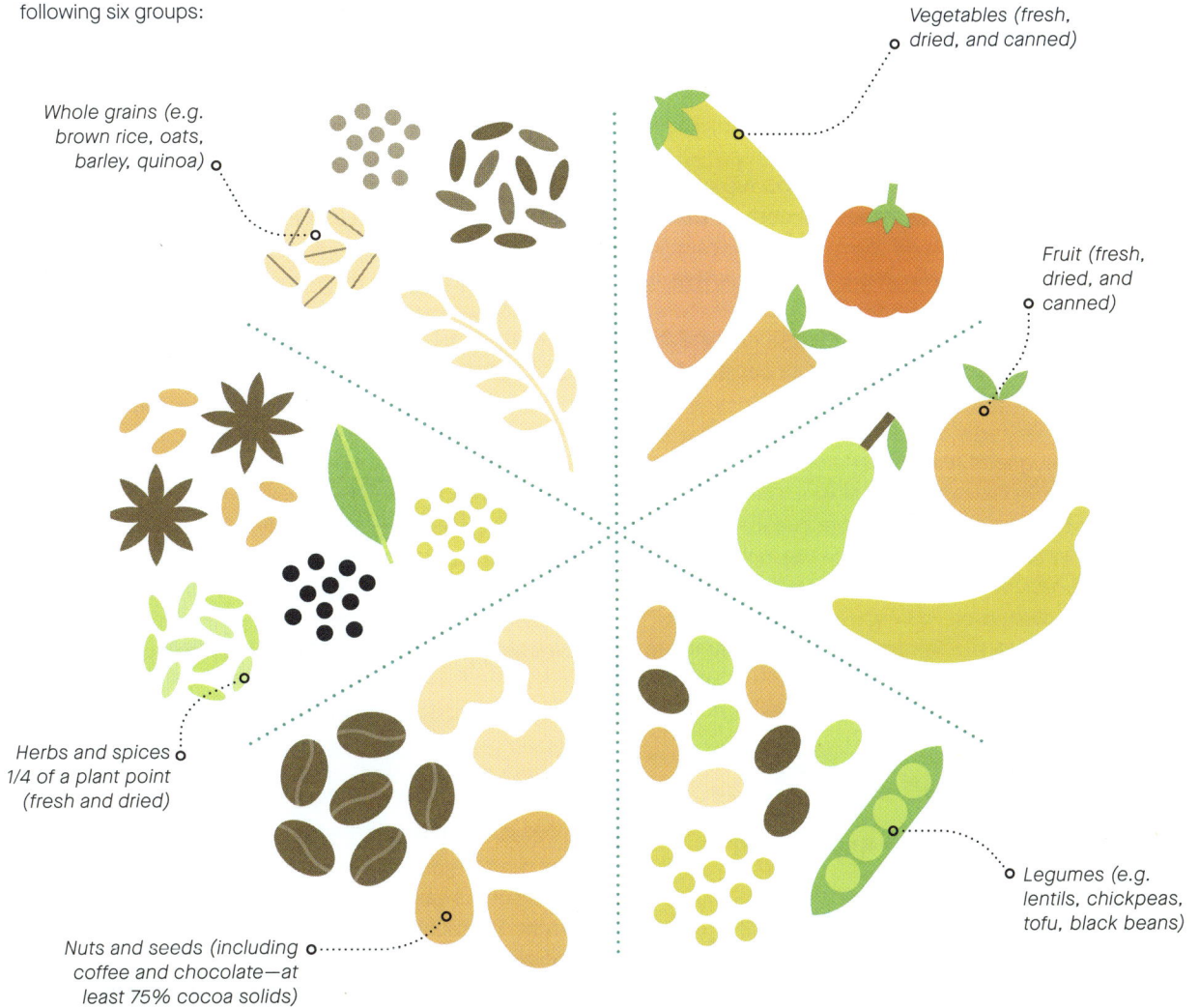

Vegetables (fresh, dried, and canned)

Whole grains (e.g. brown rice, oats, barley, quinoa)

Fruit (fresh, dried, and canned)

Herbs and spices 1/4 of a plant point (fresh and dried)

Legumes (e.g. lentils, chickpeas, tofu, black beans)

Nuts and seeds (including coffee and chocolate—at least 75% cocoa solids)

Your plant point count

Each recipe in chapter 3 (page 88) includes a "plant point" count per serving. This is an easy way for you to quickly check and cross-reference how many plant servings a recipe contains and consider your tally of plant points per week.

Including any plant serving counts for a plant point, while dried herbs and spices each count for a quarter.

Nutritional info per serving

Fiber 6.9g
Protein 12g
Plant Points 5.25

Can UPFs be linked to cancer?

In recent years, there has been growing concern about the potential link between UPFs and cancer. While it's important to approach this topic with sensitivity and avoid creating unnecessary fear and claims that UPFs cause cancer directly, it's equally important to understand the current scientific evidence on how UPFs may influence cancer risk.

One of the most-researched connections between UPFs and cancer surrounds red meats and processed meats. Classified as a "class 1 carcinogen" by the International Agency for Research on Cancer (IARC), processed meats are understood to increase the risk of colorectal cancer. This classification means there is strong evidence that processed meats can cause cancer in humans. Red meat is currently classified as a "class 2A carcinogen". A 2020 study analyzed data from over half a million UK adults over seven years and found a significant association between red and processed meat consumption and an increased risk of bowel cancer.

Specifically, individuals consuming an average of 2¾oz (79g) of processed and red meat daily had a 32% higher risk of developing bowel cancer compared to those who ate less than (⅓oz (11g) per day. The American Institute for Cancer Research stated that eating more than 18oz (500g) of red meat weekly can increase your cancer risk, and advised people to limit consumption of red meat to three servings per week and to eat little, if any, processed meat, while the UK government recommends consuming no more than 2½oz (70g) per day of red or processed meat. This research serves as a reminder that even moderate consumption of red and processed meat can still pose a significant health risk.

Nevertheless, processed meats are not the only UPFs that may be linked to cancer. There is research to suggest that high consumption of other UPFs (sugary beverages, fast foods, certain snack foods) might also be associated with an increased risk of developing various cancers. However, it's important to note that this is only a risk in the case of frequent and repeated overconsumption. Eating processed meat occasionally as part of a balanced diet is not likely to place your health at significant risk.

Why might UPFs contribute an increased risk in cancer?

- Many UPFs are high in refined sugars, unhealthy (saturated) fats and additives, which can promote chronic inflammation in the body, a known risk factor for the development of cancerous cells.

- UPFs are often calorie-dense and low in nutrients which may contribute to an increase in obesity. Obesity is a well-established risk factor for several cancers, including breast, colorectal and pancreatic cancers.

- UPFs can affect insulin regulation, leading to insulin resistance, which is linked to an increased risk of certain cancers.

- UPFs often contain synthetic chemicals, some of which may disrupt hormonal balance or induce oxidative stress, both of which can contribute to cancer risk.

Diet and lifestyle are key to health

Cancer is complex; it's still being researched and there are some cancers we know very little about, but it is becoming clear that diet plays an important role in our overall health. UPFs, however, are just one component of a much bigger picture. Cancer is a multifactorial disease, influenced by a combination of genetic, environmental, and lifestyle factors. Therefore, while reducing UPF intake may lower cancer risk, it is equally crucial to consider other aspects of diet and lifestyle, such as maintaining a healthy weight, exercising regularly, and avoiding known carcinogens like tobacco and alcohol.

The more we research and learn on this topic the better but, in the meantime, it's necessary to err on the side of caution when you come across sensationalist headlines linking UPFs and cancer. There is still no concrete data to say UPFs on their own cause chronic illness. Your overall lifestyle and genetics will still be more of a determining factor. Always consult your doctor as your first point of call if you are concerned.

The IARC carcinogen classifications

The IARC classifies substances to show whether they are suspected to cause cancer or not, based on the strength of evidence*.

Group 1 — Carcinogenic to humans

- Smoking
- Exposure to sun
- Alcohol
- Processed meat

Group 2A — Probably carcinogenic to humans

- High-heat frying
- Steroids
- Night shift work
- Red meat

Group 2B — Possibly carcinogenic to humans

- Aloe vera whole leaf extract
- Gasoline
- Gasoline engine exhaust
- Pickled vegetables

Group 3 — Carcinogenicy not classifiable

- Coffee / Tea
- Magnetic fields
- Fluorescent lighting
- Polyethylene

Group 4 — Probably not carcinogenic to humans

Caprolactam, which is used in the manufacture of synthetic fibers

However, it's important to note that some substances are not confirmed to cause cancer in humans and the evidence is often weak or based on animal studies.

Are UPFs harming the environment?

There is no denying that more needs to be done to address the impacts of climate change. What we eat and how food is produced has a direct impact on greenhouse gas emissions—about one-third of all human contributions to greenhouse gases can be linked to food.

Two clear solutions to these issues are to eat more whole foods and to switch to a plant-based diet. This does not necessarily mean following a vegan diet; it simply means reducing the amount of animal products (meat and dairy) we consume, and prioritizing our plant intake (see pages 54–55).

Although animal products are still responsible for the highest greenhouse gas emissions, compared to plant-based and low-calorie processed products, UPFs can also be linked to significant intensive agricultural and livestock practices that pose risks to the sustainability of the food system.

A global perspective

Many of the ingredients in UPFs, such as palm oil, sugar, soy, corn, and wheat are linked to large-scale deforestation and habitat destruction. Palm oil plantations contribute significantly to the loss of biodiversity in tropical regions, while soy farming is associated with deforestation in the Amazon (although it's still a better option environmentally than meat).

This diverts land away from growing diverse, nutrient-rich crops, leading to a less sustainable and less resilient food system. Large monocultures needed for UPF production also require high levels of fertilizers and pesticides, which contribute to soil degradation and water pollution. Depleted health of soil contributes to the decrease of the biodiversity we require on this planet.

Many UPFs are made with ingredients that are sourced from around the world, adding to their carbon footprint. Ingredients are transported over long distances, and the finished products themselves are often shipped to various markets, leading to high emissions from transportation. The reliance on global supply chains for

How are greenhouse gases produced?

The largest proportion of food-related greenhouse gases comes from agriculture and land use.

- Methane from cattle's digestive process.
- Nitrous oxide from fertilizers used for crop production.
- Carbon dioxide from cutting down forests for the expansion of farmland.
- Other agricultural emissions like manure management, rice cultivation, burning of crop residues, and the use of fuel on farms.

A much smaller proportion of food-related greenhouse gases are caused by...

- Refrigeration and transportation of food.
- Industrial processes, such as the production of paper and aluminum for packaging.
- The management of food waste.

UPF production also makes the food system less resilient to disruptions. UPFs are often packaged within single-use plastics, contributing to the growing global plastic waste crisis. These plastics are difficult to recycle and frequently end up in landfill or our oceans, where they contribute to pollution, threaten marine life, and take hundreds of years to break down. In 2020, packaging waste accounted for around 40% of the total plastic produced globally, with food packaging being a major contributor.

It is important to do what you can for the health of our environment. When you decrease your consumption of UPFs, you will be helping the environment as well.

Should I be worried about microplastics?

Microplastics can enter our food supply through multiple avenues. They are found in packaged and processed foods that have been exposed to plastic during manufacturing, packaging, and storage. For instance, food stored in plastic containers or heated in plastic in microwaves may lead to microplastic leaching, especially if the plastic is exposed to high temperatures. The linings of cans and disposable paper cups can also leach significant levels of microplastics into foods, like canned soups, and beverages, like hot coffee. Bottled water has also been shown to contain much higher levels of microplastics than tap water. In addition to plastic packaging, seafood (especially shellfish) has been found to be a source of microplastics, since these organisms can ingest microplastics in their marine environments.

A recently published study by the National Institutes of Health has raised alarming concerns about the presence of microplastics in the human brain. Researchers found that the brain is now, on average, 0.5% plastic by weight—a number that has been increasing over time. The study also revealed that brain samples from 2024 contained about 50% more microplastics compared to those from 2016, suggesting that the concentration of plastic in our brains is continuously rising. Given the higher levels of microplastics found in the brains of individuals with dementia, this finding is concerning. This highlights the potential links between plastic pollution and neurological health which must be further researched in the future.

Research on microplastics and human health is still in the developmental stage; however, based on studies so far, it seems that exposure to microplastics could have adverse health effects. In fact, scientists have found microplastics present in almost every single tissue in the body. Microplastics are often made with or contain chemicals like phthalates, bisphenols, and other additives that can act as endocrine disruptors, potentially affecting hormone function. Some microplastics also carry toxic pollutants adsorbed from the environment, which could contribute to oxidative stress, inflammation, and cytotoxic effects when ingested. Research has suggested that the average adult ingests between 39,000 and 52,000 microplastic particles each year through food, water, and even air, but this is even said to be an underestimate.

Tips for reducing microplastic exposure:

1. **Limit plastic use in food storage and heating.**
2. **Choose tap water over bottled water.**
3. **Avoid plastic and plastic-lined packaging.**
4. **Consume seafood mindfully.**

Which foods produce the most greenhouse gas emissions?

Animal-based foods generally have a much higher carbon footprint than plant-based foods, with meat and dairy producing significantly more emissions. This is largely due to the resources required for farming, land use, and methane production from livestock. Red meat, particularly beef, have the highest emissions, making them among the most resource-intensive foods to produce. In contrast, plant-based foods tend to have a lower environmental impact, as they require fewer resources for farming, transportation, and packaging.

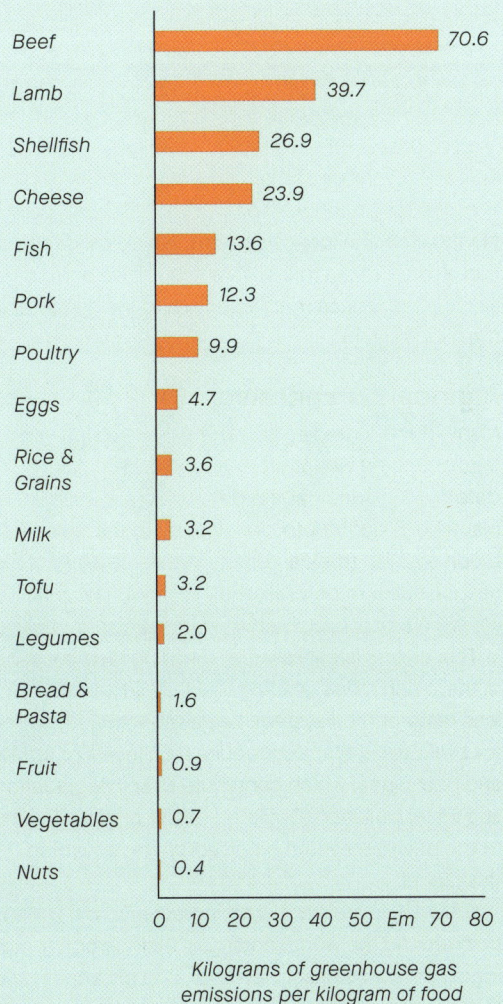

Food type

Food type	Emissions
Beef	70.6
Lamb	39.7
Shellfish	26.9
Cheese	23.9
Fish	13.6
Pork	12.3
Poultry	9.9
Eggs	4.7
Rice & Grains	3.6
Milk	3.2
Tofu	3.2
Legumes	2.0
Bread & Pasta	1.6
Fruit	0.9
Vegetables	0.7
Nuts	0.4

0 10 20 30 40 50 Em 70 80

Kilograms of greenhouse gas emissions per kilogram of food

How to build a

Let's get started on turning knowledge into action! Incorporating healthier habits into your daily life, for yourself or your family, can feel overwhelming at first, but in this chapter you'll focus on practical steps to help you build a strong foundation. You'll learn how to create a nutritionally balanced plate that works for you, plan and write shopping lists that truly serve your week, and explore simple swaps to reduce UPFs in your diet without feeling deprived. We'll also dive into tips for recognizing those "grab-and-go" items that support your goals, breaking down what's really inside the food you're buying.

UPF-free life

How to understand food labels

A lot of food waste occurs due to consumers not understanding the information on the packaging, especially date labels. You should always inspect products before consuming them, paying attention to things like appearance, texture, and smell. If it looks or smells "off," or has an unusual texture or flavor, it's best to remain on the side of caution and discard the item.

How to navigate ingredients lists

To put it simply, the catchphrase "if you don't recognize it, don't eat it," has elements of truth but is overall false, and part of a bigger issue with the rise of fearmongering surrounding food.

If a food or drink product has two or more ingredients (including any additives), then they must be listed on the packaging. Ingredients must be listed in order of weight, with the main ingredient first; so, the words you read first are those that make up the majority of the item. For example, if you look at a package of spiced mixed nuts, nuts should be the first ingredient listed, whereas spices, herbs, and any sugar added should be lower down on the list. On the flip side, if you look at a bag of candy, then sugar will likely be the first ingredient listed. Knowing the hierarchy of ingredients lists allows you to make more informed decisions when buying food.

In the EU and UK any words highlighted in bold, underlined, or in capital letters, are allergens (not UPFs!). In the US, they either do the same, or they sometimes list allergens under a separate "contains" statement on the label. These are highlighted in some way simply to make it easier for consumers to quickly check if a product is suitable for them.

Commonly listed allergens

- Gluten-containing cereals (like barley, oats, wheat, and rye)
- Crustaceans (like shrimp, crab, and lobsters)
- Eggs
- Fish
- Lupins (legumes like peanuts, lentils, peas, chickpeas, green beans, and mung beans)
- Milk
- Mollusks (like mussels, oysters, and clams)
- Nuts (tree nuts like almonds, hazelnuts, walnuts, Brazil nuts, cashews, pecans, pistachios, macadamia nuts)
- Other allergens (celery, mustard, sesame seeds, soybeans, and sulphur dioxide or sulphites at levels above 10 milligrams per kilogram or per liter)

Knowing the hierarchy of ingredients lists allows you to make informed decisions when buying food.

What are the key elements on our food packaging?

Food packaging is commonplace and we might not be in the habit of considering what information is included. However, familiarizing ourselves with the key elements on our food packaging will empower us to make informed choices around ingredients and food safety.

Use by / Best by
These labels indicate the date by which the manufacturer recommends using the product for optimal quality and freshness. Unlike expiration dates, "use by" or "best by" dates are not safety dates, and products can often be consumed safely after these dates have passed as long as they've been stored properly.

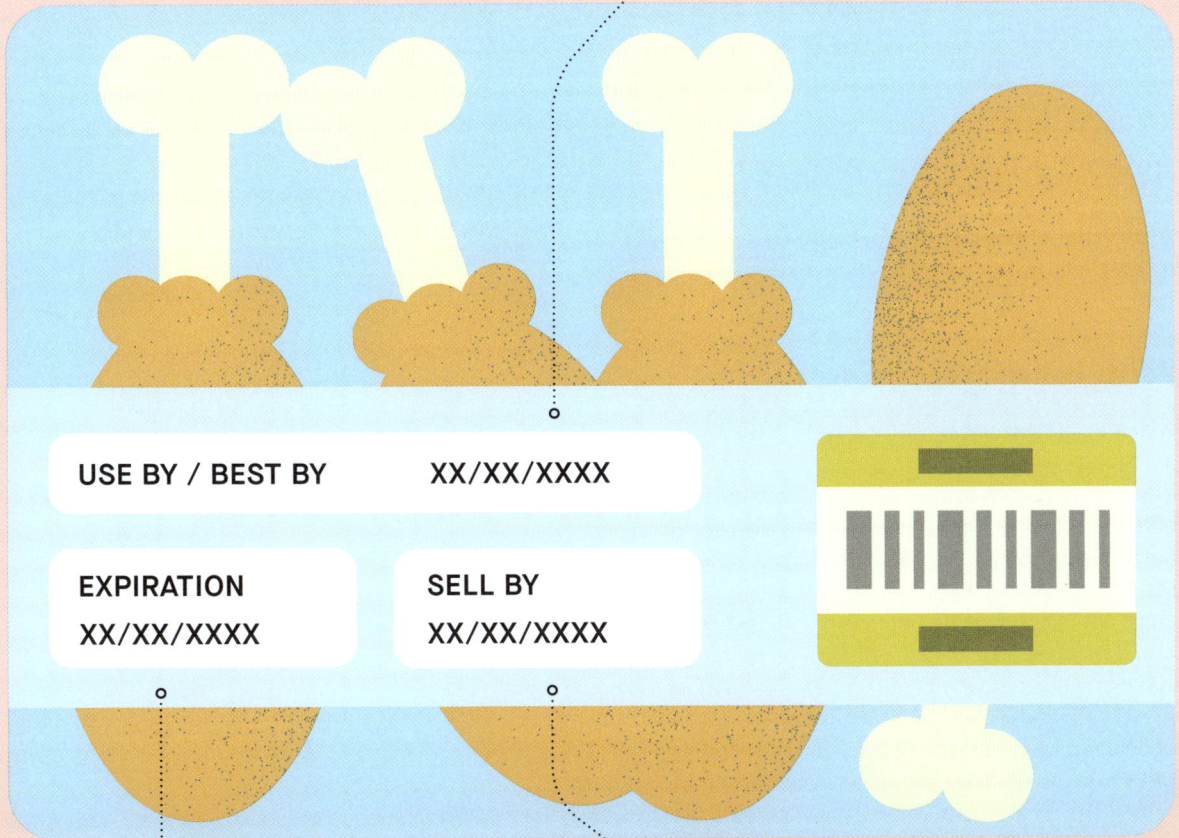

USE BY / BEST BY   XX/XX/XXXX

EXPIRATION
XX/XX/XXXX

SELL BY
XX/XX/XXXX

Expiration
This indicates the last date on which the manufacturer guarantees the product's safety and quality. After this date has passed, the product may be unsafe to eat and should be thrown out. Other factors such as temperature or exposure to oxygen once a packet is open can also impact this date and speed up the process. While these dates are only estimates, it is best to adhere to the advice.

Sell by
This label is usually printed on perishable items like meat, dairy products, and bakery items. It indicates the date by which the store should sell the product to ensure it remains fresh and safe to eat for a reasonable period afterward. If you see a product with a sell by date that has already passed, it doesn't always mean it's no longer safe to eat—just inspect the product to ensure it hasn't spoiled.

Don't fear scientific words

All food is made from chemicals—even whole foods. A strawberry is a comparatively simple food item; however, what you may not know is that a strawberry is actually a "multiple fruit" that consists of many tiny individual fruits embedded in a fleshy receptacle. The specks, which are commonly considered seeds, are the true fruits, called achenes, and each of them surrounds a tiny seed. A strawberry is a healthy item of food full of nutrition, but, if you pull it apart on a scientific level, the words may appear alarming. Do you need to know this? You probably don't, but it is important to recognize that there is a lot of nuance and complicated science behind all foods. Therefore, to pick out individual components or scientific words on ingredients lists doesn't make too much sense in isolation.

As is evident, there is a lot of confusion when it comes to ingredients lists. People often assume that all processed foods contain additives or artificial "extras"—however, this isn't always the case. For example, shelf-stable or UHT (ultra-high temperature) milk and frozen foods are both processed, and yet neither of them needs extra chemicals added during production. Reading ingredients lists correctly and understanding the hierarchy within them can be extremely helpful in deciphering the sugar, salt, and fat content of food items, while having a basic understanding of food additives (page 26) keeps us informed of what we're putting into our bodies. However, fixating on the words themselves is not the best guide to whether a food item is beneficial for your health on a day-to-day basis. Exceptions to this rule are if you have an allergy, intolerance, condition, or ethical reason that requires you to look out for certain ingredients. There will always be scientific terms that you don't understand used in ingredients lists. The key is to educate ourselves to the best of our ability so that we can make informed decisions about what we eat.

Food education is important

Online, unqualified wellness influencers would look at some of the ingredients below and label these items as "toxic," which is fearmongering at its finest. However, the cultures contained in yogurt benefit our gut, and the niacin, iron, riboflavin, thiamin, and folic acid in wheat cereal are fortifiers added to increase health (page 28).

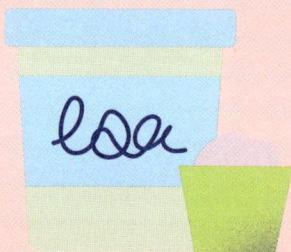

Raspberry yogurt: Live yogurt* (86%) (Milk), Sugar, Raspberries (3%), Apple purée (2%), Honey, Corn starch, Natural flavoring, Natural color (Anthocyanins), Concentrated lemon juice, Gelling agent (fruit pectin), Tapioca starch.
[*Contains Cultures: S. Thermophilus, L. Acidophilus, Bifidobacterium] o···········o *Cultures beneficial for healthy gut bacteria*

Wheat Cereal: Wholegrain Wheat (95%), Malted barley extract, Sugar, Salt. **[*Contains Niacin, Iron, Riboflavin, Thiamin, Folic acid]**
Folic acid included to keep people healthy o···········o

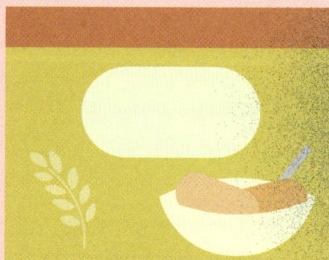

Getting familiar with "unusual" ingredients

Here are some words commonly found in ingredients lists and what they actually mean.

Ascorbic acid
Another name for vitamin C.

Beta carotene
Another name for vitamin A.

Folic acid
Synthetic form of folate (vitamin B9).

Lecithin
Natural emulsifier found in foods like soybeans and eggs that helps blend ingredients that don't naturally mix.

Pectin
Natural fiber found in fruit, often used as a gelling agent in jams and gelatins.

Aspartame
Artificial sweetener (page 41). Aspartame is one of the most common artificial sweeteners and is about 200 times sweeter than sugar. It is also used in some medications and chewable vitamins.

Maltodextrin
Used as an artificial sweetener, stabilizer, and thickening agent in processed foods. It can cause rapid spikes in blood sugar levels due to its high glycaemic index, which may be particularly harmful to individuals with insulin resistance or diabetes.

Sodium benzoate
Used as a preservative in foods. While sodium benzoate alone is not considered unsafe, when it is consumed alongside ascorbic acid (vitamin C) the acidic environment of the stomach can cause the two to react together and form small amounts of benzene—a substance that is classified as a class 1 carcinogen (page 57).

Monosodium glutamate (MSG)
This flavor enhancer, commonly known as "MSG" has been used by manufacturers for decades to create an umami, savory flavor that activates glutamate receptors in your brain. There has been a lot of misinformation surrounding MSG (despite it being approved as safe by the FDA and The European Food Information Council). The misinformation surrounding MSG is so prevalent, that manufacturers often hide it inside foods labeled as one of the following different names:

- Hydrolyzed protein
- Autolyzed yeast
- Monosodium salt
- Monohydrate
- Monosodium glutamate monohydrate
- Sodium 2-aminopentanedioate
- Monosodium L-glutamate monohydrate
- Sodium glutamate monohydrate
- UNII-W81N5U6R6U
- L-glutamic acid
- Flavor enhancer

Sodium nitrate
Used as a preservative in foods such as cured meats. The WHO has classified processed meats as a "class 1 carcinogen" (page 57). This risk comes from the sodium nitrates—when exposed to extreme heat or an acidic environment (such as the stomach), nitrates found within processed foods can change into nitrosamine in the body. Nitrosamine is a known carcinogen.

Glycerol
Added to foods and drinks to keep products moist, preserve, or sweeten them, or to change their texture. Following several cases of glycerol intoxication in children, the UK's Food Standards Agency (FSA) issued guidelines to food manufacturers and retailers regarding levels of glycerol in edible products. Glycerin (or glycerine) is a closely related ingredient used in pharmaceuticals, such as cough syrup.

How to be aware of nutritional health claims

Nutritional claims on food packaging can be incredibly misleading, leaving consumers confused about what is genuinely "healthy". While there are strict rules governing these food health claims, the way that these claims are presented on packaging often creates what we call a "health halo" around products.

For example, a branded "protein granola" might state on the package that it is a "good source of protein," meaning that it contains 10-19% of the Daily Value (DV) for protein per serving. However, to achieve its appealing taste, this granola might also contain significant amounts of added sugar. Increasing protein content can sometimes affect texture or taste, making the product drier or less palatable, so manufacturers may add sugar or syrups to improve mouthfeel and sweetness. Comparatively, a supermarket own-brand granola may have nearly the same protein content but with less sugar, making it the healthier overall choice of granola, as well as often being cheaper. Similarly, protein bars frequently highlight their high protein content but often fail to mention their high levels of salt, fat, or sugar, distracting consumers from looking into the actual nutritional values further. Because protein bars often use protein isolates or powders, which can be dry or chalky, manufacturers add sugar and syrups to improve texture and taste.

These examples show how nutritional claims and "health halos" can often distract consumers so that they don't notice the less healthy ingredients in a product. It's always worth checking the full nutritional breakdown on the back of the packaging instead of just trusting what's written on the front. Always check the nutritional breakdown of branded and unbranded products—you may be surprised which is actually better for you.

Don't be tricked into making unhealthy choices

Based on real products, these figures showing protein and sugar content are a good example of when a small increase of protein doesn't justify an even larger increase in sugar, or the additonal cost ("health branded" products often cost significantly more than own-brand products). It's unusual to be deficient in protein so, in this case, it makes far more sense to stick with "normal" granola and get our protein from other wholefood sources.

Branded protein granola

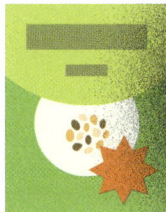

Protein per 100g = **13g**

Sugar per 100g = **18g**

Supermarket own-brand granola

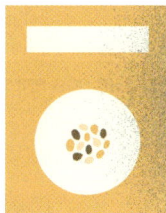

Protein per 100g = **10g**

Sugar per 100g = **13g**

Don't let "health halos" confuse you!

The wording of nutritional claims can be very confusing for consumers. It can be hard for anyone in the supermarket to understand the differences between the phrases "low sodium," "very low sodium," "sodium free," or "reduced sodium". Here are some of the most common nutritional terms in Europe and the US, and what they mean. For more detail on specific US guidelines, check the FDA "Regulatory Requirements for Nutrient Content Claims".

Low fat
No more than 3g fat per serving.

Fat-free
No more than 0.5g fat per serving.

Low saturated fat
The sum of the saturated fat and trans-fatty acids in the product cannot exceed 1.5g per 100g and the sum of saturated fat and trans-fatty acids cannot exceed more than 10% of total energy.

Saturated fat-free
The sum of saturated fat and trans-fatty acids cannot exceed 0.1g of saturated fat per 100g or 100ml.

Reduced sugar
At least 25% less sugar per serving when compared to the non-reduced food.

Sugar-free
No more than 0.5g sugar per serving.

No added sugar
Does not contain any added mono- or disaccharides or any other food used for sweetening properties. If sugars are naturally present in the food, the label must state "contains naturally occurring sugars".

Low sodium
No more than 140mg sodium per serving.

Very low sodium
No more than 35mg sodium per serving.

Sodium free
Less than 5mg sodium per serving.

Reduced sodium
At least 25% less sodium per serving when compared to the non-reduced food.

Good source of fiber
Contains at least 10% of the Daily Value (DV) for fiber per serving (about 2.5g).

High in fiber
Contains at least 5g fiber per serving.

Good source of protein
Contains 10-19% of the Daily Value (DV) for protein per serving—about 5-9.5g of protein per serving.

High in protein
Contains 20% or more of the Daily Value (DV) for protein per serving—10g or more of protein per serving.

High in monounsaturated fat
At least 45% of the fatty acids present in the product derive from monounsaturated fat, under the condition that monounsaturated fat provides more than 20% of the total energy of the product.

High in polyunsaturated fat
At least 45% of the fatty acids present in the product derive from polyunsaturated fat, under the condition that polyunsaturated fat provides more than 20% of the total energy of the product.

High in unsaturated fat
At least 70% of the fatty acids present in the product derive from unsaturated fat, under the condition that unsaturated fat provides more than 20% of energy of the product.

Calorie free
Contains less than 5 calories per serving.

Low calorie
Contains 40 calories or less per serving (serving size greater than 30g).

Reduced calorie
Contains at least 25% fewer calories per serving when compared to the regular-calorie food.

Light or Lite
One-third fewer total calories or 50% less fat per serving compared to the regular food. If more than half the calories are from fat, the fat content must be reduced by 50% or more.

Understanding seasonal eating

Seasonal eating is important to embrace when trying to reduce our UPF consumption, since fruit and vegetables that are in season are packed with flavor, making them more appealing to our taste buds. They're also packed with nutrients, which is better for our health.

The idea of "seasonal eating" simply means that you eat produce that is grown and harvested locally or close to where you live, and you also eat this produce during the season that it has been harvested.

For example, for someone living in the UK, consuming British asparagus in the month of May would be considered seasonal eating. If you live in Peru, eating avocados during the summer months is seasonal eating. However, the key here is that if you live in the UK and you also eat avocados during the summer months, this is NOT seasonal eating, since the avocados were not grown or harvested locally.

"Global seasonality" is based on where the food is produced and refers to food that is produced in season but not necessarily consumed where they were harvested.

Eat seasonally and locally to reduce your UPF intake

There's no need to get overwhelmed by what you can and can't eat—simply start small by buying a produce calendar for your local region/country and sticking it up on your kitchen wall. By being more aware of what is in season throughout the year and available locally to you, you're more likely to make more informed choices.

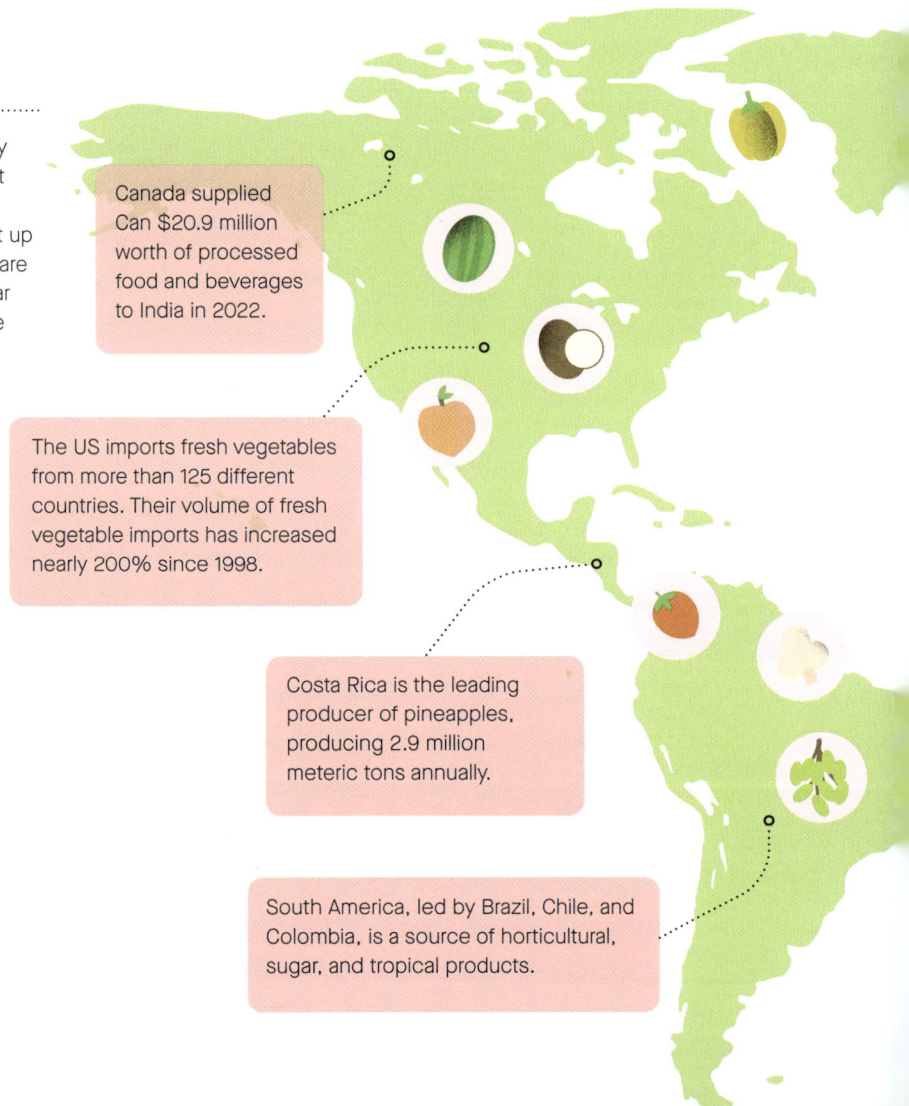

Canada supplied Can $20.9 million worth of processed food and beverages to India in 2022.

The US imports fresh vegetables from more than 125 different countries. Their volume of fresh vegetable imports has increased nearly 200% since 1998.

Costa Rica is the leading producer of pineapples, producing 2.9 million meteric tons annually.

South America, led by Brazil, Chile, and Colombia, is a source of horticultural, sugar, and tropical products.

"Local seasonality" is based on where the food is produced and then consumed. This refers to foods that are harvested and eaten locally during the natural growing season.

When possible, you should aim to eat fruit and vegetables produced in your country. However, global food systems don't usually support this notion. For instance, in 2023, the Netherlands was the largest exporter of fresh tomatoes to the UK during the summer months, when UK domestic production of tomatoes is also at its greatest. In 2022, Mexico supplied 69% of the United States' vegetable imports and 51% of its fresh fruit imports by value. So even when produce is in season locally to where you live, it can be easy to fall into the trap of buying imported items. It's also worth noting that some fruits and vegetables, such as bananas, can only grow in certain regions due to climate suitability.

Generally speaking, plants contain more nutrition when picked at the height of their season, and we know that this declines over time after harvesting. One study found that many fruits and vegetables lose phenolics, vitamin C, and anthocyanins (antioxidants that fight free radical damage and oxidative stress in the body) after 15 days of cold storage. They're also often much more affordable when in season, which makes them a better option than cheap convenience products. In addition, they have less of an environmental impact, due to decreased transportation.

Although seasonal eating should become the norm to foster a healthier food system globally, it's just one of the ways you can reduce your UPF intake.

In 2020, 42 countries accounted for 90% of the UK's imported food supply.

The Netherlands has nearly 24,000 acres of crops flourishing within its extensive greenhouse facilities—an area nearly twice the size of Manhattan.

Cereals and oil crops together account for more than 50% of the value of Russia's total agri-food exports.

In 2023, the largest exporters of fresh vegetables to the UK were Spain (32%) and the Netherlands (25%).

China is by far the largest producer of cucumbers, accounting for just over 81% of global production in 2022.

In 2021–2022, imports from Singapore to the UK increased more than any other country.

New Zealand is the UK's main source of fresh seafood, dairy products, and meat.

How to build a balanced plate

Understanding how to build a balanced plate will help you navigate the food choices you make at home and on-the-go. When possible, striving to include key nutrients and managing serving sizes is key to a healthy lifestyle.

Everyone has slightly different nutritional and portion requirements based on things like age, physical metrics, energy expenditure, and profession, but if you follow these general guidelines, you'll be on the right track to building a balanced plate.

- Choose **one** protein source—e.g. fish, chicken, pork, tofu, legumes
- Choose **one** healthy fat source— e.g. nuts, seeds, avocado, olives, healthy oils
- Choose **one** carbohydrate source—e.g. starchy root vegetables, grains, fruit

- Choose up to **four** different-colored vegetables—the more color on your plate, the better!
- Choose a **combination** of herbs and spices—you may not realize that these also contribute toward your plant points (page 54).

If you're unsure about what your personal serving size should be for each meal, the simplest way to gauge this is by using your hands! See the guide below to roughly figure out how much of each food item should feature on your plate.

Once you've used these formulas to build your plates a few times, it will become second nature. Of course, when eating in a restaurant, you can't ensure you're consuming a balanced plate, but that's fine. What's important is that you make good food choices when at home or packing lunch boxes for work or school.

Your hand is your portion tool

Use this "handy" guide to figure out your personal serving size for each meal.

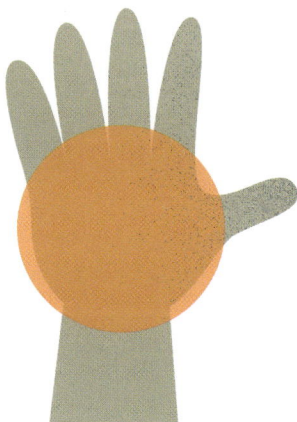

A serving of
protein = 1 palm

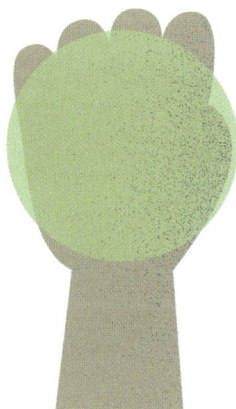

A serving of
vegetables = 1 fist

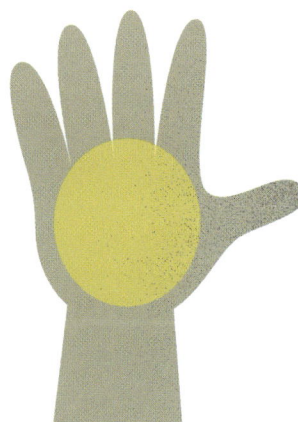

A serving of carbs
= 1 cupped hand

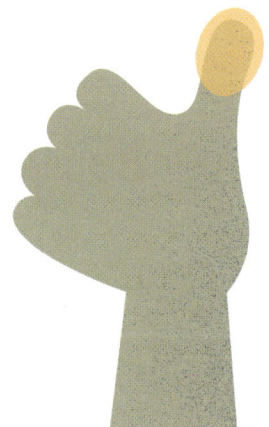

A serving of healthy
fats = 1 thumb

What does a balanced plate look like?

If you follow the formulas on this page and aim to eat 30 different plants a week (page 54), building balanced plates will get easier and easier. Turn to page 88 for plenty of balanced recipe ideas.

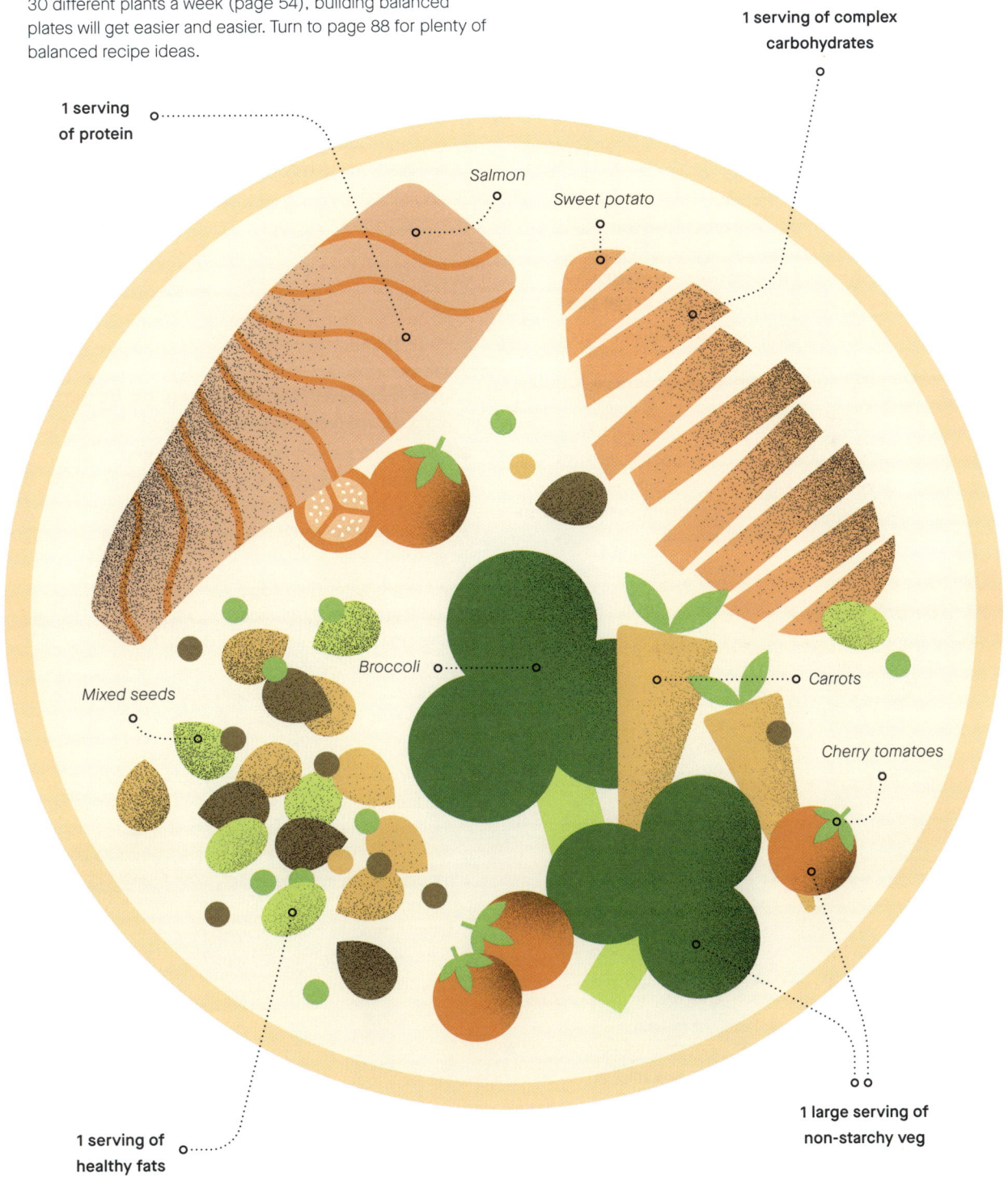

1 serving of complex carbohydrates

1 serving of protein

Salmon

Sweet potato

Broccoli

Mixed seeds

Carrots

Cherry tomatoes

1 serving of healthy fats

1 large serving of non-starchy veg

How to write a UPF-free shopping list

Whether you visit the supermarket every week, buy your groceries online, or go to the store every day after work, the principles of healthy eating remain the same. Focus on your five food groups—fruit and vegetables, carbohydrates, dairy or plant-based alternatives, protein, fats—and have a rough idea of your meal plan before going to the store. Temptation is everywhere in stores, with deals and offers often promoting UPF items over healthier whole foods.

It can be hard to break your regular shopping habits, whether that's regularly going to the grocery store, or filling your weekly shopping basket on autopilot. Taking a moment to consider your grocery shop makes it easier to maintain healthy habits during the week.

Shopping tips

- Never shop without a list!
- Plan your meals for the week. When are you going to be in? Would it be handy to have leftovers for the next day? Are there members of your family who might not be in on certain days?
- Always check your pantry, fridge, and freezer and cross reference with your shopping list before you leave the house.
- Are you a paper and pen person, or a phone notes person? There are now apps and other helpful tools to help with your shopping list, so find the one that works for you.
- Try shopping online. Sometimes, when not overwhelmed with visual choice and in-your-face marketing, we can make more sensible food choices. Say goodbye to impulse-purchases and stick to your list.
- Stock up on one item each week to make the task of building a healthy pantry less overwhelming and expensive.

STEP 1: fruit and vegetables

- **Eat the rainbow!** Ensure you select lots of different-colored vegetables since this is one of the easiest ways to ensure you're eating a variety of nutrients.
- **Count.** Fresh produce goes off quickly, so only buy what you need to last you for the next week.
- **Think seasonal.** Try to only buy fruit and vegetables that are in season in your local area (page 68) for the cheapest prices and most nutrients.
- **Shop for your needs.** Prepackaged picked lettuce will go off more quickly than a whole lettuce. But if you need lettuce for a particular recipe, it's better to buy some prewashed bagged greens for ease, and to avoid food waste.
- **Don't just buy for the fridge.** Remember that frozen, canned, jarred, and dried options exist for a lot of fruit and vegetables. They should last for a long time and are really convenient when you need a simple, quick dinner. Just remember to check the ingredients list to make sure they don't have any added salt, sugar or syrups.
- **Save it for the weekend.** Instead of buying cheap processed/ultra-processed convenience products more often, it's preferable to buy better-quality, minimally processed or unprocessed products infrequently. For example, ditch juice from concentrate and buy 100% fruit juice instead. It doesn't need to be consumed every day, so why not save it for the weekend?

STEP 2: carbohydrates

- **Good grains.** Stock up on grains that will keep for a long time in your pantry. This includes items like pearl barley, quinoa, brown rice, bulgar wheat, and wholewheat pasta.
- **Bread.** If buying bread, try to buy freshly baked whole wheat bread without additives. When you get home, simply slice it and store it in the freezer.

STEP 3: dairy and plant-based alternatives

- **Make it last.** Always check the use-by dates when buying dairy and select the farthest date you can find to ensure you're purchasing the freshest product possible.
- **Read the labels.** Sometimes "light" or "low-fat" products can contain additives and added sugars. Read the labels on all dairy products to ensure there aren't added sugars, colors, or flavors.
- **Add flavor at home.** Opt for unflavored dairy products and add your own flavorings at home in the form of honey or fruit.
- **Dairy-free is fine!** If opting for dairy-free milks, find more information on page 35.
- **Don't be worried about adapting to your needs.** If necessary, shelf-stable or powdered products are completely fine to use. Just be sure to check the ingredients lists don't contain too many ingredients.

Take a moment to consider your grocery shop and build healthy habits during the week.

STEP 4: protein

- **Eat more legumes.** If possible, aim to reduce animal consumption and replace some of your protein with legumes, like lentils and beans.
- **Go big.** Purchase legumes in large bags or cans, since they store well and are cheaper to buy in bulk.
- **Check out the freezer aisle**. Visit the frozen section of the supermarket for meat and fish. Products are often cheaper here, and their nutrients are preserved through freezing.
- **Get those omega-3s.** Don't forget that lots of oily fish, like mackerel, sardines, and anchovies, can often be bought in cans. Look for those packed in olive oil.
- **Give soy a try.** Soybeans, tempeh, or tofu are cheaper than meat and fish and contain good amounts of beneficial protein.

STEP 5: fats

- **Liquid gold.** Opt for extra-virgin olive oil as your everyday oil choice for dressings and salads, since it's full of antioxidants and unsaturated fats. It's a little expensive, but ultimately worth it. Buy it in larger quantities for the most cost-effective option.
- **High-heat cooking.** Pick up some avocado oil for when you're roasting, frying, or cooking anything using high heat.
- **Beware of misleading labels!** Many fat spreads marketed as "low-fat" or "heart-healthy" are full of ultra-processed ingredients. Choose minimally processed options, like those made from olive oil, if you prefer a spreadable alternative to butter.
- **Quality matters.** In the case of oils and butter, buy the best-quality fats you can afford to ensure you are consuming the healthiest option.

How to prioritize home-cooked meals

For lots of people, cooking can seem like a chore if you don't have reliable recipes you can turn to, especially if you work long hours, have to do shift work, or have a hectic family life. With so many convenience items available to us, it's easier than ever to fall into the trap of relying on UPFs at every mealtime. (As a working mom of two, I am no stranger to the daily demands of a busy life, and even as a nutritionist I don't always have the time to cook from scratch!)

The best thing you can do is make incremental changes that will make cooking and eating more straightforward. As well as using the simple recipes in chapter three (page 88), here are 10 helpful habits that you can introduce to enable you to make better food choices for you and your family, so that you can reduce the number of times you turn to UPFs.

1 Prioritize breakfast

Always try to make breakfast from scratch, whether the night before so you can grab-and-go the next day, or quickly in the morning to set you up for whatever comes your way. Turn to page 90 for some of my favorite recipes for starting the day right.

2 Simplify

Never underestimate the power of a baked potato cooking away in the oven as you get changed after work, put the kids to bed, or finish up some emails. Simple but balanced meals, or one-pan dishes that you can throw in the oven require minimal time, cooking skill, and washing up. Turn to page 139 and 161 for some simple yet nutritional traybakes.

3 Utilize your weekends

Set aside an hour to prep vegetables for the week ahead. Simply chop and slice your veggies; then store them in sealed containers in the fridge or freezer for quick and easy cooking on week days.

4 Cook once, eat twice

If it's something that will keep for a few days, always cook more food than you need so you have leftovers for lunch or dinner the next day. My rainbow rice bowl (page 117) is perfect for a packed lunch and my veggie-loaded lasagna (page 151) can be portioned up and frozen for easy homemade convenience meals.

5 Stay hydrated

Drinking water helps with digestion, regulating hunger levels, and keeps you thinking straight. This means you'll be less likely to reach for UPFs in the form of snacks and carbonated drinks.

6 Try meal planning

Plan your meals for the week ahead to save yourself time, brain power, and money. By buying only what you need for the meals you've planned, you'll avoid picking up unnecessary UPF options (see opposite).

7 Rely on your pantry

Ensure that you always have quick "base" carbohydrate options in the pantry (like quinoa, brown rice, or brown pasta) and protein sources (like canned beans, lentils, and canned fish). Add some roasted veggies and a handful of nuts and seeds, and you've got a variety of balanced dinners for almost zero effort.

8 Make meals work for you

Only got 30 minutes to spare? Then prioritize recipes that take less time to make. There's a whole section of "30-minute heroes" on page 128 for when you're limited on time but want to ensure you're cooking balanced meals.

9 Sauce prep

Some of the most common UPFs we consume on a daily basis are sauces and spreads, so turn to page 202 for homemade versions of your most-loved condiments. Make them in advance and store them in the fridge for easy access.

10 Make friends with your appliances

Microwaves, air fryers, and slow cookers can all save you time and money, making it easier to rely on home cooking more often. Find out which appliance is best suited to you on page 76.

Make incremental changes that will make cooking and eating more straightforward.

How to meal plan

Meal planning is a great tool for eating healthily, reducing food waste, and saving you cooking time during the week. Simply follow these four steps for stress-free meals.

1. Take time to plan
Use the recipes in chapter three (page 88) to plan your meals for the week.

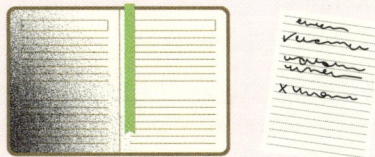

2. Do your food shopping
Use the shopping list guidance on page 72 to plan your shopping.

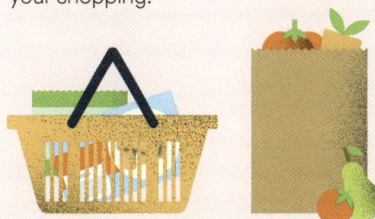

3. Prep and cook
Carve out cooking time on a Sunday to prep your meals for the week.

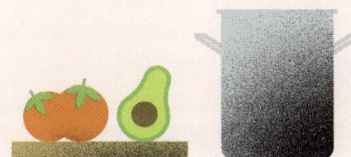

4. Store it safely
Portion and store your prepped meals in the fridge or freezer (page 84).

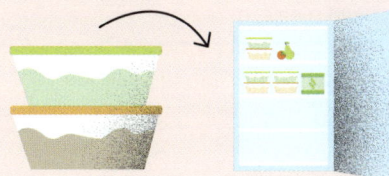

Make the most of your kitchen

When trying to reduce consumption of UPFs, it's important to give yourself the best chance of making nutritionally balanced home-cooked meals. To do this you need to ensure that your kitchen works for YOU. Having useful pieces of equipment and appliances is key to making cooking easy and enjoyable.

Figure out which appliances work for your cooking needs based on budget, cooking time, and how many people you regularly cook for. Cooking from scratch not only helps you to reduce your UPF consumption and therefore eat more healthily, but it also saves you money. By ensuring you have basic cooking equipment and an understanding of how different appliances can work for your space and budget, there's no reason why you can't create wholesome, nutritious food every day.

Oven

Most ovens range from 2000 to 5000 watts, which makes them more energy-intensive than air fryers. The reason ovens are more expensive to use is that they heat a larger space and are often on for longer periods.

Having useful items of equipment and appliances is key to making cooking easy and enjoyable.

However, this larger capacity can make them more cost-efficient for batch cooking or cooking for families, so it's best to adapt based on the quantity of food you are cooking.

Stovetop

Induction stovetops are the most energy- and cost-efficient stoves to cook with. They work by passing current through copper coils below the surface to heat only the cookware, resulting in less wasted heat and faster cooking times. In contrast, **electric** stovetops heat the cooking surface using electricity, and **gas** stovetops use an open flame, both of which are less efficient and lead to slightly higher energy costs.

Microwave

Microwaves use less energy in general than other appliances in the kitchen because because they heat food directly rather than the entire oven space. However, the actual cost varies quite a lot depending on the power (wattage), which often ranges from 500W to 1500W.

Air fryer

Air fryers use more energy per minute than people think; however, it's important to note that the time taken to cook food products is usually less than it would take in a conventional oven, meaning the overall cost may work out to be cheaper.

Slow cooker

Slow cookers use far less energy than most other kitchen appliances, even when left on for eight hours. This means they won't cost you much. They are a useful tool for getting comforting home-cooked food on the table on even the busiest of days.

Equipment

To make cooking from scratch as easy as possible, ensure that your kitchen has these handy tools.

Essentials

Baking dish

Spatula

Wooden spoon

Whisk

Tongs

Vegetable peeler

Sieve or Colander

Electric hand blender

Box grater

Digital scale

Measuring spoons

Mixing bowl

Stockpot

Frying pan

Roasting pan

Sharp knives

Nice to have

Meat thermometer

Mortar and pestle

Blender

Food processor

Rolling pin

Casserole dish

Easy UPF swaps

If you are looking to reduce the number of additives, salt, sugar, and fat you eat (which more often than not go hand in hand with the consumption of convenience items) here are some simple swaps you can make when shopping and eating. You can find even more helpful ideas for making healthy food choices in the recipe section on page 88.

Did you know?

Spices are a great way to boost your plant-based food intake, and they even count toward your goal of 30 plants a week (page 54). Even in small amounts, they are rich in antioxidants and offer a burst of flavor, making it easy to add variety to your diet while supporting your health.

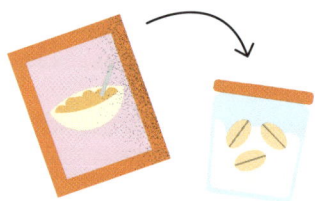

Cereals

Swap sugary, UPF breakfast cereals, that are full of additives and added sugar, with homemade overnight oats (page 92) or granola (page 95). You can add fresh fruit, nuts, and/or nut butter to these too, to give your body the perfect balanced start to the day.

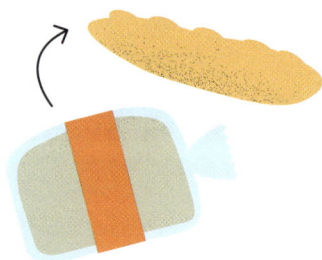

Bread

Instead of picking up a prepackaged loaf of bread containing emulsifiers, preservatives, salt, and sugar, switch to a freshly baked whole wheat or sourdough bread that is made without the addition of these ingredients. Remember, these breads will go stale faster than those containing preservatives; to counteract this, simply slice the loaf and store it in the freezer so you can grab slices as and when you need them. If you want to make your own bread, try my soda bread (page 97), cottage cheese bread (page 110), or yogurt flatbreads (page 179).

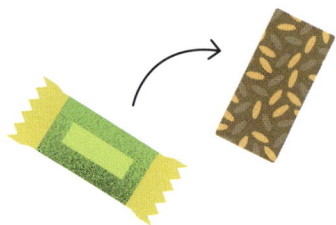

Snack bars

Instead of snacking on prepackaged cereal bars, which are high in added sugar and other unnecessary ingredients, try making your own granola bars at home using oats, honey, nuts, and dried fruit. The coconut, date, and orange energy balls on page 197 are a perfect pre- or post-workout snack, while the chocolate, peanut, and date bars on page 194 are always on hand when you need that chocolate fix!

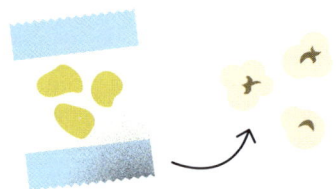

Packaged snacks

Instead of reaching for a bag of chips, crackers, or sweetened popcorn as a mid-afternoon snack, try making your own snacks and store them in airtight containers in the pantry for easy access throughout the week. Homemade popcorn is so easy to make and allows you to add only essential flavorings, or you could try miso-roasted nuts (page 181) or seedy crackers (page 175).

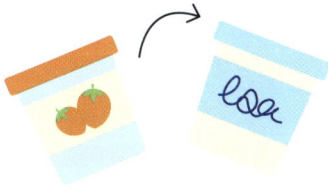

Yogurt

Sweetened, flavored, low-fat, or "light" yogurts are often classed as UPFs due to the many ingredients they contain. Switch them out for plain or Greek yogurt, which is simply made from milk and strains of "good" bacteria. Top it with fresh fruit or a drizzle of honey if you still need sweetness.

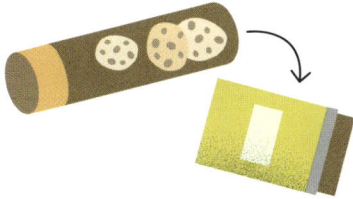

Sweets, chocolate, and prepackaged cookies

While we all enjoy a sweet treat every now and then, these items are best consumed in moderation. Try snacking on dark chocolate, dates, homemade fruit roll-ups (page 198), or homemade oaty cookies (page 201) instead. If you really want some candy, try to choose a brand that uses natural, and fewer, ingredients (always check the label!).

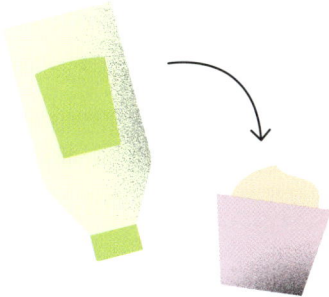

Sauces and spreads

Condiments like ketchup and mayo are household favourites, but they are often full of preservatives and additives to keep them staying fresh for months. These food items are actually incredibly easy to make at home yourself, which means you can be in complete control of what you put into your body. Try my spiced ketchup (page 206), aquafaba mayo (page 207), chilli and mint hummus (page 174), pesto (page 211), tartare sauce (page 208), nutty chocolate spread (page 205), chia and berry jam (page 204), and a selection of salad dressings (page 213) for easy homemade swaps.

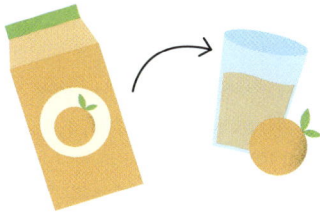

Fruit juice and soda

Fruit juices from concentrate, those with added sugars, and sodas are all full of additives, artificial colorings, and preservatives. Switch to a freshly squeezed fruit juice (1 serving is just 3½fl oz/100ml), or simply add a slice of lemon or cucumber, or some berries, to a glass of still or sparkling water. If you're struggling to give up soda, wean yourself off by mixing a little cordial (which is still high in sugar) into a glass of sparkling water.

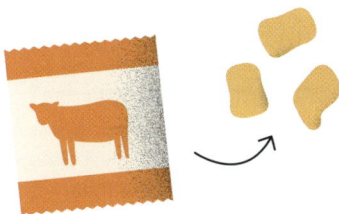

Processed meat products

Processed meats contain additives to keep them fresh for longer and maintain flavor, and are thought to be linked to an increased risk in cancer (page 56). Therefore, it's best to avoid these products when possible. Try making your own chicken nuggets using ground chicken, or switch out the meat entirely for a plate packed full of protein from beans and lentils, like my triple protein dal (page 152) or protein-packed green fritters (page 126).

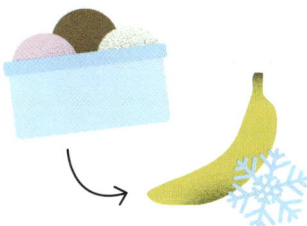

Ice cream

Most store-bought ice cream is heavily processed and full of synthetic chemicals to keep it smooth, frozen, and delicious. "Soft serve" is one of the worst culprits. When buying ice cream, sorbet, or gelato, check to ensure that the ingredients list only contains egg, sugar, milk, and cream. If you want to make a quick banana ice cream, blend frozen bananas with a splash of milk or yogurt. Or try making the ice pops on page 192.

The UPF-free pantry

How do we know if our most-used store-bought staples are benefiting our health? Here's a handy guide to some common ingredients so that you're able to identify hidden UPFs and make informed decisions about what you buy, cook, and eat.

Products like this contain varying levels of processing depending on their brand, ingredients, and shelf life.

Although many are UPFs, the intent isn't to demonize these products – they're convenience items for a reason! Don't be too hard on yourself – a bit of jam or ketchup isn't the end of the world. But hopefully this will encourage you to stop and think next time you're shopping, and either choose to select a less processed product, or have a go at making some of them yourself where possible.

Common store-bought pantry staples

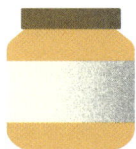

Nut butters

Nut butters are an excellent source of healthy (unsaturated) fats, protein, and micronutrients like magnesium and vitamin E. To avoid UPFs, choose those that are made with 100% nuts and have no added oils, sugar, or salt.

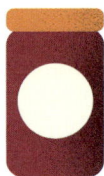

Jams and preserves

Jams, jellies, and preserves are delicious because they're high in sugar! This doesn't mean you shouldn't enjoy them, but just be mindful of the sugar content and consume them in moderation. Jams and preserves from some brands contain significantly less sugar than others, so it's worth comparing a few jars. For a healthier homemade alternative, try the recipe on page 204.

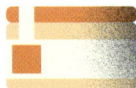

Miso

Miso is a fermented soy product rich in umami flavor and gut-friendly probiotics. Look for unpasteurized miso to maximize its probiotic benefits as the pasteurized versions are heat-treated and will contain only minimal beneficial bacteria. However, be mindful of the high salt content of miso. Reduced salt versions are available, but are not essential if you consume miso in moderation.

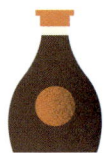

Soy sauce

Soy sauce provides a rich source of umami, but is very high in salt. Opt for low-salt versions and check for natural brewing processes that avoid using synthetic additives. Tamari is a good gluten-free alternative with a similar flavor profile to soy sauce, and is often less processed with fewer ingredients.

Stock and gravy

Premade stock and gravy is convenient, but is often high in salt and artificial flavorings. Where you can, choose organic, low-salt options, or make your own.

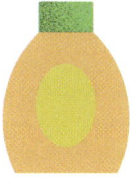

Honey

When it comes to honey, opting for high-quality, raw, local varieties or Manuka honey offers far more benefits than the processed, plastic-bottled versions, which are often pure sugar with little to no nutritional value. While Manuka honey can be pricey, its unique properties and health benefits make it a worthwhile investment for those seeking a natural, nourishing sweetener. Manuka honey is renowned for its unique antibacterial properties, which are attributed to its high levels of methylglyoxal (MGO). This compound gives Manuka honey its potent ability to help fight bacteria and support immune health. Additionally, it has anti-inflammatory properties and can aid in wound healing and digestive health. This sets it apart from regular honey, which lacks these benefits after high levels of processing.

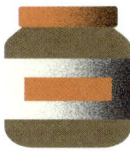

Chocolate spreads

Many chocolate spreads are highly processed and high in sugar and palm oil. Look for options with a high percentage of cacao and made with natural sweeteners or minimal added sugars. Nut-based spreads with cacao are a better alternative for a more nutrient-dense option. Find a recipe for homemade chocolate spread on page 205.

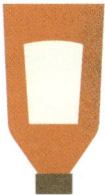

Ketchup

Store-bought ketchup often contains added sugars, salt, and preservatives. When possible, choose reduced-sugar or naturally sweetened options, and check that whole tomatoes are the first thing listed in the ingredients list. Don't be fooled by fancy-looking jars of ketchup since they often contain more sugar than generic brands! Find a recipe for homemade ketchup on page 206.

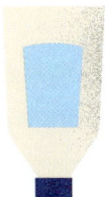

Mayonnaise

Store-bought mayonnaise is inevitably a highly processed condiment and should be consumed in moderation. While it's easy to make a less processed version from scratch using simple ingredients like eggs, oil, and lemon juice, homemade mayo won't stay fresh for long. For store-bought options, just be mindful of serving sizes, since it's a calorie-dense addition to meals. Find a recipe for homemade mayo on page 207.

Cooking pastes

Cooking pastes like curry, tomato, or garlic pastes are handy but can contain added sugar, salt, and preservatives. Look for products with minimal ingredients, focusing on pure herbs and spices, or make your own cooking pastes for a fresher alternative.

Dried herbs and spices

Dried herbs and spices are an inexpensive and convenient way to enhance flavor and, in turn, often mean you can add less salt to a meal. They also count toward your goal of 30 different plants a week (page 54). Check labels to avoid those mixed with anticaking agents or fillers.

How to reorganize your pantry

If you want to reduce your UPF intake and get more creative in the kitchen, rethinking how you store your dry goods is going to make a huge difference. There is nothing more therapeutic than a pantry clear-out. If you want to take things a step further, you can use airtight containers to sort and store ingredients, too. Just remember that the more visible the ingredients, the more likely you are to use them, which is why glass or clear containers work best. If the containers you use are opaque, it's even more important to label everything clearly.

Life is busy and it can be tough to eat well if the environment you inhabit is in a state of disarray and chaos. A bit of mess is inevitable, especially if you have children, but when your kitchen pantry has structure and there is a clear food system in place, it will enable you to make sensible choices most of the time. Psychology of nutrition plays a surprisingly large role when it comes to the way we organize and arrange our kitchen. One study found that when living in a chaotic food environment, consumption of items such as crackers and carrots were not impacted, but items like cookies were overconsumed when compared to living in a tidy food environment. It's also likely that our childhood influences our food decisions, and even the way we store our food. To break this cycle and form better food habits, the change has to come from you. This pantry clear-out and reset is going to make a huge difference to your life, allowing for a calmer cooking experience and better food choices.

STEP 1

Remove all the dry goods from your pantry and check that they are not past their due dates.

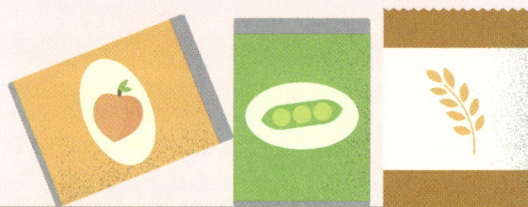

STEP 2

Group together all the **dry** staple grains and carbohydrate bases. These are grains, legumes, pastas, nuts, and seeds that are simple to cook and/or add to a dish as a side, or as an extra boost of protein or fat. Place these back in the pantry together on one shelf with the packages clearly visible, or in labeled airtight containers. I make sure I always have the following:

- Quinoa
- Bulgar wheat
- Pearl barley
- Spelt
- Brown rice
- Wholewheat pasta
- Red lentils
- Mixed nuts and seeds

STEP 3

Now group cans or jars of **cooked** legumes, beans, and animal protein and allocate a shelf to store them all on. Try to have a selection of the following:

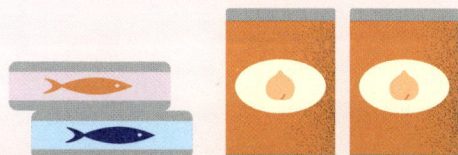

- Lima beans
- Kidney beans
- Black beans
- Chickpeas
- Lentils
- Sardines
- Mackerel
- Anchovies
- Tuna (choose skipjack or yellowfin for more sustainable options)

STEP 4

Now do the same for any canned fruit and vegetables, ensuring they also have their own shelf. Things like:

- Tomatoes
- Corn
- Pumpkin
- Fruit chunks (in water, not in syrup!)

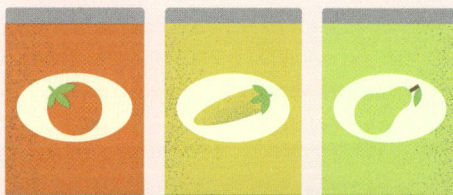

STEP 5

Next, sort out all the goods that would fit into "the baking section" or "the breakfast section" and store them together somewhere that is easily accessible. As in STEP 2, it may be useful to store certain items in labeled airtight containers. This selection will, of course, vary from person to person, but here is what I usually have on hand:

- Breakfast cereals
- Oats
- Flax or chia seeds
- Baking powder
- Baking soda
- Whole wheat flour
- All-purpose flour
- Dried fruit
- Salt
- Sugar
- Extra-virgin olive oil
- Infused/flavored oils
- Nut butters
- Tahini
- Honey
- Maple syrup
- Jam (keep in the fridge once open)

STEP 6

It's useful to have a few snacks to hand for the family or quick lunch additions. These get their own shelf too. These are the items I buy most often:

- Wholegrain crackers
- Popcorn kernels
- Dark chocolate (at least 75% cocoa solids)
- Medjool dates
- Spiced nut mixes or crispy chickpeas

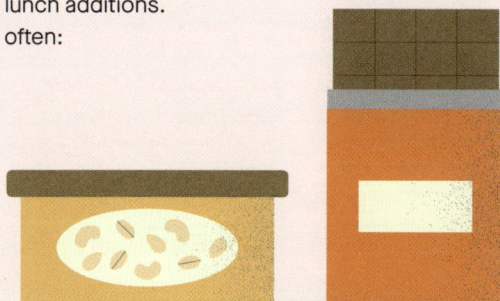

Love your freezer

New clients at my clinic are asked the same question at nearly every initial consultation: **can you list every item in the bottom drawer of your freezer?** Often, the answer is no!

Our freezer tends to be a space we use with good intention but with very little organization. Items get forgotten about and, instead of decreasing food waste, we create a home for forgotten foods. In fact, the freezer is an incredibly useful tool for preserving home-cooked leftovers, reducing food waste, and ultimately stopping us from reaching for convenient UPFs.

There is also countless research looking at the nutritional variances between frozen and fresh produce. Research suggests that freezing blueberries shortly after harvest preserves most of their antioxidants. One study found that, even three months after freezing, blueberries did not show any significant difference in anthocyanin content when compared to their fresh counterparts. Additionally, some research has found that the vitamin C content of frozen blueberries is higher than that of fresh.

Fresh fish is a rich source of omega-3 fatty acids, vitamin D, and protein. However, like most other foods, the nutrient content can decline over time if the fish is not handled correctly during transportation or consumed shortly after being caught. Freezing fish immediately likely preserves its omega-3 and nutrient content. One study analyzed the stability of omega-3 and other lipids in fish when frozen and found that most of the omega-3 in the frozen fish was still nutritionally available three months after freezing.

Don't take your freezer for granted

Having a freezer is a privilege. In the UK, an estimated 480,000 households, or 1.2 million adults and children, are missing at least one large household appliance (washing machine and/or fridge-freezer). Turn to page 18 to read more about how privilege impacts food choices.

How to make friends with your freezer

- **Set it to the correct temperature.** In order to prolong the life of your frozen items, the recommended temperature for freezers is 0°F (-18°C).

- **Label your shelves/drawers.** This may sound strange, but by organizing your freezer into different sections, you'll be more likely to use it properly and know what's inside. Use the guide opposite for optimal freezer organization.

- **Portion control.** Divide leftovers into individual portions before freezing them so that you can easily grab as many servings from the freezer as you need, rather than having to defrost the whole batch (and therefore potentially wasting it). Think of these as your own homemade convenience meals, which are so much better for you than the UPF alternatives.

- **Label your leftovers.** Once something is frozen it can be hard to tell what it is. Always label the containers that you store leftovers in so that you're more likely to reach for them.

- **Follow freezing and defrosting advice.** Always check food packaging for freezing guidance and remember that food can be frozen right up until midnight on the "use by" date printed on the label.

- **Consider these handy frozen veg tips.** To avoid soggy vegetables when cooking them from frozen, defrost your vegetables overnight in a colander set over a bowl in the fridge. This helps drain excess water so they cook with a better texture and consistency. While items such as frozen chopped onions are technically processed since they've been pre-chopped for you, they're just as nutritious as fresh ones and save you loads of time in the kitchen!

How to organize your freezer

Make your freezer more user-friendly by roughly dividing it into the following sections:
· vegetables, herbs, stock, bread
· fruit, homemade ice pops, ice cream
· fish, meat, sauces, leftovers

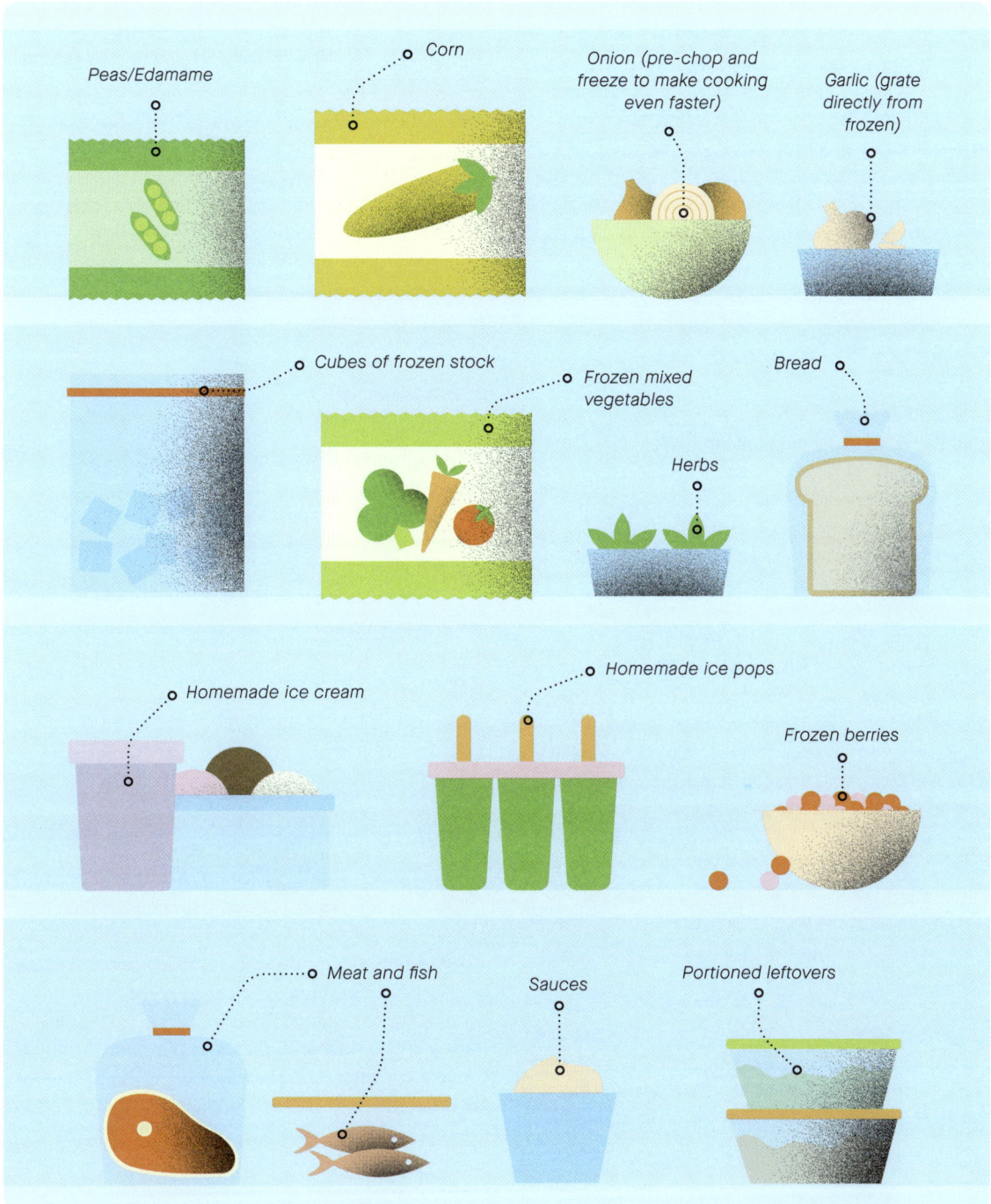

Peas/Edamame

Corn

Onion (pre-chop and freeze to make cooking even faster)

Garlic (grate directly from frozen)

Cubes of frozen stock

Frozen mixed vegetables

Herbs

Bread

Homemade ice cream

Homemade ice pops

Frozen berries

Meat and fish

Sauces

Portioned leftovers

How to avoid UPFs when out and about

On-the-go items are often where UPFs sneak into our diets, purely because convenience foods are made to be easily transportable, sit on shelves for extended periods, and remain palatable. With a little planning and creativity, you can enjoy wholesome, nutritious food on-the-go or in your lunch box that keeps you satisfied and energized throughout the day without the need to always reach for UPF items.

Plan ahead

One of the best ways to steer clear of UPFs is to plan ahead. By taking a few moments to think about your meals for the week, you can ensure that you have the ingredients and time to prepare healthier options. The term "meal prep" is often associated with gym-goers who strictly monitor their intake of food groups. However, meal prepping can be a really powerful tool for everybody. Check out the meal planning guide on page 75, then try preparing several packed-lunch options that will last you through the week. Homemade salads (try the recipes on pages 112, 114, and 119), grain bowls (page 117), or wraps are great choices that are easy to assemble quickly and store well. If you have a microwave at your office, you can also prep hot things that travel well, like soup (pages 121, 122), stews (pag 158), and dal (page 152).

If you often skip breakfast, before you leave the house try prepping overnight oats (page 92) or some muffins (pages 100, 105) the night before, which you can easily grab and take to work with you. This will help reduce the habit of purchasing a UPF convenience product from somewhere en route. Kicking this habit can prevent the spike in blood glucose levels that contribute to a mid-morning slump, and potentially increase the urge to reach for something else just a few hours later.

Prepare portable, nutrient-dense meals

One of the reasons we reach for UPFs is their portability. Lunch often needs to be something we can grab quickly and eat on-the-go. To avoid this trap, prepare meals that are easy to pack and transport (try the salads on pages 112 and 114). Give yourself a helping hand by ensuring you have some glass jars or sealable containers that you can store and transport your prepped food in.

Cook from scratch

Cooking from scratch allows you to control what goes into your food, avoiding additives and preservatives commonly found in processed or UPF meals. Even something as simple as a sandwich can be much better for you when made at home using fresh ingredients. Swap store-bought staples, which often contain emulsifiers and preservatives, for homemade versions in the "sauces and essentials" section (page 202).

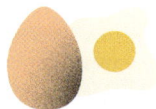

Rethink your protein source

As mentioned in more detail on page 38, prepackaged deli meats, sausages, and other processed protein options are major culprits when it comes to the overconsumption of UPFs. Instead, try to cook with whole, minimally processed proteins like chicken breast, eggs, tofu, or legumes. Roasting some chickpeas, baking chicken breasts, pan-frying marinated tofu, or preparing a batch of boiled eggs at the start of the week can give you easy, versatile protein options for salads.

Make simple swaps

Avoiding UPFs doesn't mean you have to give up your favorite lunch foods entirely, but simple swaps can make a big difference to your total UPF intake. For example, instead of buying store-bought soup (which may contain emulsifiers, preservatives and flavor enhancers), make a batch of homemade soup using fresh vegetables and broth (try the recipes on pages 121 and 122). Instead of using processed wraps that contain many additives, try making easy flatbreads (page 179) at home for use throughout the week. Small changes like this can have a positive impact on your health over time. Find more ideas for easy UPF swaps on page 78.

Make your own salad dressings and toppers

Salad dressings and sauces are common sources of UPFs, often loaded with additives like emulsifiers, stabilizers, and added sugars. The same goes for delicious toppings that add an extra punch of texture and flavors to store-bought salad bowls. Making a batch of your own dressings (page 213) and salad or soup toppers (page 214), and storing them in the fridge at home or at work, is an easy way to add healthy extra flavor and variety to your lunches.

Choose whole grains

Bread products can be a hidden source of UPFs (page 36) and can contain emulsifiers, preservatives, and added sugar. If you can't avoid buying bread at the supermarket, always try to choose bread, wraps, and other similar products made only with whole grains and other natural ingredients (always check the label). Even better, try to make your own bread at home using the recipes on pages 97 and 110, or buy from local bakeries that use traditional methods and minimal ingredients.

If bread is a regular part of your lunch, try switching things up occasionally by making wholegrain salads using things like quinoa or buckwheat—try my quinoa Niçoise salad on page 112 to get you started.

Choose your drink wisely

Soft drinks, sugary juices, flavored coffee, and processed energy drinks are loaded with UPFs, including artificial sweeteners, preservatives, and coloring agents. Sticking to water is the healthiest way to hydrate and one of the easiest ways to reduce UPF intake. Invest in a good nonplastic water bottle so that you always have it to hand and are less tempted to purchase an ultra-processed drinks when on the go.

Ditch the packaged snacks

UPFs often find their way into our lunches through snacks like chips, crackers, or cookies. To avoid this, opt for whole foods that are naturally nutrient dense. Swap chips for a small portion of nuts or seeds (page 181), and instead of packaged granola bars, try making your own using oats, honey, and nuts. Not only does this eradicate unnecessary added ingredients, but it is also cheaper than buying small packs of bars. Fresh fruit is another great option to satisfy sweet cravings without reaching for highly processed desserts.

Minimize, don't demonize

Wraps are often considered UPFs due to the preservatives added to extend their shelf life. Without these preservatives, wraps go off quickly and aren't as shiny and soft. When choosing wraps, it's best to go for whole wheat, since it offers more fiber and nutrients. It's also wise to select wraps that don't contain added palm oil. If you can't, however, it's not a major health concern—it's just a bonus if you can avoid it. You can find wraps in supermarkets that are made with just wheat, water, extra-virgin olive oil or avocado oil, and salt, which aren't classified as UPFs. These are the best options, but keep in mind that they are more expensive. They will also go off faster because they contain no additives. Buying them in bulk and freezing them is a great solution for keeping them fresh.

Recipes to

The food we eat is undeniably important for how we feel and perform every day, as well as for how we age and reduce our risk of disease. Most of us are aware that when we eat "well" – however that looks to us—we reap the benefits.

For this reason, I've created recipes that replace your usual go-to UPFs both at home and on-the-go. I've also calculated the **plant point**, **fibre** and **protein** content of each meal. Plant points are a positive way to assess your meal—every herb, spice, variety of vegetable, pulse, or even dark chocolate can contribute (page 34). This system is a refreshing change from the typical focus on restriction in most nutrition books. Instead, it encourages what you can add to your diet, rather than what you should eliminate.

I've also included pantry essentials found in many households—from ketchup and spreads to dressings—and even delicious alternatives to the classic cookies we love to dunk in our tea!

Some recipes are air-fryer friendly. Look out for the symbol at the top of the page and refer to the notes for alternative cooking instructions.

unprocess your plate

Whether you're rushing out the door at the crack of dawn, feeding the kids before school, or simply not a breakfast person, these recipes will help you rediscover the joy of the first meal of the day—no matter how much time you have. As an avid breakfast eater (with two very hungry little mouths to feed every morning), skipping this meal is not an option for me.

While it's a myth that every adult needs to eat breakfast every single morning, the choices you make when you do enjoy that first bite are incredibly important. Ideally, you want a balanced meal that's rich in fibre, nutrients, and protein to fuel your body with steady energy for the day ahead.

Some grab-and-go store-bought breakfast options are improving nutrition-wise, like overnight oat (instant oatmeal) pots and yogurt alternatives, but they often come at a premium price and still contain added ingredients for preservation and shelf life. The simplest way to make a healthier choice—and save time reading labels in a rush—is to prepare your breakfast the night before or batch cook something over the weekend for the week ahead.

Start the day right

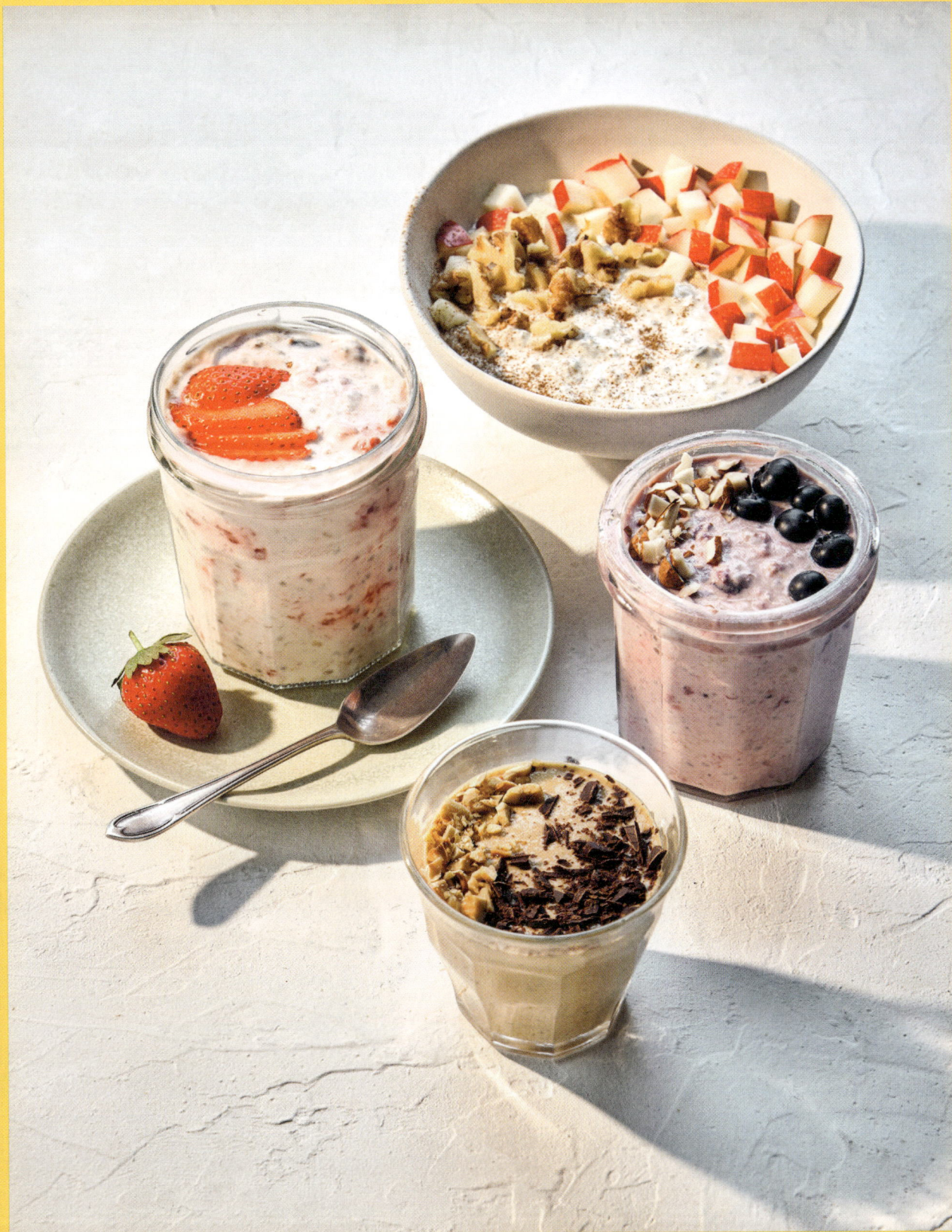

Overnight oats (4 ways)

Store-bought instant porridge or oat (oatmeal) pots often have a variety of additives included, which there is no need to consume when you can create your own version at home in a matter of minutes, ready for the next morning. Oats are a wonderful way to start the day, providing us with beta glucan, which is known to support heart health. Pictured on page 91.

Serves One   **Prep** 5 mins   **Cook** 0 mins

Base mixture

**Makes 500g (18oz):
enough for 10 servings**

350g (12½oz) rolled (old fashioned) oats

30g (1oz) chia seeds or flaxseeds

120g (4½oz) mixed seeds (I use a mix of pumpkin, sunflower, and sesame seeds)

1. Simply mix together the ingredients for the base mixture, then choose one of the four flavor variations.

Strawberries and cream

50g (1¾oz) base mixture (see left)

100ml (⅓ cup) milk of your choice

5 fresh (or frozen and defrosted) strawberries, 4 mashed + 1 sliced

1–2 tsp honey or maple syrup (optional)

2 tbsp thick yogurt of your choice

2 tbsp double (heavy) cream or vegan alternative

1 tsp almond or peanut butter

1. The night before you intend to eat, add the base mixture and milk to a jar or container, then cover and place in the fridge.

2. The following morning, stir the mashed strawberries into the base mixture. Add the honey or maple syrup (if using), yogurt, cream, and nut butter and stir again. Top with the sliced strawberry and enjoy.

Nutritional info per 100g

Fibre 8.8g
Protein 22g
Plant Points 8

Berry blast

50g (1¾oz) base mixture (see left)

100ml (⅓ cup) milk of your choice

4 tbsp fresh (or frozen and defrosted) raspberries, blackberries, and blueberries, plus extra to serve

½ small ripe banana

4 tbsp thick yogurt of your choice

1 tbsp chopped almonds

1. The night before you intend to eat, add the base mixture and milk to a jar or container, then cover and place in the fridge.

2. The following morning, mash the berries and the banana together with a fork in a small bowl, then stir this, along with the yogurt, into the soaked base mixture. Top with the chopped almonds and a few extra berries and enjoy.

Nutritional info per 100g

Fibre 9.3g
Protein 21g
Plant Points 11

Chocolate and coffee

50g (1¾oz) base mixture (see opposite)

100ml (⅓ cup) milk of your choice

1 shot (25ml/1fl oz) espresso, cooled

1–2 tsp honey or maple syrup (optional)

4 tbsp thick yogurt of your choice

1 small square of dark (bittersweet) chocolate (at least 72% cocoa solids), chopped

1 tbsp chopped roasted hazelnuts

1. The night before you intend to eat, add the base mixture and milk to a jar or container, then cover and place in the fridge.

2. The following morning, add the soaked base mixture, espresso and honey or maple syrup (if using) to a blender and blitz until smooth. Add the yogurt and briefly mix again to combine. Top with the chopped chocolate and hazelnuts and enjoy.

Apple, tahini, and cinnamon

50g (1¾oz) base mixture (see opposite)

100ml (⅓ cup) apple juice or milk of your choice

1 small apple, cored

⅛ tsp ground cinnamon, plus an extra pinch to serve

1–2 tsp honey or maple syrup (optional)

4 tbsp thick yogurt of your choice

1 tsp tahini (optional)

1 tbsp chopped walnuts

1. The night before you intend to eat, add the base mixture and apple juice or milk to a jar or container. Grate in half the apple (reserving the other half for the following day) and stir in the cinnamon, then cover and place in the fridge.

2. The following morning, stir in the honey or maple syrup (if using), the yogurt and the tahini. Chop the remaining apple into small chunks and place on top of the oats, then sprinkle with the chopped walnuts and a little extra cinnamon before enjoying.

Note For a warm topping, place the chopped apple, honey or maple syrup, and cinnamon in a microwaveable bowl, cover with cling film (plastic wrap), then microwave on high (900W) for 1–1½ minutes until soft. Spoon this over the soaked oats.

Nutritional info per 100g

Fibre 7.8g
Protein 20g
Plant Points 8

Nutritional info per 100g

Fibre 9g
Protein 23g
Plant Points 9.25

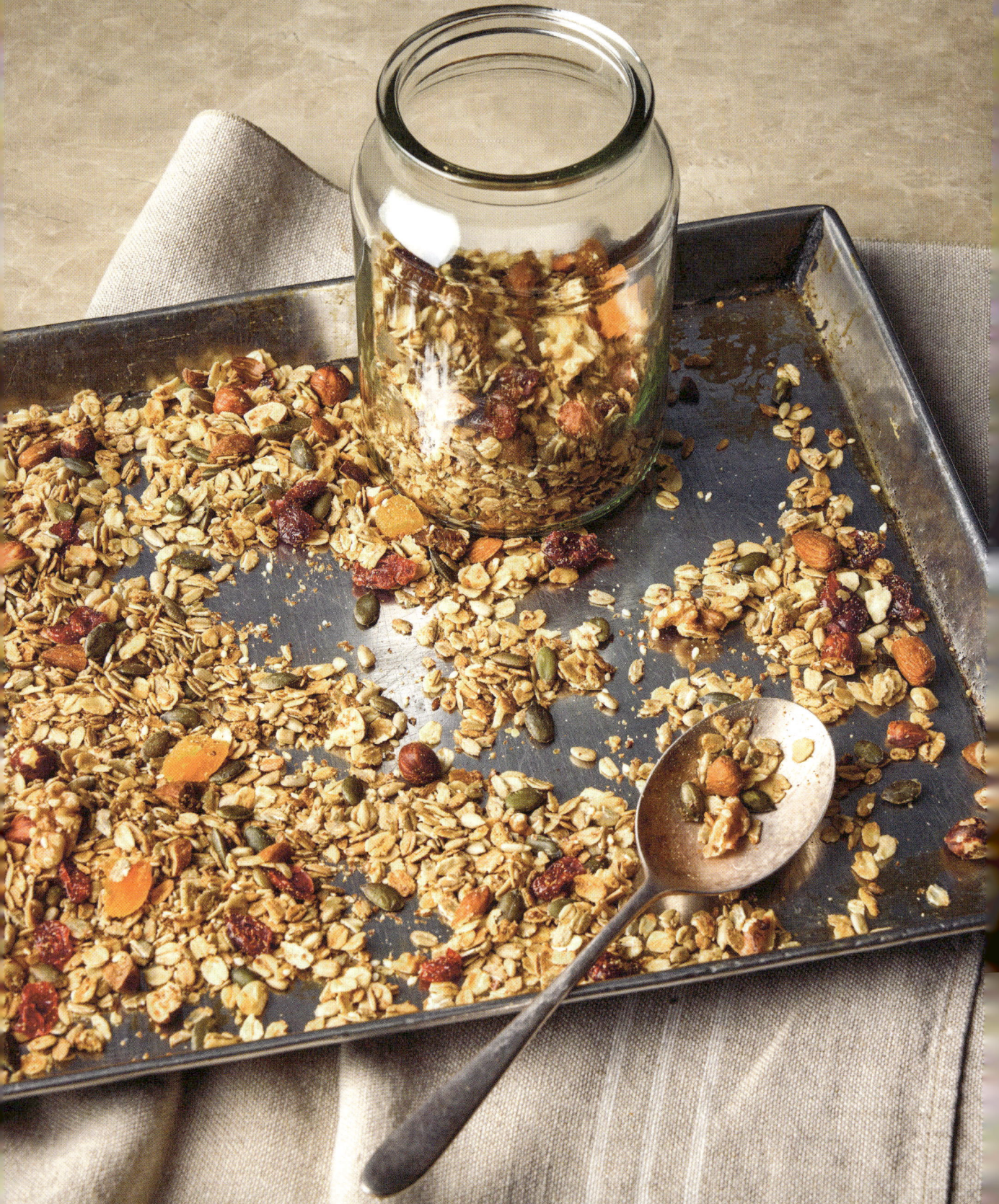

Seedy granola

Nutritional info per 40g portion

Fibre 3.3g
Protein 5.3g
Plant Points 15.25

Makes about 800g (3¼lb)

Prep 25 mins

Cook 40 mins

175g (6½oz) jumbo (old fashioned rolled) oats

175g (6½oz) barley, spelt, or rye flakes (or simply use more oats)

150g (5½oz) nuts, roughly chopped (I use a mix of almonds, hazelnuts, pecans, and walnuts)

150g (5½oz) seeds (I use a mix of pumpkin, sunflower, sesame, and flaxseeds)

1 tbsp ground cinnamon, nutmeg, ginger, or cardamom (or a mix) (optional)

50g (5 tbsp/1¾oz) coconut oil

100g (⅓ cup/3½oz) maple syrup

4 tbsp almond or peanut butter (optional)

75g (2¾oz) organic* dried fruit, roughly chopped (I use a mix of dried apricots, figs, dates, cranberries, and sour cherries)

Sea salt

* Select organic dried fruit to ensure it doesn't contain additives like sulphur dioxide.

This is such an adaptable recipe that you can make based on what you have in your store cupboard or your personal preferences for flavor and crunch. I love it, as it provides my family and me with lovely healthy fats and fibre for the day ahead. Serve as it is with your preferred milk, or top with fresh fruit and yogurt.

1. Preheat the oven to 160°C/140°C fan/325°F and line your largest baking sheet with baking paper (parchment paper).

2. Mix all the dry ingredients in a large bowl.

3. Melt the coconut oil in a small saucepan over a low heat (or melt in the microwave for 30 seconds). Stir in the maple syrup, nut butter (if using), and a pinch of salt, then mix until fully combined. Pour over the dry ingredients and stir until everything is nicely coated.

4. Spread out in an even layer on the baking sheet and bake for 30–35 minutes until golden, stirring and tossing occasionally so that it cooks evenly.

5. Leave to cool on the tray, then stir in the dried fruit.

6. Store in an airtight container at room temperature for up to 1 week.

Note You can cook this using your air fryer too! Heat the air fryer to 160°C/325°F and air fry for 10–12 minutes, tossing occasionally. You may need to air fry the granola in two batches depending on the size of your air fryer, for ultimate crispness. It will crisp up further as it cools.

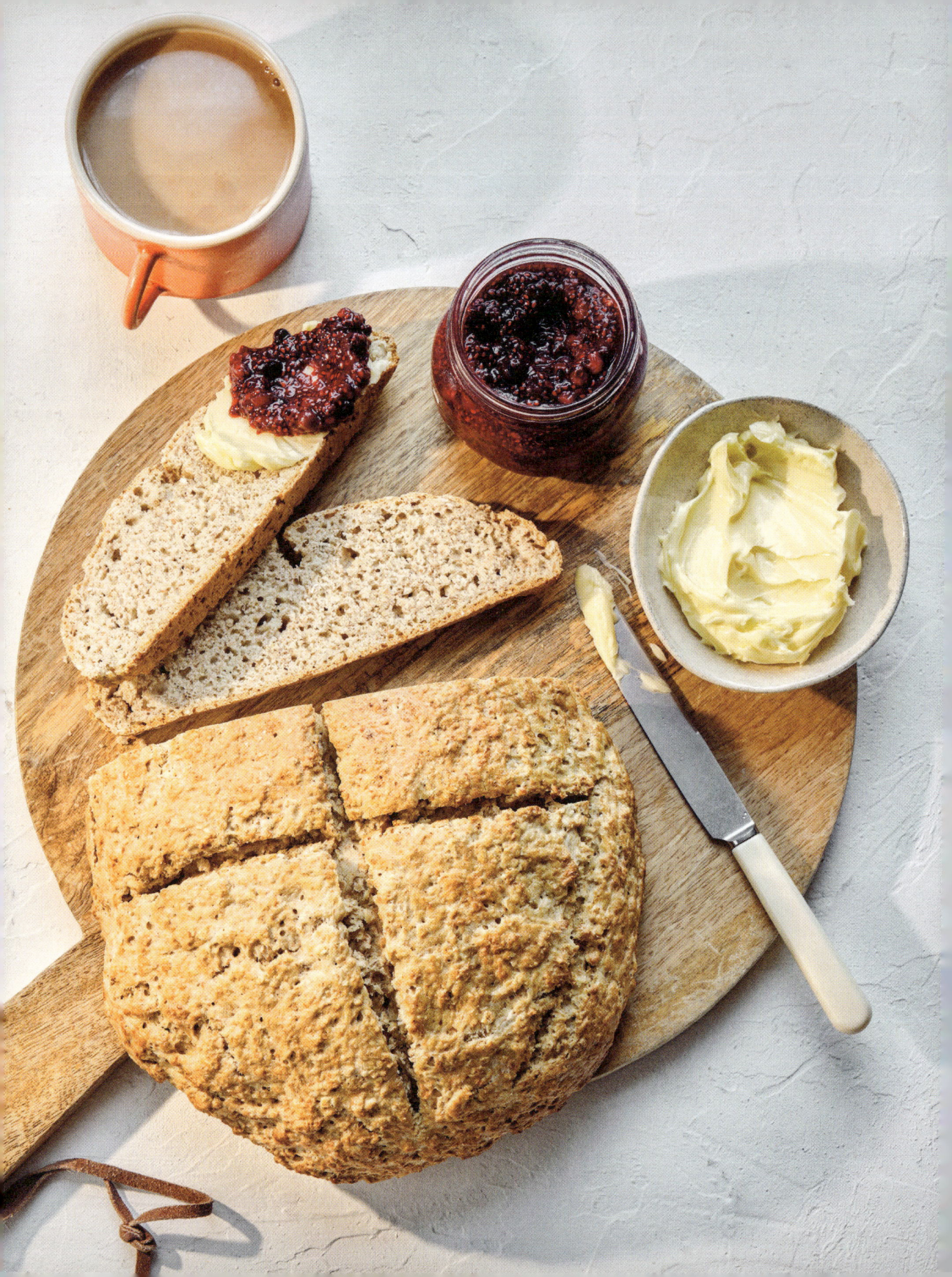

Soda bread

Makes 1 loaf   **Prep** 5 mins   **Cook** 45 mins

120g (4½oz) rolled (old fashioned) oats

250g (1¾ cups/9oz) all-purpose flour, plus extra for dusting

250g (1¾ cups/9oz) wholemeal (whole wheat) flour

1 tsp bicarbonate of soda (baking soda)

1 tsp sea salt

30g (2 tbsp/1oz) cold unsalted butter, diced (or use vegan alternative)

500ml (generous 2 cups/ 18fl oz) buttermilk (or use plain yogurt or soy milk), at room temperature, plus extra for brushing

Bread is food for the soul and has been consumed for thousands of years. Recently, we have of course commercialized it and added lots of extra ingredients that can cause it to be classed as a UPF, high in not just additives but sugar and salt too. Luckily, making your own bread at home is easier than you think—you don't even need yeast—and it can be ready in under an hour from start to finish. If you prefer, you can simply use all all-purpose flour or all wholemeal flour.

1. Preheat the oven to 200°C/180°C fan/400°F and line a baking sheet with baking paper (parchment paper).

2. Combine all the dry ingredients in a mixing bowl. Add the butter, then rub it into the dry ingredients using your fingertips until the mixture resembles breadcrumbs. Pour in the buttermilk, then work everything together lightly with your fingers until you have a loose, wet dough.

3. Flour your hands, shape the dough into a ball, then transfer it to the lined baking sheet. Brush the surface of the loaf with a little extra buttermilk, then cut a deep cross on the top with a sharp knife.

4. Bake for 40–45 minutes, or until golden and the loaf sounds hollow when you tap the base.

5. Transfer to a wire rack to cool a little before slicing. This is best eaten on the day it is made, but it can be stored in an airtight container at room temperature for up to 5 days, or sliced and stored in the freezer (see Note below).

Note Once my bread has cooled, I like to slice it and store it in the freezer to keep it fresher for longer. I simply grab as many slices as I need the night before and allow them to defrost overnight, ready to make toast the next morning. You get more beneficial resistant starch once you freeze and reheat bread, which is great for gut health!

Feel free to experiment with this bread by adding organic dried fruit, spices, or herbs!

Spelt and oat pancakes

Nutritional info per portion

Fibre 6.9g
Protein 12g
Plant Points 5.25

Serves 4   **Prep** 15 mins   **Cook** 15 mins

For the pancakes

100g (3½oz) jumbo or rolled (old fashioned) oats

100g (¾ cup/3½oz) spelt, wholemeal (whole wheat), khorasan, or einkorn flour

350ml (1½ cups/12fl oz) milk of your choice, plus extra if needed

2 eggs or 2 flax eggs (see Note on page 100)

1 tbsp maple syrup

Butter, coconut oil, or other neutral oil, for frying

Greek or coconut yogurt, to serve (optional)

For the fruit topper

2 eating apples, such as Braeburn, Gala, or Pink Lady, cored and cut into chunks

150g (5½oz) frozen blackberries (or other frozen berries of your choice)

2–3 tbsp dark brown sugar or maple syrup

½ tsp ground cinnamon

Zest of ½ orange, plus juice of 1 orange

Not to be reserved just for pancake day, these pancakes are a proper family-pleaser. Try loading them with the fruit topper below or dollop them with my chia and berry jam (page 204) or nutty chocolate spread (page 205). If you're short on time, you can make this batter in a blender or food processor, but do note that the pancakes will likely turn out a little chewier in texture if so. If you prefer smaller, fluffier pancakes, simply add 1½ teaspoons of baking powder when adding the flour and add smaller dollops of batter to the pan when frying.

1. To prepare the batter for the pancakes, place the oats in a blender and blitz to a fine powder. Transfer to a large mixing bowl along with the flour and make a well in the centre. In a separate bowl, whisk together the milk, eggs, and maple syrup, then gradually pour this into the well of flour, whisking constantly, until you have a batter the consistency of single (light) cream (you may need to add a little extra milk if the batter is too thick). Set aside for at least 10 minutes to rest while you prepare the fruit topper.

2. Combine all the fruit topper ingredients in a small saucepan set over a medium heat and bring to a simmer. Reduce the heat and leave to gently bubble away for 8–10 minutes until the apple is tender.

3. To cook the pancakes, place a medium non-stick frying pan (skillet) or crêpe pan over a medium–high heat and add a little butter or oil (just enough to lightly coat the base of the pan). When hot, add 3–4 tablespoons of your batter and swirl to coat the base of the pan. Cook for 1–2 minutes, then gently flip the pancake and cook the other side for a further 1–2 minutes. Remove from the pan and keep warm in a low oven while you cook the remaining pancakes, adding a little more butter or oil to the pan between each one.

4. Serve the pancakes with the warm fruit topper and a dollop of yogurt, if you like.

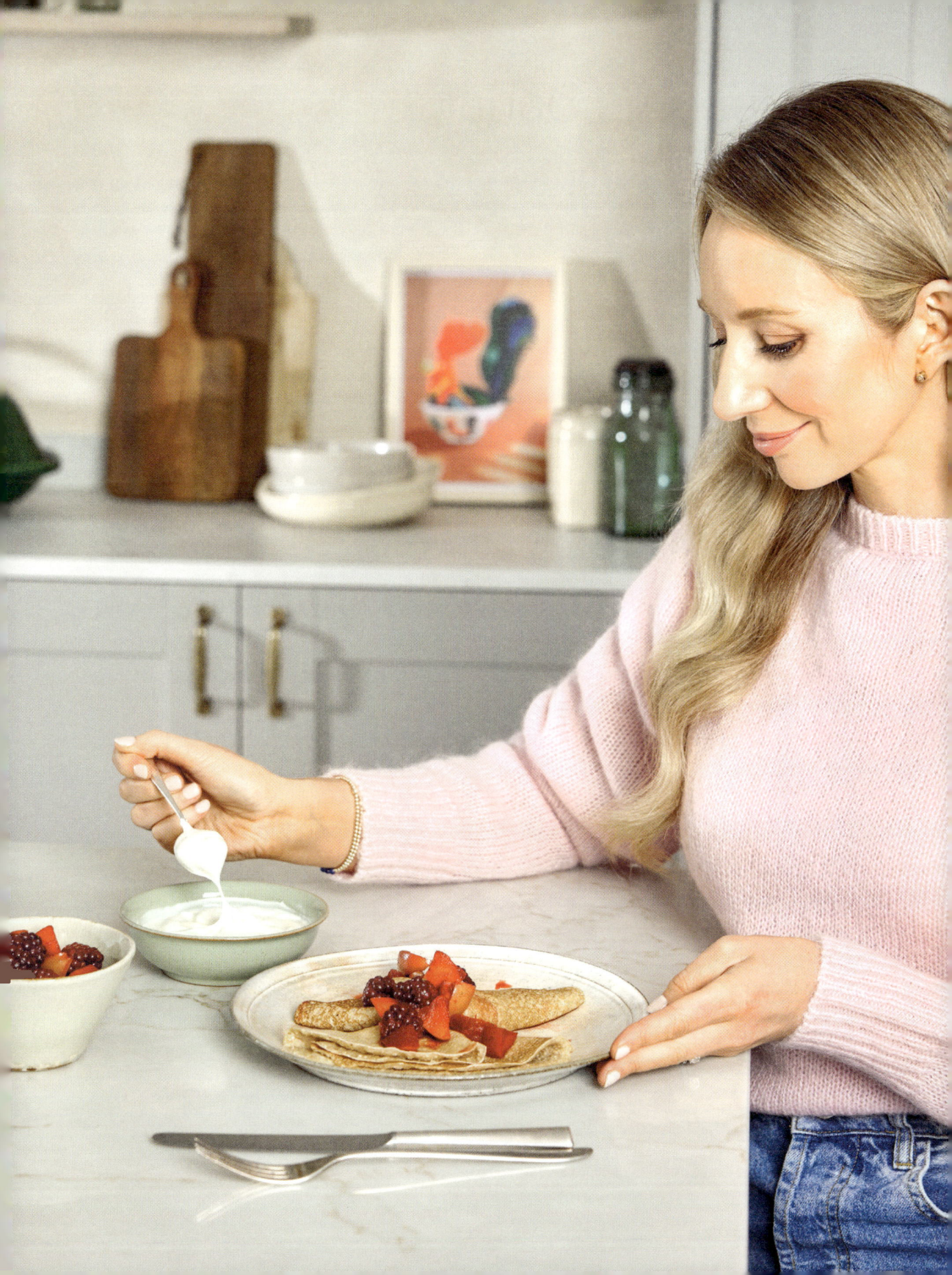

Wholesome banana muffins

Nutritional info per muffin

Fibre 3.2g
Protein 8.1g
Plant Points 7.75

Makes 12   **Prep** 10 mins   **Cook** 25 mins

250g (9oz) ripe bananas
(about 3 medium bananas)

125g (½ cup/4½oz) smooth
peanut butter

125g (½ cup/4½oz) plain
yogurt or coconut yogurt

60g (6 tbsp/2oz) olive oil
or rapeseed (canola) oil

50g (4 tbsp/1¾oz)
muscovado or
coconut sugar

2 eggs or 2 flax eggs
(see Note below)

160g (scant 1¼ cups/5½oz)
wholemeal (whole wheat),
spelt, or oat flour (or a mix)

1 tsp baking powder

½ tsp bicarbonate of soda
(baking soda)

½ tsp salt

1 tsp ground cinnamon

¼ tsp ground nutmeg

50g (1¾oz) raisins, soaked
in just-boiled water for
5 minutes (optional)

50g (1¾oz) walnuts,
chopped (optional)

40g (1½oz) seeds (I use
a mix of pumpkin and
sunflower seeds)

These are packed with nutritious ingredients while still feeling like a breakfast treat—perfect for those that want something they can take to work with them. If you'd like to use oat flour for these, simply pulse oats in a blender or food processor until you have a fine powder. Do note, using all oat flour can make the texture of these muffins a little dense, so I'd recommend using half oat flour and half wholemeal or spelt flour instead.

1. Preheat the oven to 200°C/180°C fan/400°F and line a 12-hole muffin pan with muffin cases.

2. Mash the bananas in a medium bowl with a fork, then stir in the peanut butter and yogurt.

3. In a separate bowl whisk together the oil and sugar, then add the eggs and whisk again until fully combined. Stir in the banana mixture, then set aside.

4. In a large mixing bowl, combine all the remaining ingredients (apart from the seeds) and stir well. Fold in the wet ingredients until just combined, then spoon the batter evenly into the muffin cases. Sprinkle the top of each muffin with some of the seeds, then bake the muffins for 20–25 minutes until risen, golden and a skewer inserted into the middles comes out clean.

5. Transfer the muffins to a wire rack to cool, then store in an airtight container at room temperature for up to 4 days.

Note To make egg-free muffins, simply replace the eggs with "flax eggs". The general rule of thumb to replace 1 egg is to use 1 tbsp ground flaxseeds combined with 3 tbsp water (then leave to rest for at least 5 minutes). So, for this recipe, you'll need to combine 2 tbsp ground flaxseeds with 6 tbsp water. Simply add to the recipe at the same point that you would add the eggs.

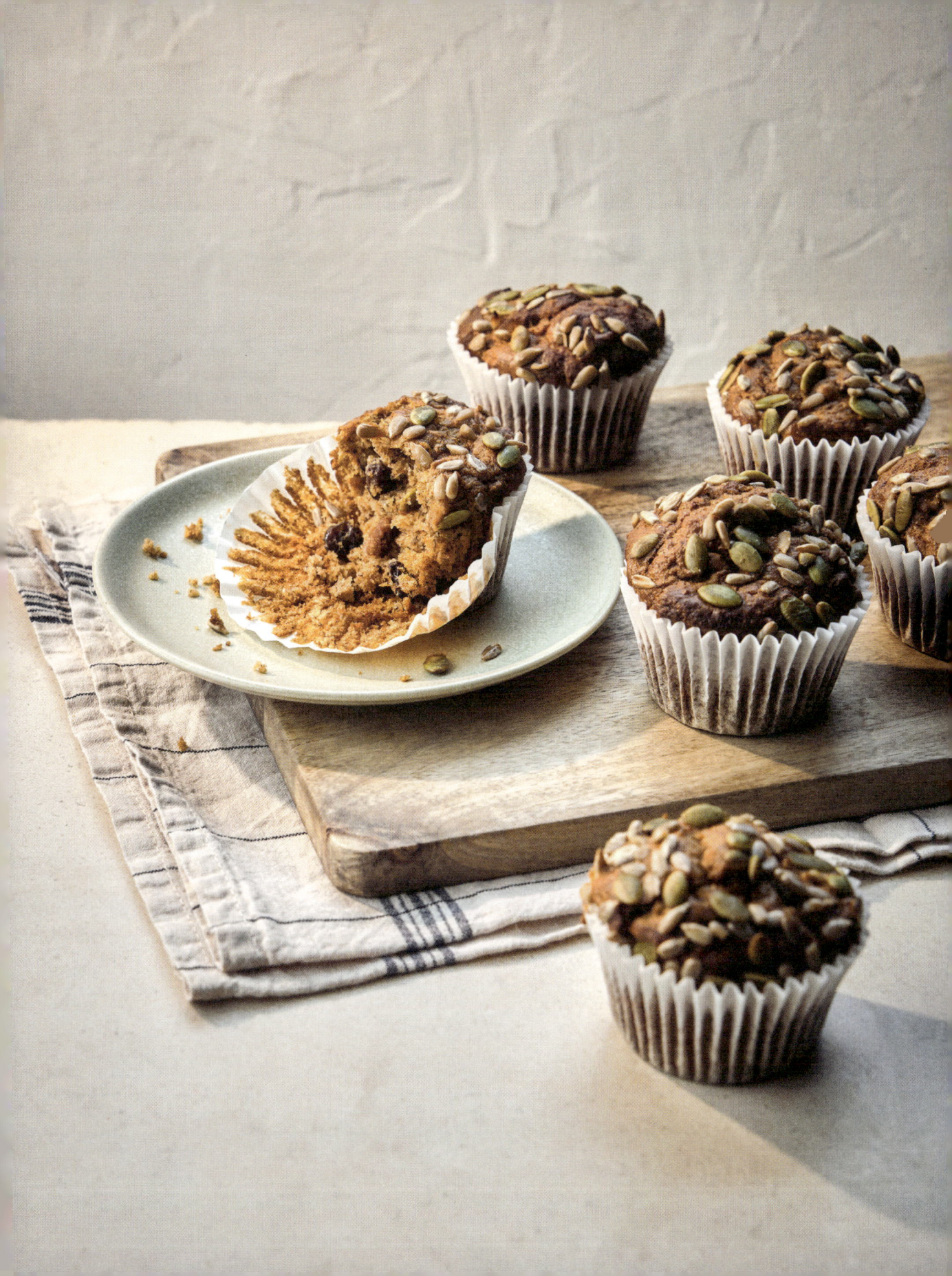

Baked beans with speedy hash browns

Nutritional info per portion

Fibre 23g
Protein 21g
Plant Points 8.5

Serves 4–6   **Prep** 10 mins   **Cook** 45 mins

For the baked beans

2 tbsp olive oil

1 onion, chopped

2 garlic cloves, chopped

1 tsp sweet paprika

1 tsp ground cumin

¼–½ tsp dried chilli flakes (optional)

3 × 400g (14oz) cans beans (I use a mix of any of the following: black beans, cannellini beans, kidney beans, butter (lima) beans, borlotti beans, pinto beans, lentils, or chickpeas), drained and rinsed

500g (18oz) passata (diced tomatoes)

2–3 tbsp tamari or soy sauce, plus extra to taste

8 small dates, pitted and finely chopped (or use 2 tbsp maple syrup)

1 tbsp balsamic vinegar (or use 1 tbsp red wine vinegar plus 1 extra date)

1 bay leaf

Sea salt and freshly ground black pepper

For the hash browns

900g (2lb) potatoes, such as Maris Piper, Russet or King Edward

1 large onion

6 tbsp olive oil

To serve

Poached eggs

Chopped chives

While there is nothing wrong with treating yourself to a can of baked beans, I want to empower you to have a go at making them yourselves, as they taste truly incredible! Use any combination of beans you fancy—you can even make them ahead for a super stress-free morning. Stored in an airtight container, they will keep for 1 week in the fridge or 1 month in the freezer.

1. To make the baked beans, warm the olive oil in a deep saucepan set over a low–medium heat then add the onion and a pinch of salt. Sweat gently for 8 minutes, then add the garlic and cook for a further 2 minutes.

2. Stir the paprika and cumin into the onions for 30 seconds, then add all the remaining baked bean ingredients, along with a big pinch each of salt and pepper. Pour in 100ml (7 tbsp/3½fl oz) of water, then bring to a simmer. Reduce the heat to low and leave to bubble gently, stirring occasionally, for about 30 minutes while you make the hash browns. Add a splash more water to the pan if it looks like it's drying out.

3. Preheat the oven to 200°C/180°C fan/400°F and place a large (preferably heavy-bottomed) roasting pan in the oven to get hot.

4. Coarsely grate (shred) the potatoes and onion into a large bowl of cold water. Stir them with your hand to rinse off some of the starch, the drain. Tip the drained potato and onion onto a clean kitchen towel, then pull up the edges and twist and squeeze it tightly over the sink to wring out as much liquid as possible.

5. Carefully remove the hot pan from the oven and add 3 tablespoons of the oil. Tilt it so the base is evenly covered, then carefully transfer the potato and onion mixture to the pan. Use a spoon to spread the mixture to a thickness of about 2cm (1 inch), trying not to compress it too much, and neaten the edges to prevent burnt bits. Drizzle the top with the remaining oil and season with salt and pepper.

6. Place the pan on the bottom of your oven for 10 minutes to get the base crispy, then move the tray to the middle rack of the oven and cook for a further 15–20 minutes until golden on top and the potato is tender. Slice into 6 or 8 pieces.

7. Check if the beans need any extra seasoning, then serve up on plates with the hash browns. Top with poached eggs, sprinkle with chopped chives, and dig in.

Note You can cook the hash brown using your air fryer too! Generously grease the base of your air fryer and heat to 190°C/375°F. Shape the potato and onion mixture into 4–6 patties then place them in the air fryer, drizzle the tops with oil, and air fry for 18 minutes. Carefully flip them, then air fry for a further 5 minutes until crispy.

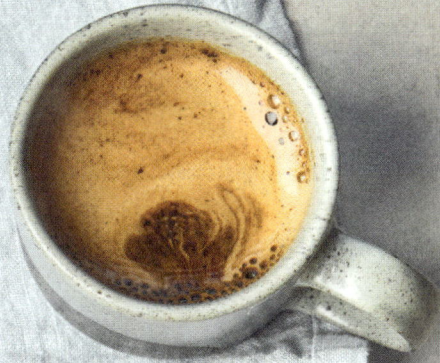

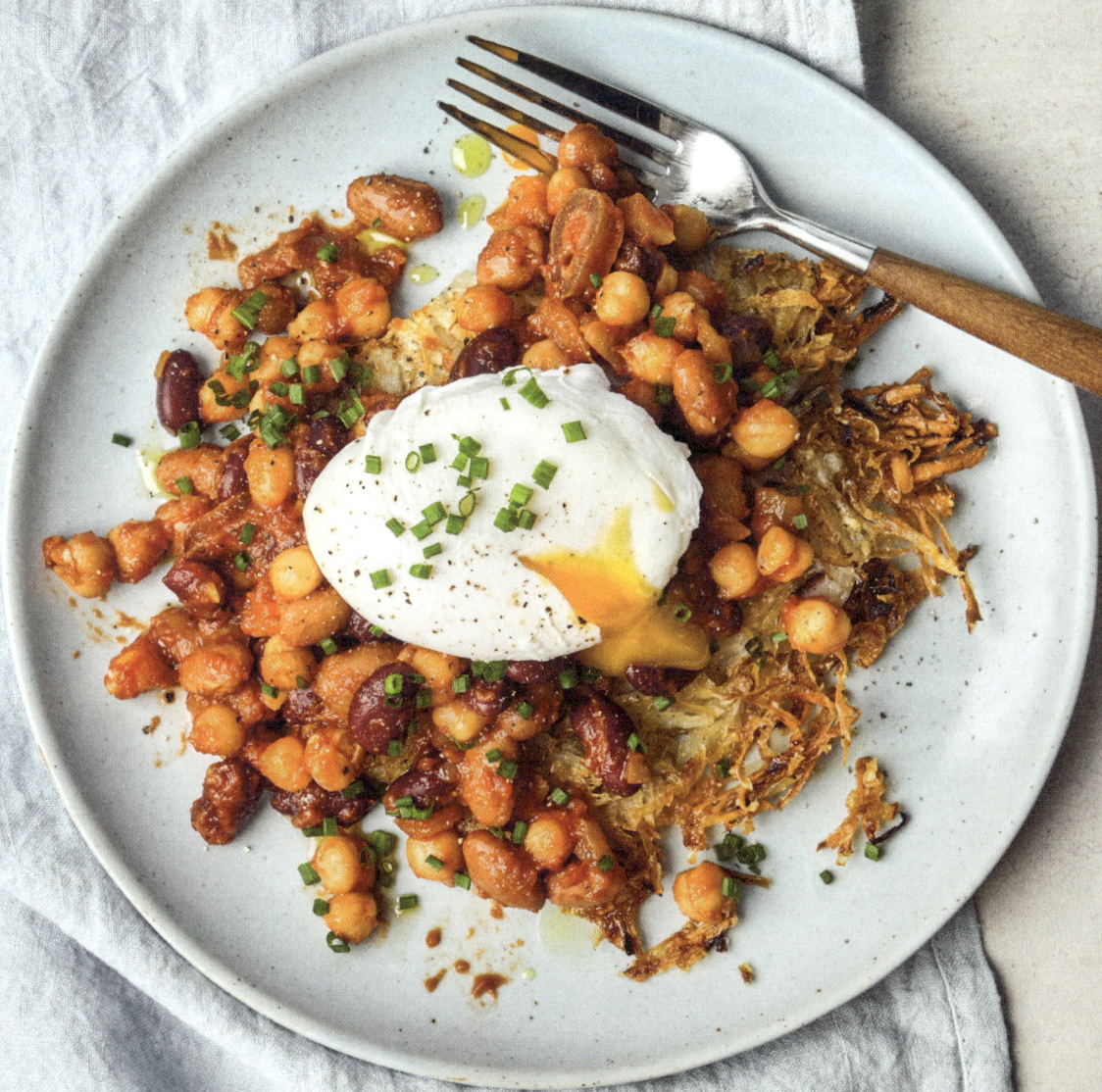

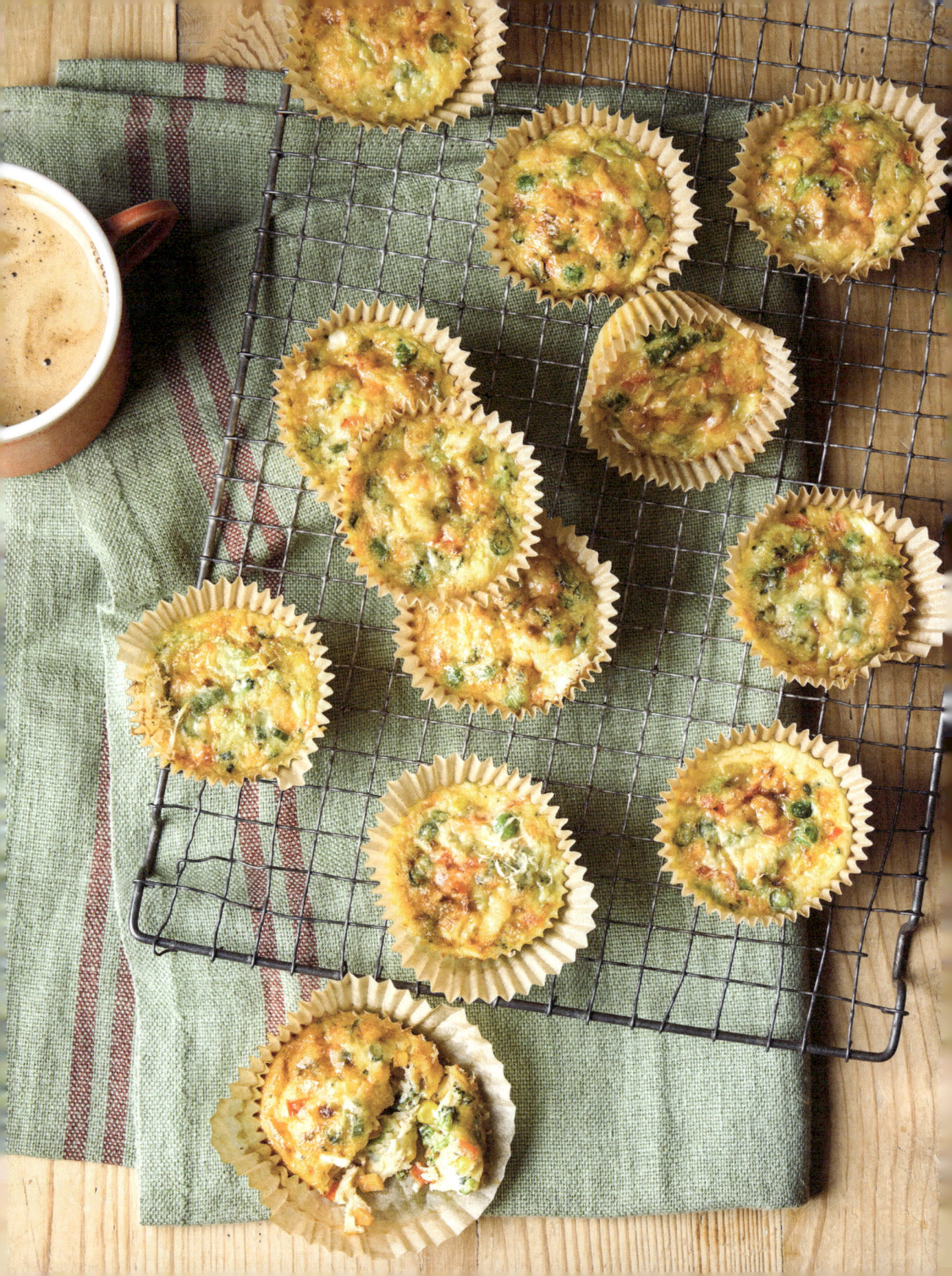

Fridge-raid omelette muffins

Nutritional info per muffin

Fibre 0.8g
Protein 6g
Plant Points 6.75

Makes 12　　**Prep** 5 mins　　**Cook** 30 mins

1 tbsp olive oil, cold-pressed rapeseed oil, or avocado oil

250g (9oz) mixed vegetables (I use a mix of broccoli, sweetcorn, frozen peas, sweet potato, red (bell) pepper, green beans, and asparagus), all finely chopped to a similar size

2 spring (green) onions, sliced

6 large eggs

1 tbsp milk

¼ tsp sweet paprika

75g (2¾oz) Cheddar, Comte, Parmesan, or Gruyère, grated

Sea salt and freshly ground black pepper

These are ideal for using up whatever vegetables you have lurking in the fridge. They are the perfect savory bite when you're running out of the door in the morning or an ideal after-school snack for hungry kids. Whatever veggies you use, just ensure they are all chopped to the same size, and you can't go wrong.

1. Preheat the oven to 200°C/180°C fan/400°F. Add paper cases to a 12-hole muffin pan.

2. Add the oil to a small frying pan (skillet) and set over a medium–high heat. When hot, add the mixed vegetables, spring onions, and a pinch of salt. Fry, stirring often, for 5–10 minutes until tender, then set the pan to one side.

3. In a large bowl, whisk the eggs with the milk, paprika, half the cheese, and some salt and pepper until well combined, then stir in the cooked vegetables. Divide the mixture evenly between the muffin cases, then sprinkle each with the remaining cheese.

4. Bake for 15–17 minutes until golden brown and cooked through. Allow to cool in the muffin pan for 5 minutes before enjoying immediately. Once completely cool, store in an airtight container in the fridge for up to 5 days.

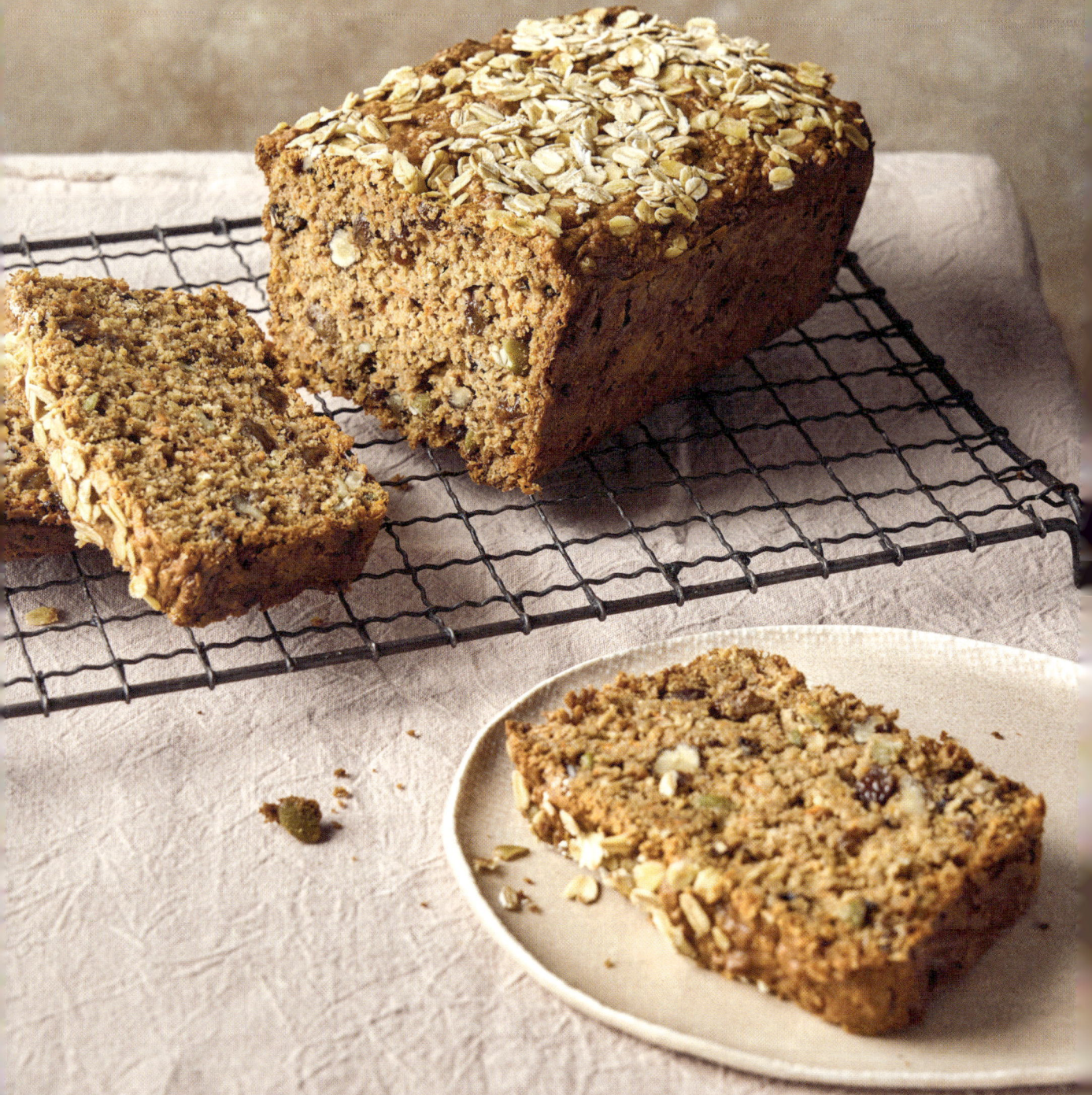

Carrot and yogurt breakfast loaf

Nutritional info per portion

Fibre 4.1g
Protein 9.6g
Plant Points 7

Makes 1 loaf (serves 8)　　**Prep** 15 mins　　**Cook** 60 mins

125g (4½oz) jumbo or rolled (old fashioned) oats, plus an extra 2 tbsp

125g (generous ¾ cup/4½oz) strong white bread flour

2 tsp baking powder

1 tsp bicarbonate of soda (baking soda)

½ tsp salt

2 tsp mixed spice (pumpkin pie spice)

1 tsp ground cinnamon

½ tsp ground ginger

Zest of 1 orange

200g (¾ cup/7oz) plain yogurt (or use soy or coconut yogurt)

80g (½ cup/2¾oz) molasses sugar, muscavado sugar or coconut sugar

80g (⅔ cup/2¾oz) olive oil

2 eggs or 2 flax eggs (see Note on page 100)

160g (5½oz) carrots (about 2 medium carrots), peeled and coarsely grated

60g (2oz) raisins or sultanas, soaked in just-boiled water for 5 minutes

50g (1¾oz) walnuts, chopped (optional)

30g (1oz) pumpkin seeds (optional)

We often crave something sweet in the morning, and a slice of this sumptuous cake is the perfect replacement for a croissant grabbed on-the-go. If you have a teenager at home, this may even entice them to wake up in the morning! Filled with fibre, plant points and protein, this delightful breakfast option means you can have your cake and eat it too! If you would like to make this vegan, simply use soy or coconut yogurt and flax eggs. You can also use this batter to make 12 muffins—simply follow the oven temperatures and cooking timings on page 100.

1. Preheat the oven to 180°C/160°C fan/350°F and line the base of a 900g (2lb) loaf pan with baking paper (parchment paper).

2. Place the oats in a blender or food processor and blitz them to a fine flour. Transfer to a large mixing bowl, then stir in the strong white flour, baking powder, bicarb, salt, and spices. Set aside.

3. Stir the orange zest with the yogurt in a small bowl and set aside.

4. Add the sugar and oil to another mixing bowl, then beat using an electric hand-held whisk for 2–3 minutes until it begins to lighten in color. Next, add the eggs one at a time, whisking for 2–3 minutes between each addition, until the mixture is thick and pale. Gently fold the yogurt into the eggs until just combined, then fold in the dry ingredients with a large metal spoon.

5. Add the grated carrots, raisins, walnuts, and pumpkin seeds (if using), then gently fold in until everything is just combined and evenly distributed.

6. Transfer the batter to the lined loaf pan, then sprinkle with the extra 2 tablespoons of oats. Bake on the middle rack for 50–60 minutes until risen, golden, and a skewer inserted into the middles comes out clean. Allow to cool in the loaf pan for 10 minutes before removing from the pan and transferring to a wire rack to cool completely. Store in an airtight container at room temperature for 3–4 days.

Lunch is often an overlooked or forgotten meal, but it is incredibly important, as eating well in the afternoon can help combat those post-work or evening cravings and leave you feeling productive and energized for the rest of the day.

Sadly, many UPF lunch options aren't the best when it comes to meeting your nutritional goals. A typical store-bought sandwich or wrap often lacks sufficient protein, vitamins, and minerals. In fact, packaged lunch options usually contain long ingredient lists filled with added salt, saturated fat, and sugar—far from an ideal, healthy choice.

These recipes have been designed to offer twists on the classic options you might normally purchase, with a nutritional boost! You don't need a long list of ingredients to make great-tasting food, but you might want to invest in a high-quality lunch box to help you stay on track with your new cooking routine.

Lunch and on-the-go

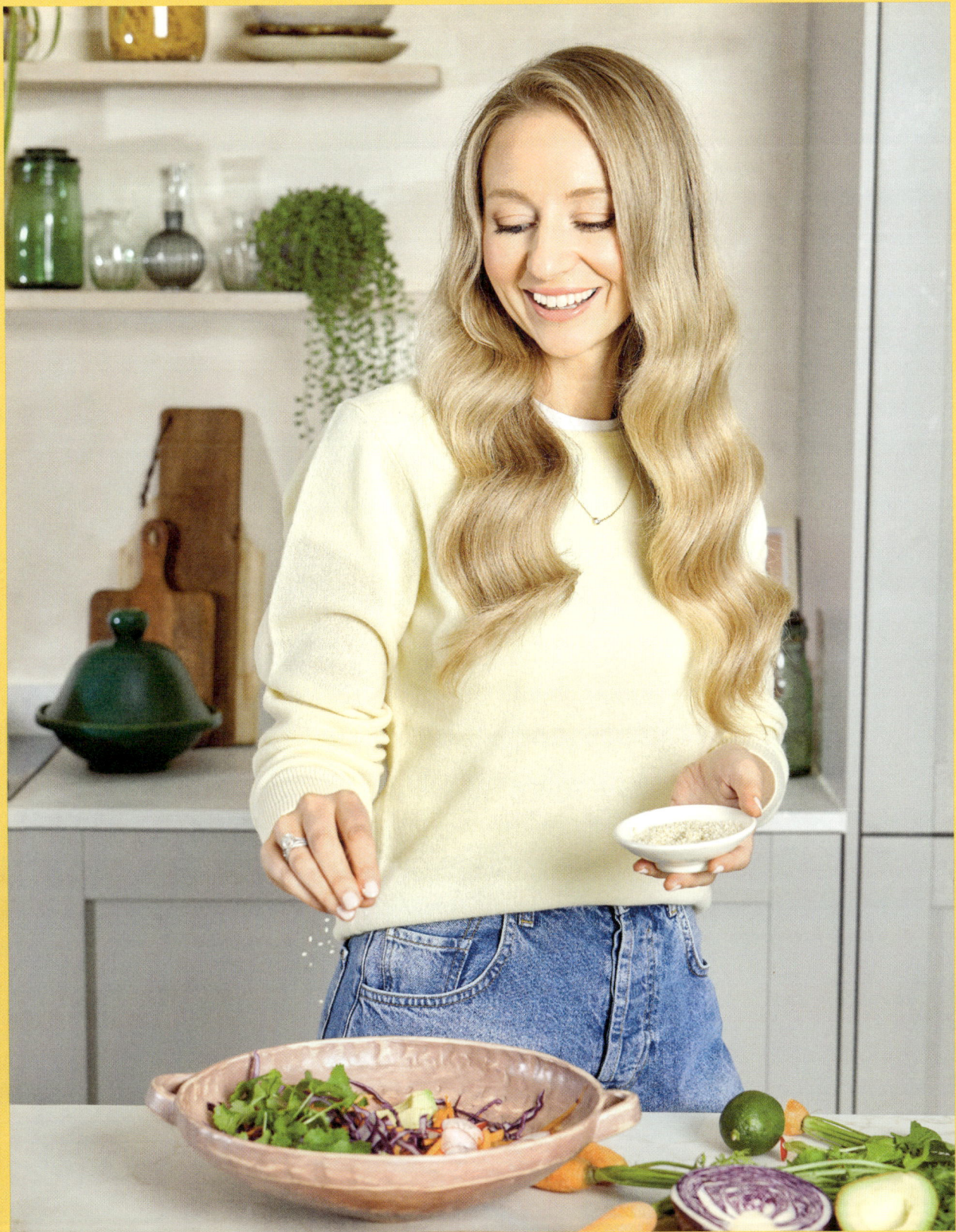

Cottage cheese bread

Nutritional info per slice

Fibre 2.8g
Protein 8.8g
Plant Points 3

Makes 1 loaf   **Prep** 5 mins   **Cook** 1 hour

200g (2 cups/7oz) jumbo rolled (old fashioned) oats

300g (1½ cups/10½oz) cottage cheese (or use a vegan alternative)

50g (5 tbsp/1¾oz) pumpkin seeds

2 tbsp flaxseeds

½ tsp salt

2 eggs

1 tsp baking powder

I bet you never thought you could get added protein from a simple loaf of bread, but now you can! Cottage cheese works wonders in this soda-bread-style loaf, even when you have no time to spare. This has been one of the most popular recipes I have created for my nutrition clients over the years.

1. Preheat the oven to 200°C/180°C fan/400°F and line a baking sheet with baking paper (parchment paper).

2. Combine all the ingredients in a large bowl, mixing well with a wooden spoon.

3. Transfer the dough to the baking sheet and use your hands to shape it into an oval loaf shape, about 5cm (6 inches) in length.

4. Bake for 50 minutes–1 hour until golden and the base sounds hollow when you tap it. Transfer to a wire rack and allow to cool completely before slicing.

5. Store in an airtight container at room temperature for up to 3 days, or slice and store wrapped in the freezer for up to 1 month (see Note on page 97).

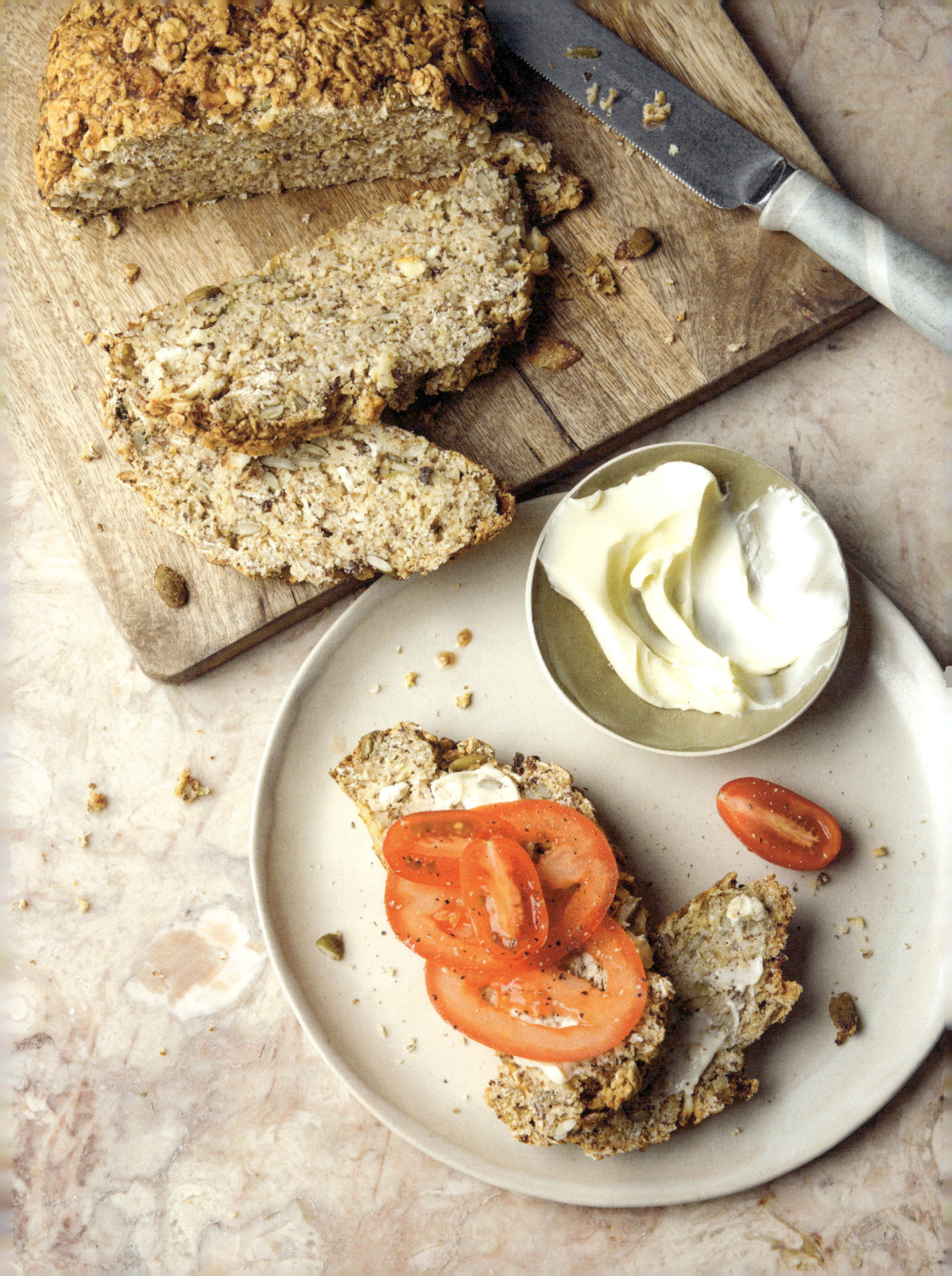

Quinoa niçoise salad

Nutritional info per portion

Fibre 13g
Protein 6.4g
Plant Points 6.75

Serves 4   **Prep** 10 mins   **Cook** 25 minutes

125g (¾ cup/4½oz) red, white or black quinoa, rinsed

250g (9oz) fresh or frozen green beans, trimmed

4 medium eggs

250g (9oz) cherry tomatoes, halved

½ large cucumber, sliced into half moons

70g (2½oz) pitted black olives, halved

220g (8oz) high-quality canned tuna in oil or brine, drained

2 tbsp extra-virgin olive oil

3 tbsp red wine vinegar

Handful of parsley leaves, finely chopped

Juice of ½ lemon

8 anchovy fillets in oil, torn in half (optional)

Sea salt and freshly ground black pepper

A fresh summer salad perfect for a packed lunch. I like to keep this very lightly dressed, as the olives and anchovies are so flavorful, but do serve with extra dressing on the side if you prefer.

There are plenty of switches you can make if you're vegan, or things you can add if you're a maximalist like me! Jarred roasted red (bell) peppers are a great addition, as is asparagus if it's in season and you're feeling fancy. New potatoes are fairly traditional when it comes to this salad and an ideal way to bulk things out, while salad leaves such as rocket (arugula), little gem or romaine lettuce can add additional crunch. Avocado and crispy chickpeas (page 214) would also work nicely.

1. Pour the quinoa into a small saucepan, add a pinch of salt, and cover with plenty of cold water. Bring to the boil, then reduce the heat to low and simmer for 15–20 minutes until the quinoa begins to unfurl and becomes tender. Drain into a sieve (strainer), then place the sieve on top of the now empty pan, cover with a kitchen towel and leave to one side to steam dry.

2. Bring a medium pan of salted water to the boil and add the green beans and eggs. Fish the beans out after 5 minutes (3 minutes for frozen) using a slotted spoon and continue cooking the eggs for a further 3 minutes. Drain and cool the beans and eggs under running cold water.

3. Combine the cooled green beans in a large bowl with the tomatoes, cucumber, olives, tuna, half the olive oil, and the red wine vinegar. Season with salt and pepper and toss very lightly, avoiding breaking up the tuna too much.

4. Transfer the quinoa to a large salad bowl and stir in the parsley, lemon juice, and remaining 1 tablespoon of oil and season lightly with salt and pepper. Toss so it's nicely coated, then pile the rest of the salad on top. Peel the eggs, cut them into halves or quarters and sit them on top of the salad. Finish by draping the anchovies on top, if you like, then serve.

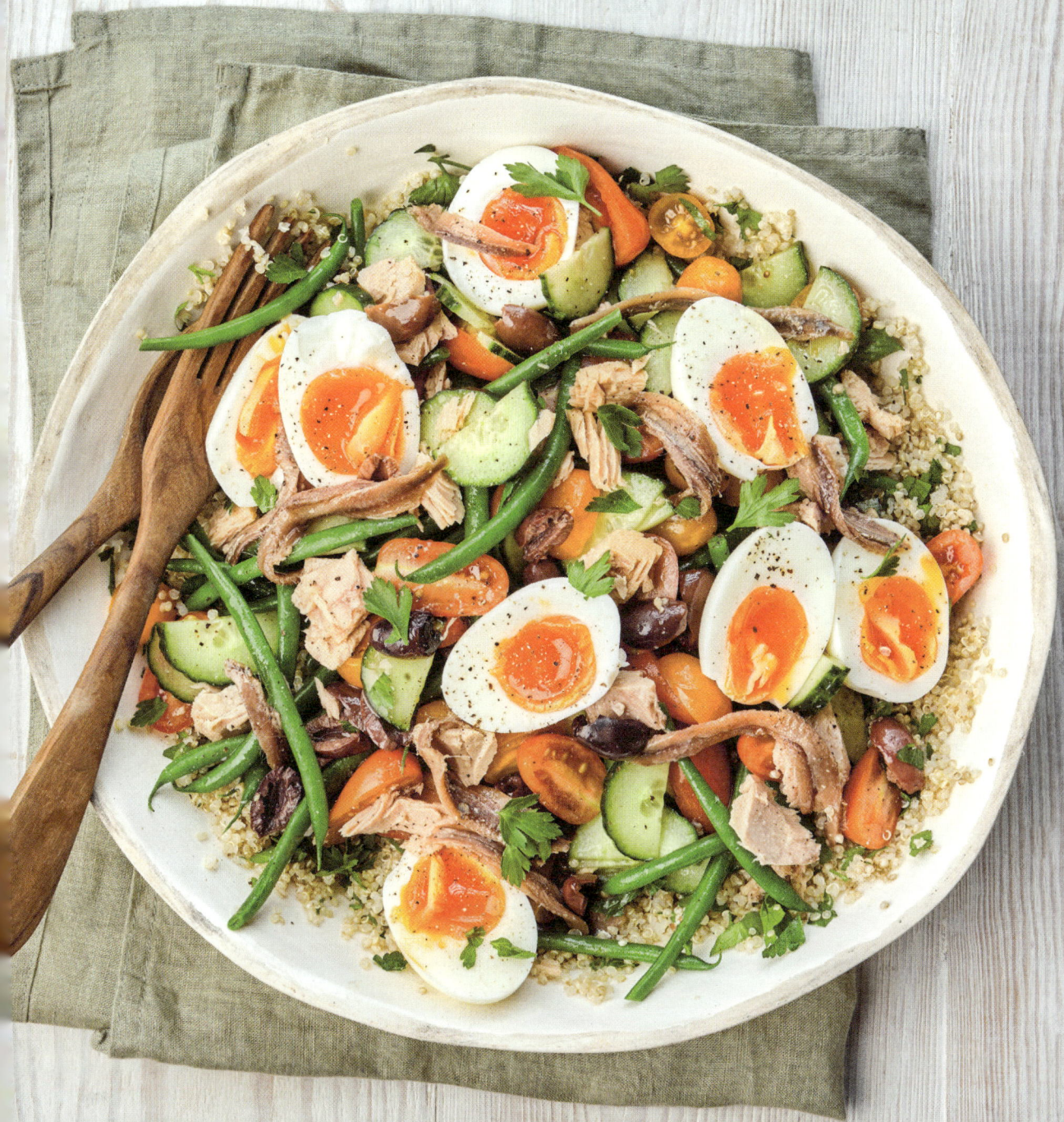

The ultimate pasta salad

Nutritional info per portion

Fibre 7.5g
Protein 7.5g
Plant Points 9.25

Serves 4   **Prep** 10 mins   **Cook** 15 minutes

250g (9oz) wholewheat penne or fusilli

70g (2½oz) walnuts

1 small garlic clove, grated

Pinch of dried chilli (red pepper) flakes (optional)

1 tbsp red wine vinegar

4 tbsp olive oil

2 spring (green) onions, finely sliced

60g (2oz) pitted black olives, roughly chopped

1 heaped tbsp capers

50g (1¾oz) sun-dried tomatoes, roughly chopped

250g (9oz) cherry tomatoes, halved

1 avocado, peeled, de-stoned, and chopped (optional)

Small handful of basil or parsley leaves, roughly chopped

60g (2¼oz) rocket (arugula)

Handful of Parmesan shavings (or use vegan alternative) (optional)

Sea salt and freshly ground black pepper

You can't go wrong with pasta and I love whipping this up for packed lunches. Perfect for the whole family, it's super-easy to prep and travels well, so it's ideal for picnics too. Don't overdo the raw garlic here—it should just be a background flavor.

1. Bring a pan of salted water to the boil and cook the pasta to al dente according to the packet instructions. Drain and rinse under cold water, then set aside.

2. While the pasta is cooking, place a small frying pan (skillet) over a medium heat. Add the walnuts and toast gently for 5–8 minutes, moving the pan constantly, until lightly colored. Allow to cool, then roughly chop.

3. Grate the garlic into a salad bowl, then add the chilli flakes, vinegar, and olive oil and whisk well to make a dressing. Stir in the spring onions, olives, capers, and sun-dried tomatoes, then season well with salt and pepper.

4. Add the pasta, cooled walnuts, tomatoes, avocado (if using), herbs, rocket, and Parmesan (if using), then toss really well. Store in an airtight container in the fridge for up to 3 days.

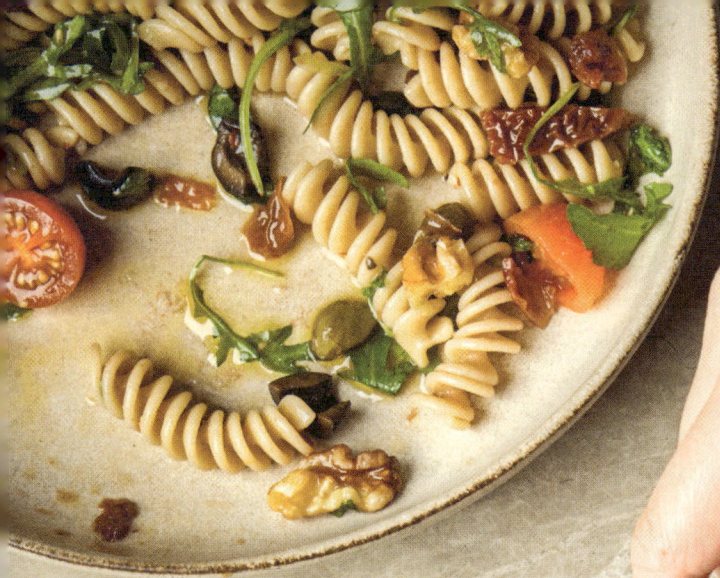

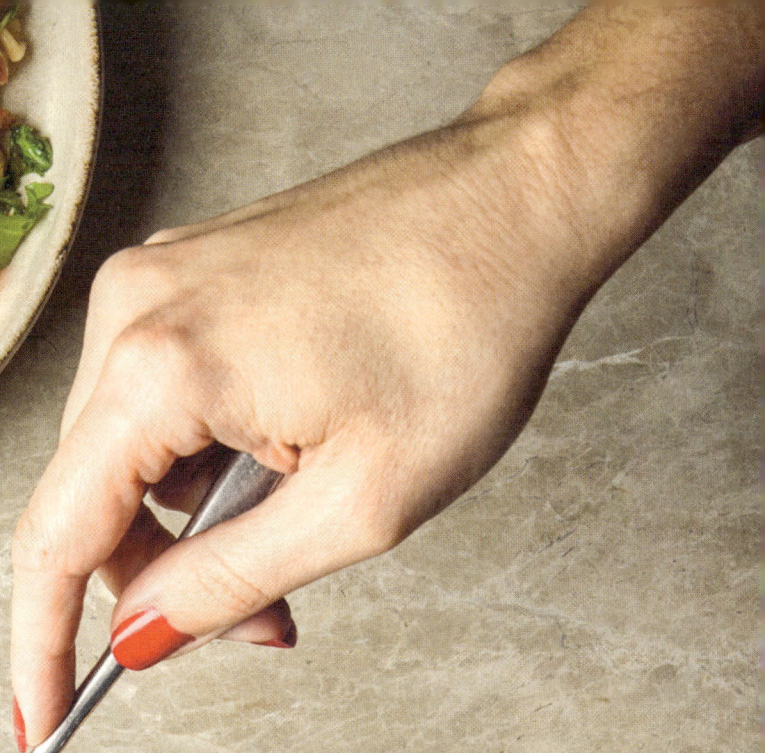

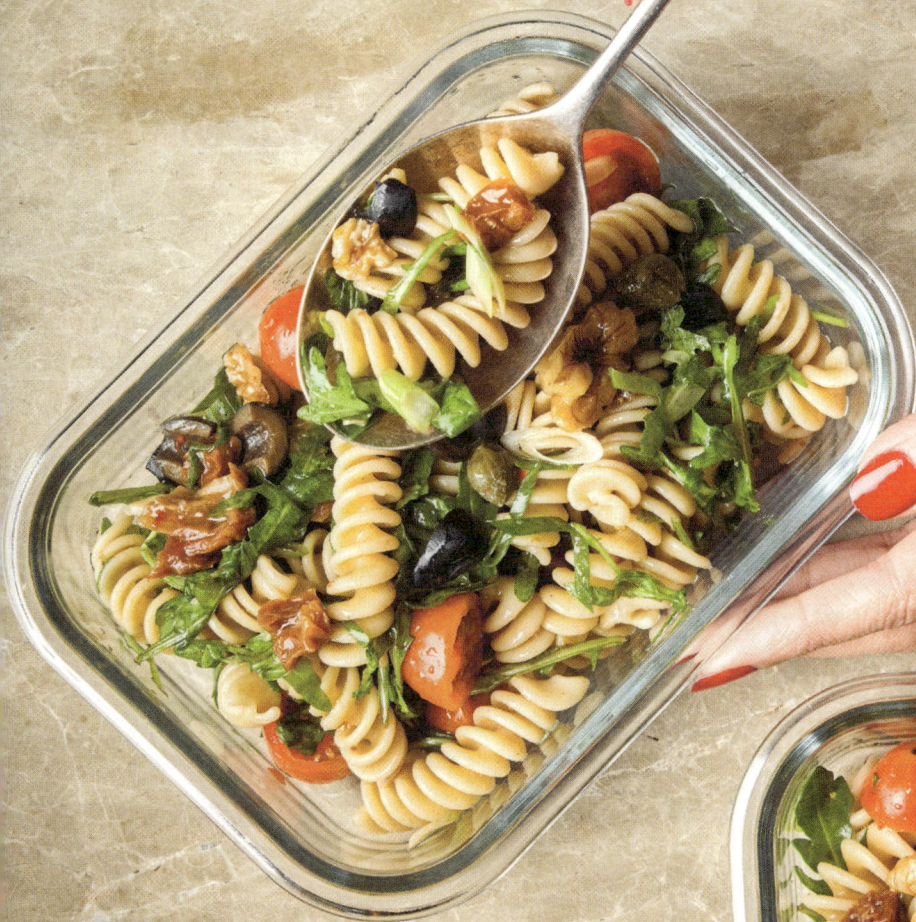

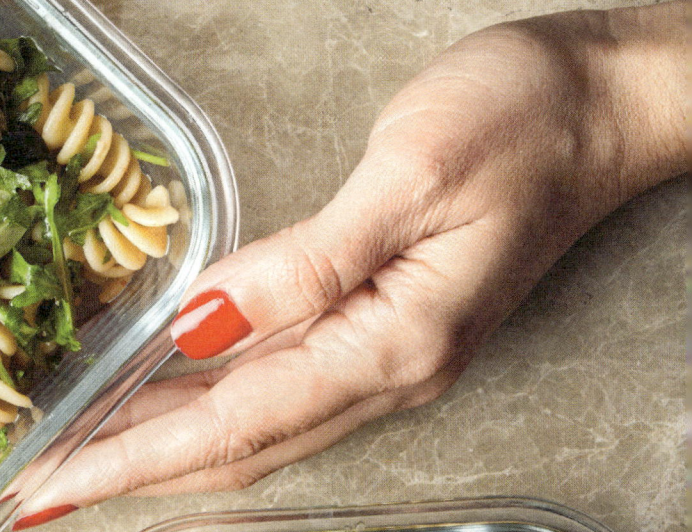

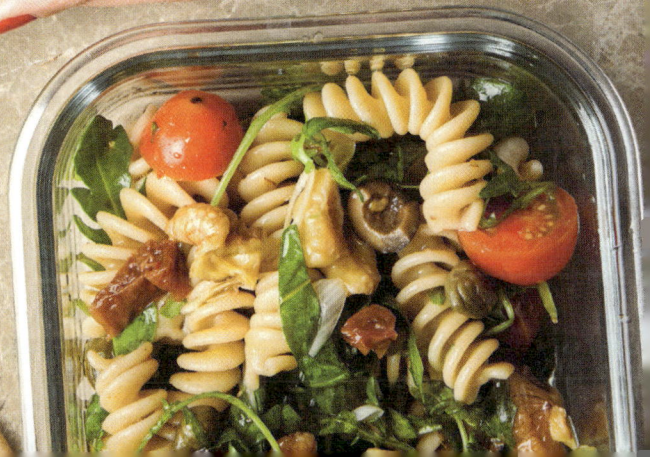

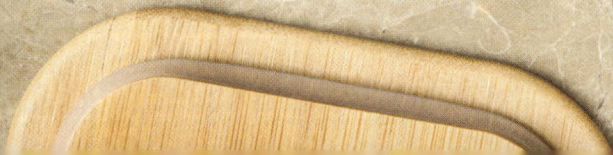

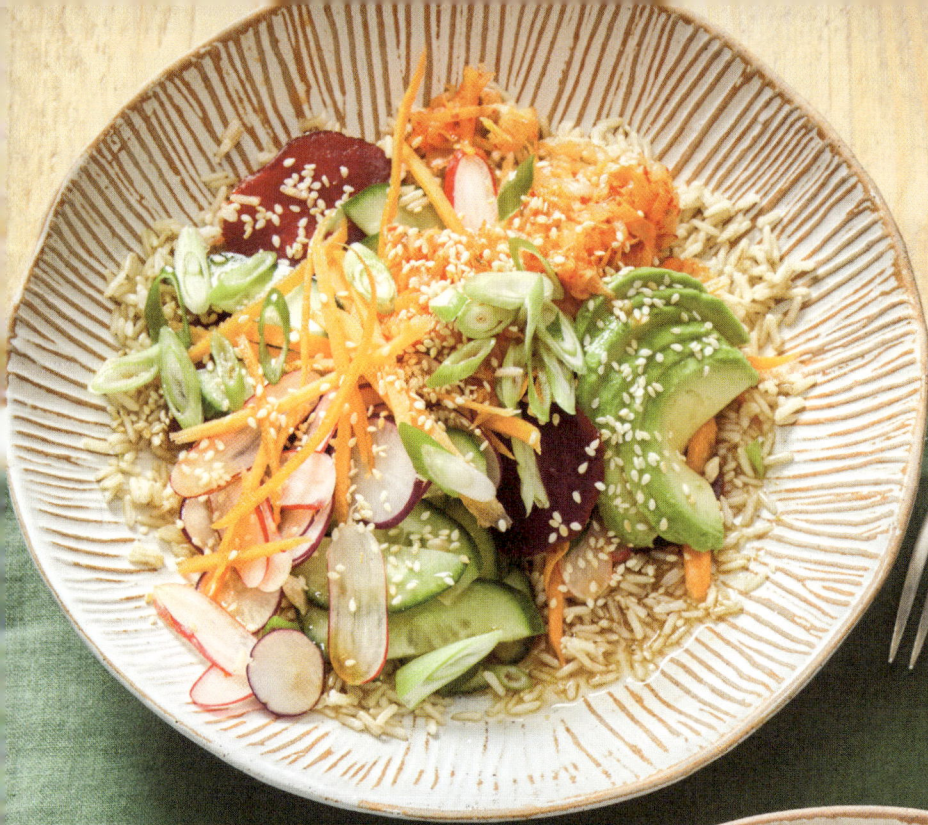

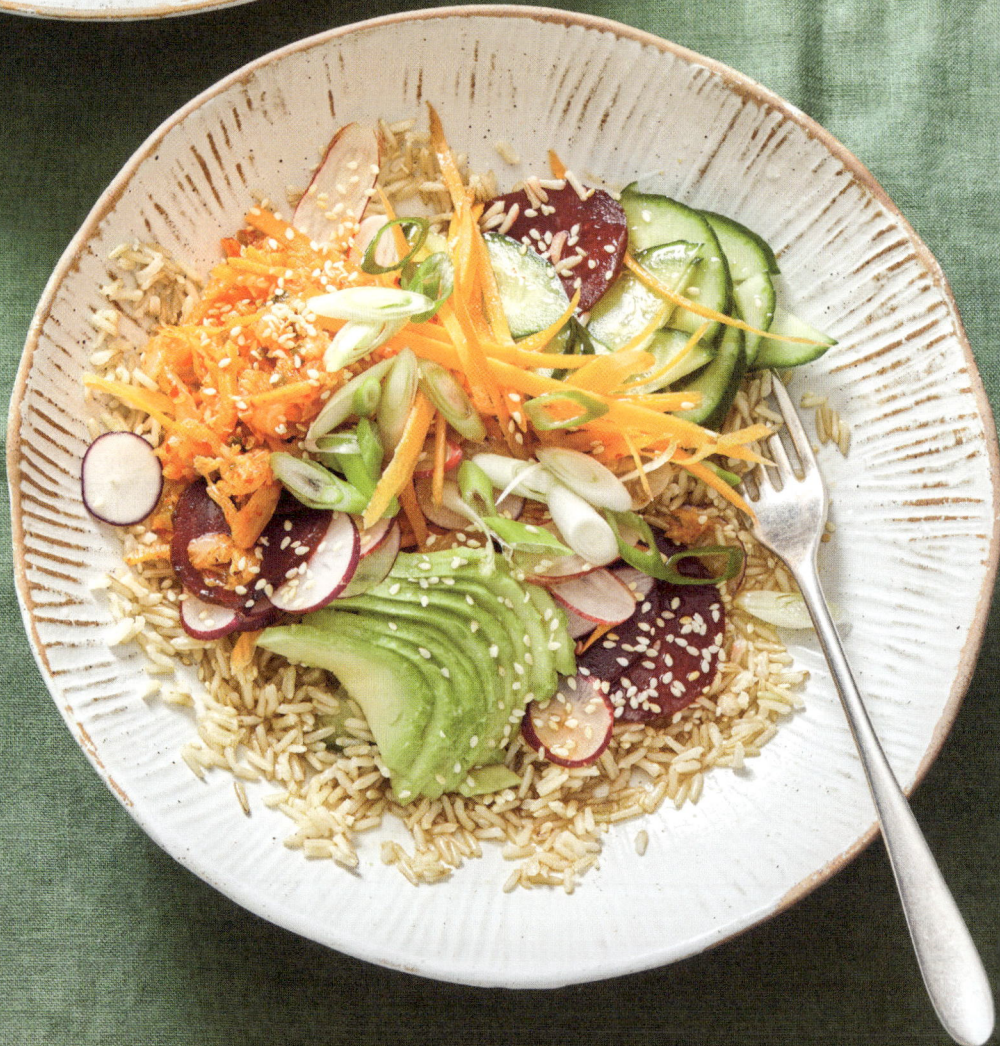

Rainbow rice bowl

Serves 2   **Prep** 15 mins   **Cook** 15 minutes

100g (½ cup/3½oz) long-grain brown rice

1 large carrot, peeled and julienned or grated

2 medium cooked vac-packed or canned beetroots (beets), sliced

⅓ cucumber, sliced into half moons

1 avocado, peeled, de-stoned, and sliced

8 radishes, sliced

4 tbsp kimchi or sauerkraut

3 tsp toasted white or black sesame seeds

2 spring (green) onions, finely sliced

For the dressing

Juice of 1 lime

1 tsp brown sugar or maple syrup

2 tbsp tamari or soy sauce

2 tbsp extra-virgin olive oil

4 tsp sesame oil

This is a very substantial dish, packed with a host of health-boosting ingredients. It's also super-adaptable, so feel free to add or swap in some of the optional additions listed below to adapt it to your tastes and add some variety to your weekly lunches.

1. Cook the rice according to the packet instructions. Drain into a sieve (strainer), then place the sieve on top of the now empty pan, cover with a kitchen towel and leave to one side to steam dry.

2. Meanwhile, prepare the vegetables and whisk together the dressing ingredients.

3. Pile the rice into a bowl (either still warm or room temperature), then add all the vegetables and the dressing. Toss well, then scatter with the sesame seeds and spring onions.

Optional additions

- Wilted baby spinach (or frozen and defrosted spinach)
- Sliced red (bell) pepper
- Shredded red cabbage
- Roasted tofu cubes
- Spicy mayonnaise (combine the aquafaba mayo on page 207 with some lime juice and your favourite hot sauce)
- Boiled eggs
- Grilled chicken
- Tuna

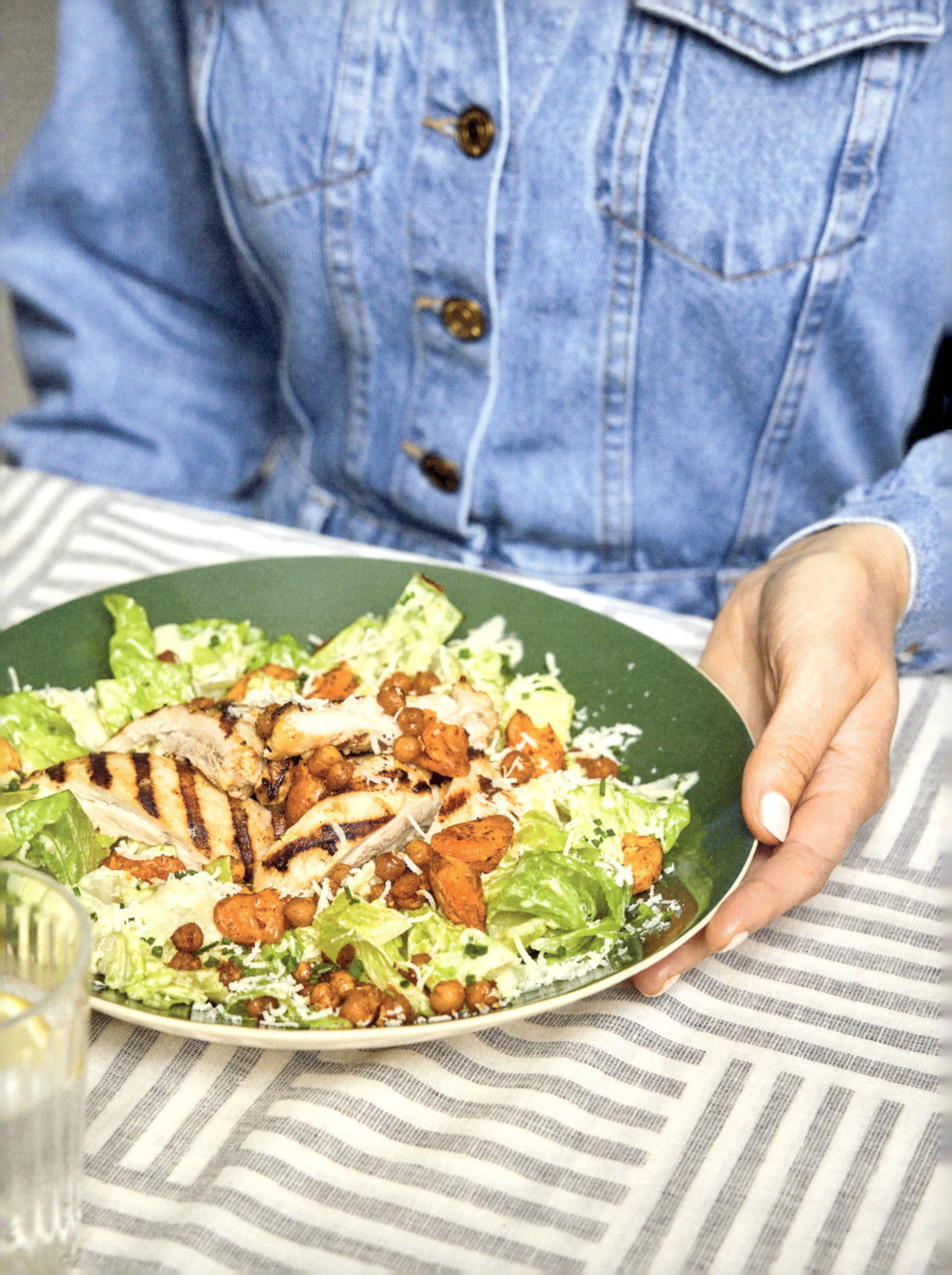

Chicken Caesar salad

Nutritional info per portion

Fibre 5g
Protein 58g
Plant Points 5

● **Serves** 4   ● **Prep** 15 mins   ● **Cook** 7 minutes

6 tbsp Greek yogurt

4 tbsp mayonnaise (see page 207 for homemade) (or use more Greek yogurt)

70g (2½oz) Parmesan, finely grated

2 garlic cloves, minced

Zest and juice of 1 lemon

600g (21oz) skinless, boneless chicken thighs

2 anchovy fillets in oil, finely chopped

2 tsp Dijon mustard

1 tsp Worcestershire sauce

1½ tbsp chopped chives

2 tbsp olive oil

2 large or 3–4 small heads of romaine lettuce, shredded

150g (5½oz) roast butter bean and chickpea sprinkle (page 214)

Sea salt and freshly ground black pepper

Caesar salad is loved by almost everyone, but it can often be disappointing when grabbed on-the-go or even ordered at a restaurant. Try making it yourself instead— that way you know exactly what's going into it and you can also ensure it's packed with deliciousness! If you want to make this vegan, substitute the anchovies for 1 tablespoon of capers, the chicken for tofu or avocado, omit the Worcestershire sauce, use coconut yogurt instead of plain yogurt, and use a vegan alternative to Parmesan.

1. Combine the yogurt, mayonnaise, about half the Parmesan, the garlic, and lemon zest and the juice in a medium bowl and season with salt and pepper. Transfer half the mixture to a salad bowl and set aside, then add the chicken thighs to the original bowl with the remaining half of the mixture. Toss well to coat the chicken, then set aside to marinate briefly while you prepare everything else.

2. Stir the anchovies, mustard, Worcestershire sauce, and chives into the salad bowl, then slowly drizzle in the olive oil, whisking constantly until it's completely combined. Season to taste with salt and pepper.

3. Set a griddle, cast-iron or non-stick frying pan (skillet) over a medium–high and let it get super-hot. Add the chicken and cook, turning occasionally, for 5–7 minutes until dark and golden on the outside and cooked in the middle (cut into the thickest piece to check if you're not sure). Remove from the pan and leave to rest for 5 minutes before slicing into thick strips.

4. Add the romaine to the salad bowl and toss with the dressing. Divide the salad between plates, then top with the warm chicken strips. Scatter over the roast butter bean and chickpea sprinkle and the remaining Parmesan, then dig in.

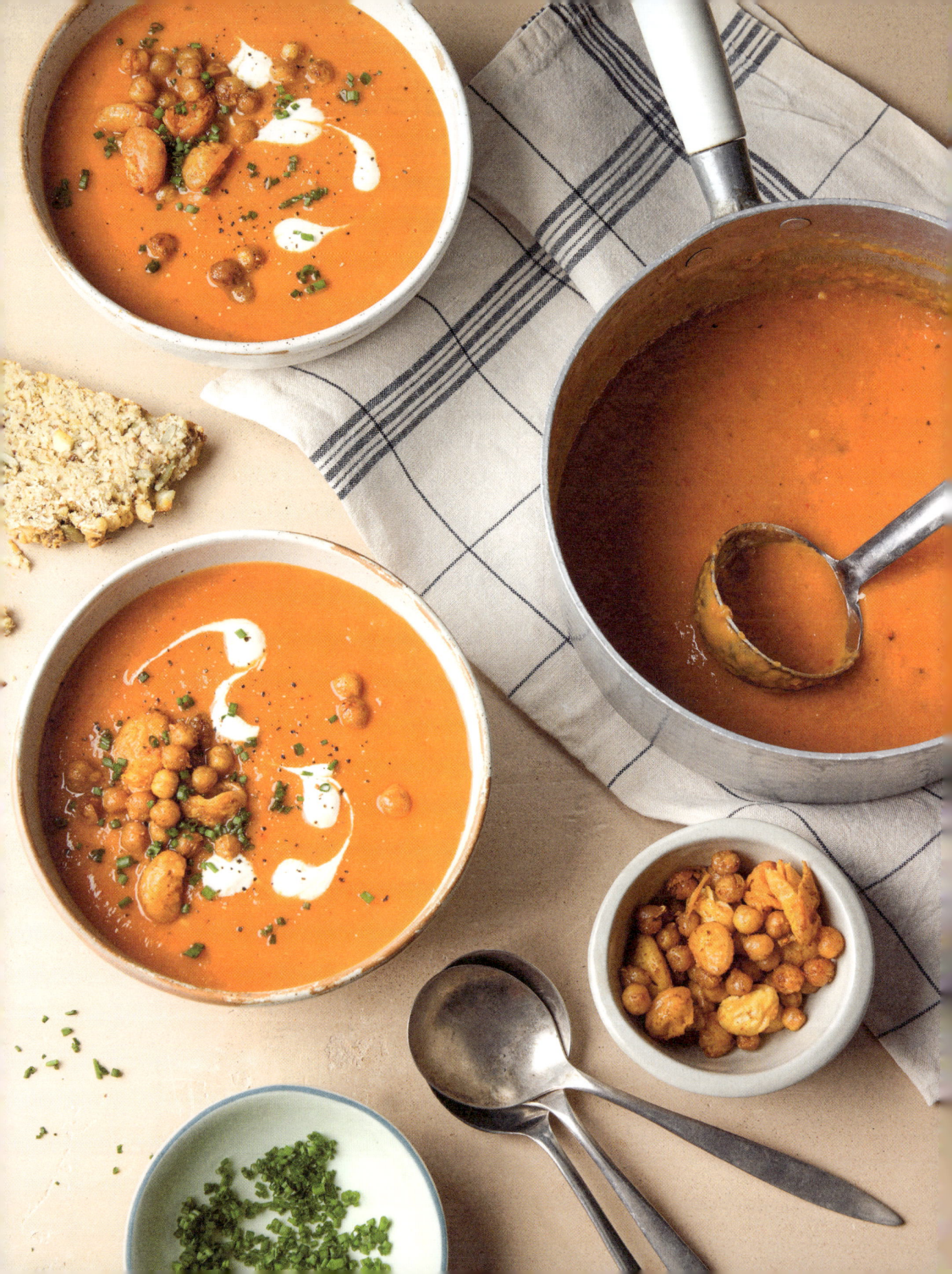

Smoky tomato, pepper, and bean soup

Nutritional info per portion

Fibre 14g
Protein 13g
Plant Points 10.25

● **Serves** 4   ● **Prep** 10 mins   ● **Cook** 40 minutes

4 tbsp olive oil, cold-pressed rapeseed oil, or avocado oil

1 onion, chopped

2 celery stalks, chopped

1 carrot, chopped

2 garlic cloves, chopped

1 tbsp thyme leaves

1 × 400g (14oz) can chopped plum tomatoes

250g (9oz) jarred roasted red (bell) peppers in brine, drained and chopped

¼ tsp dried chilli (red pepper) flakes (optional)

1 tbsp maple syrup, plus extra if needed

1 tbsp tamari or soy sauce

1 tsp sweet paprika, plus extra if needed

1 × 400g (14oz) can white beans, drained and rinsed

850ml (3½ cups/30fl oz) hot chicken or vegetable stock

Sea salt and freshly ground black pepper

To serve

4 tbsp sour cream, Greek yogurt or coconut yogurt

100g (3½oz) roast butter bean and chickpea sprinkle (page 214)

Chopped chives

This is delicious served with cottage cheese bread (page 110) for dunking. It's a great recipe for batch cooking—simply double the quantities.

1. Warm the oil in a large deep pan set over a medium heat, then add the onion, celery, carrot, and a pinch of salt. Gently fry for 8–10 minutes until the vegetables are tender, then add the garlic and thyme and continue cooking for another 2 minutes until fragrant.

2. Add all the other soup ingredients, season with 1 teaspoon of salt and plenty of black pepper, then bring to a simmer and cook for 30 minutes.

3. Once the soup is ready, use an electric hand-held blender to blitz until smooth. Add a little boiling water from the kettle if you'd like it looser, then have a taste and add more salt, pepper, paprika, or maple syrup if you feel it needs it.

4. Transfer the soup to bowls, then dollop over some sour cream and scatter with the roast butter bean and chickpea sprinkle and the chopped chives.

5. Store in an airtight container in the fridge for up to 1 week or in the freezer for up to 1 month.

Note Try stirring leftover soup through cooked pasta to add a bit of variety to your weekly meal plan.

Optional additions

· Grated Cheddar
· Crumbled feta
· Cooked small pasta

Super green soup

Nutritional info per portion

Fibre 7.8g
Protein 12g
Plant Points 11

● **Serves** 4–6   ● **Prep** 10 mins   ● **Cook** 25 minutes

4 tbsp olive oil, cold-pressed rapeseed oil, or avocado oil

1½ tsp fennel seeds

1½ tsp coriander seeds

1 large leek, outer layer discarded and roughly chopped

2 celery stalks, chopped

4 garlic cloves, chopped

275g (9½oz) celeriac (celery root) or potatoes, peeled and chopped into 1cm (½ inch) cubes

150g (5½oz) broccoli, head and stalk, roughly chopped

1.25 litres (5 cups/40fl oz) hot chicken or vegetable stock

125g (4½oz) frozen peas

125g (4½oz) spinach or watercress (frozen and defrosted is fine too)

Handful of parsley, chopped, plus extra to serve

Handful of dill, chopped, plus extra to serve

2 tbsp tahini (optional)

4–6 tbsp Greek or coconut yogurt

4 tbsp tamari seeds (page 214), to serve

Sea salt and freshly ground black pepper

This is a very unfussy soup packed full of vegetables and it tastes great. Add whatever green veg you have to hand or needs using up—I've listed a few ideas below to bulk out the soup, or for toppers to add crunch. I like to add a little tahini to enrich this and add some plant iron, but you can always leave this out if you like. You can also leave it chunky instead of blending it to mix things up. I often serve this topped with tamari seeds (page 214) or a dollop of pesto (page 211), with cottage cheese bread on the side for dipping (page 110).

1. Warm the oil in a large deep pan set over a medium heat, then add the fennel and coriander seeds. Wait for 30 seconds, then add the leek, celery, and a pinch of salt and gently fry for 6–8 minutes until the vegetables are tender. Add the garlic and continue cooking for another 2 minutes until fragrant.

2. Add the celeriac or potato, the broccoli, and 1 teaspoon of salt and gently fry for 2 minutes. Add the stock to the pan, cover and simmer for 10 minutes, or until the celeriac or potatoes are just tender.

3. Add the peas and spinach or watercress and push them under the liquid. Bring back to a simmer and cook for a further 2–3 minutes, then take off the heat and stir in the herbs and tahini (if using).

4. Use an electric hand-held blender to blitz until smooth. Taste and adjust the seasoning – it'll probably need quite a bit of salt and pepper.

5. Transfer the soup to bowls, then swirl in dollops of yogurt and sprinkle over the tamari seeds and some extra herbs.

Note Try stirring leftover soup through cooked pasta to add a bit of variety to your weekly meal plan.

Optional additions

· Cavolo nero or kale (Tuscan or curly kale)
· Fennel
· Courgette (zucchini)
· Cauliflower
· White beans
· Cooked small pasta
· Cooked quinoa
· Cooked brown rice

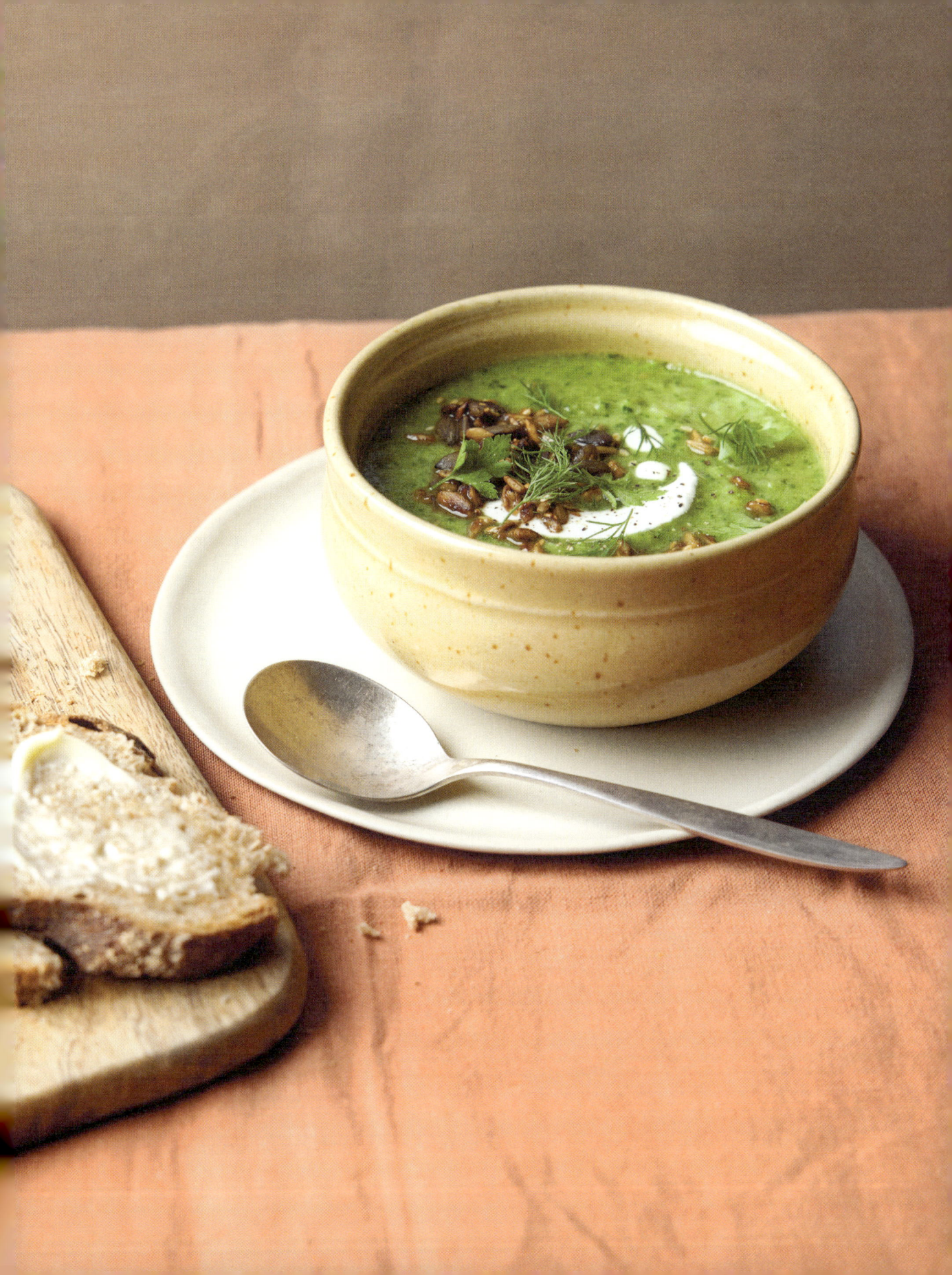

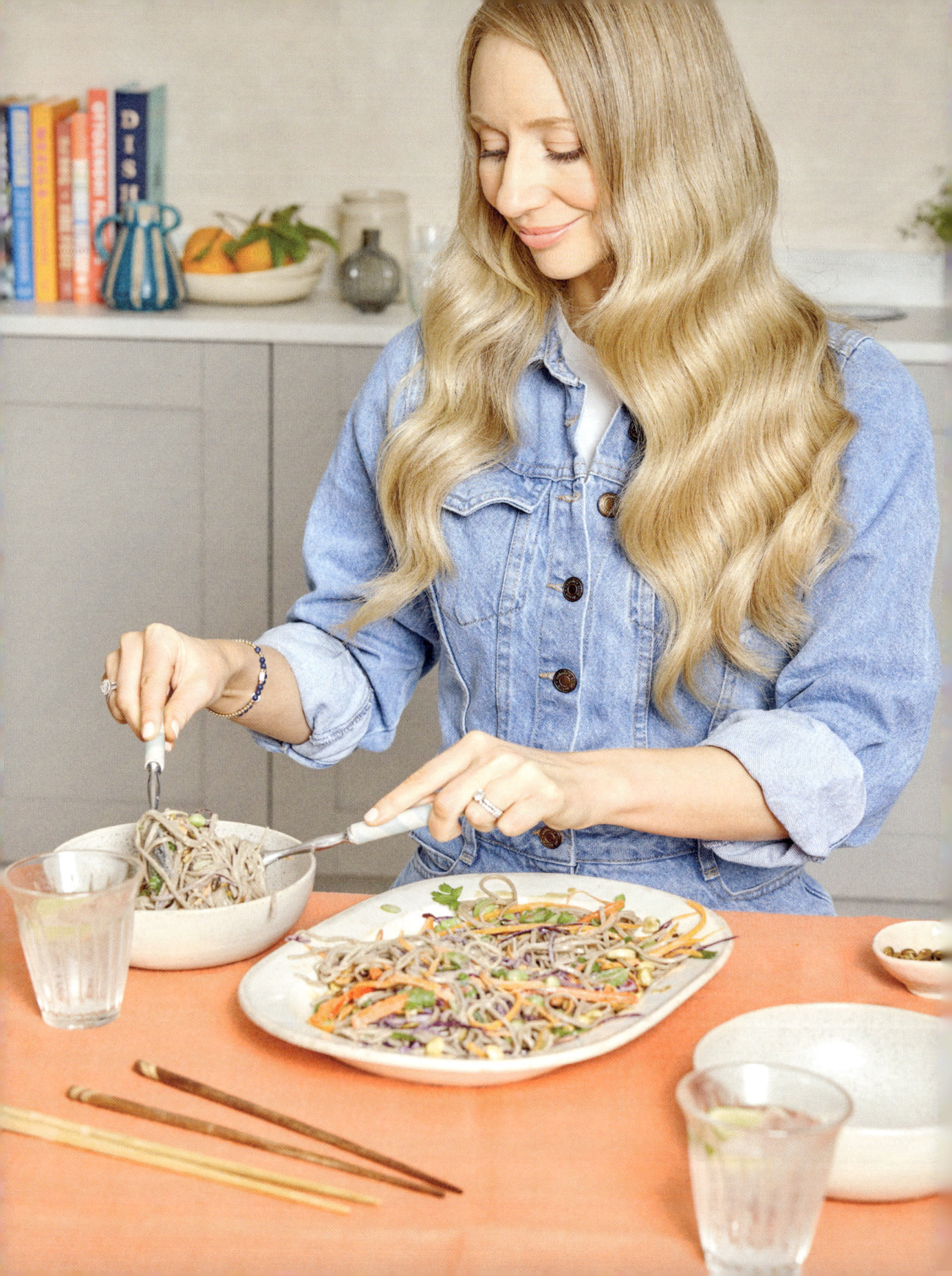

Tahini noodle salad

Nutritional info per portion

Fibre 11g
Protein 22g
Plant Points 13

Serves 4   **Prep** 10 mins   **Cook** 5 minutes

180g (6½oz) soba, brown rice, or egg noodles, or wholewheat spaghetti

100g (3½oz) frozen edamame or peas, defrosted

3 spring (green) onions, thinly sliced

2 small carrots, peeled and julienned or grated

½ red, orange or yellow (bell) pepper, deseeded and thinly sliced

150g (5½oz) red or white cabbage or little gem or romaine lettuce, very finely shredded

Handful of coriander (cilantro) leaves, roughly chopped

Handful of mint leaves, roughly chopped

70g (2½oz) roasted peanuts, chopped (or use cashews, walnuts, or almonds)

60g (2oz) tamari seeds (page 214), to serve

For the dressing

4 tbsp tahini or smooth peanut butter

1 garlic clove

1 tbsp sesame oil

2½ tbsp tamari or soy sauce, plus extra to taste

1½ tbsp maple syrup

Juice of 1 lime (or 2 tbsp white wine vinegar)

Sea salt and freshly ground black pepper

Brilliant for picnics and packed lunches, I promise that cold noodles are super satisfying and the perfect carrier for a variety of colorful veggies. You can also add cooked chicken or tofu to bulk this up and add extra protein, plus whatever else you fancy from the optional additions listed below.

1. Bring a pan of salted water to the boil and cook the noodles according to the packet instructions. Drain into a colander and rinse under cold water until cool. Set aside.

2. Next, make the dressing. Spoon the tahini into a large salad bowl, grate in the garlic, then stir in the rest of the ingredients to make a thick paste. Using a fork, slowly whisk in 2–3 tablespoons of cold water until you have a dressing the thickness of single (light) cream. Have a taste and a little extra tamari or soy sauce, and some salt and pepper, if needed.

3. Add the noodles to the bowl, along with the rest of the salad ingredients, and toss with your hands until everything is nicely coated in the dressing. Sprinkle with the tamari seeds and serve.

Optional additions

· Sliced cucumber
· Sliced radishes
· Chopped avocado
· Canned sardines
· Flaked smoked mackerel
· Grilled or roast chicken
· Roast tofu cubes
· Cooked prawns (shrimp)
· Chilli oil

Green fritters with whipped herby cottage cheese

Nutritional info per portion

Fibre 5.1g
Protein 13g
Plant Points 6

Serves 4　　**Prep** 10 mins　　**Cook** 10 minutes

For the fritters

100g (½ cup/3½oz) cottage cheese, ricotta, Greek yogurt, or coconut yogurt

Zest of 1 lemon

100g (3½oz) frozen peas, defrosted

75g (2½oz) spinach (frozen and defrosted is fine too)

3 tbsp milk of your choice

125g (4½oz) chickpea (gram) flour (or use wholemeal/ whole wheat or spelt flour)

1 tsp baking powder

2 eggs or 2 flax eggs (see Note on page 100)

3 spring (green) onions, finely sliced

Olive oil, cold-pressed rapeseed oil, or avocado oil, for frying

Sea salt and freshly ground black pepper

For the whipped herby cottage cheese

Juice of ½ lemon

1 small garlic clove, grated

200g (1 cup/7oz) cottage cheese, ricotta, Greek yogurt, or coconut yogurt

2 tbsp grated Parmesan (or use vegan alternative)

3 tbsp olive oil

Handful of parsley leaves, roughly chopped

Handful of mint leaves, roughly chopped

These fritters are full of wholesome greens and protein, surprisingly substantial, and an easy way to pack nutrition into your day. Eat with the herby sauce and a salad for lunch or with a poached or fried egg, as I've done here, for brunch. If using a yogurt for the dip instead of cottage cheese, don't blitz it in the blender as it will loosen too much—just stir it into the other ingredients at the end.

1. First, make the whipped herby cottage cheese. Add all the ingredients to a blender or food processor (see intro) with some salt and pepper, and 2 tablespoons of water, then blitz until smooth. Check the seasoning, then transfer to a small bowl and set aside.

2. Without cleaning out the blender, make the fritters. Place the cottage cheese, lemon zest, half the peas, the spinach, milk, flour, baking powder, eggs, and ¼ teaspoon of salt in the blender and blitz briefly until you have a thick green purée. Gently stir in the spring onions, remaining peas, and a little salt and pepper to create a chunky batter.

3. To cook the fritters, set a medium non-stick frying pan (skillet) or crêpe pan over a medium–high heat and coat the base of the pan in a fine layer of oil. Spoon in heaped tablespoons of batter and gently push down with the back of the spoon. Cook the fritters for 1–2 minutes until you can see a few air bubbles on the surface, then gently flip them and cook the other side for a further 1–2 minutes until golden brown on both sides. Keep warm in a low oven while you cook the remaining batter, adding a little more oil when the pan looks like it needs it.

4. Once all the fritters are cooked, serve them up with dollops of the whipped herby cottage cheese (I also like to add a poached or fried egg for added protein). Store the fritters and dip separately in airtight containers in the fridge for up to 4 days. The fritters reheat well in the microwave.

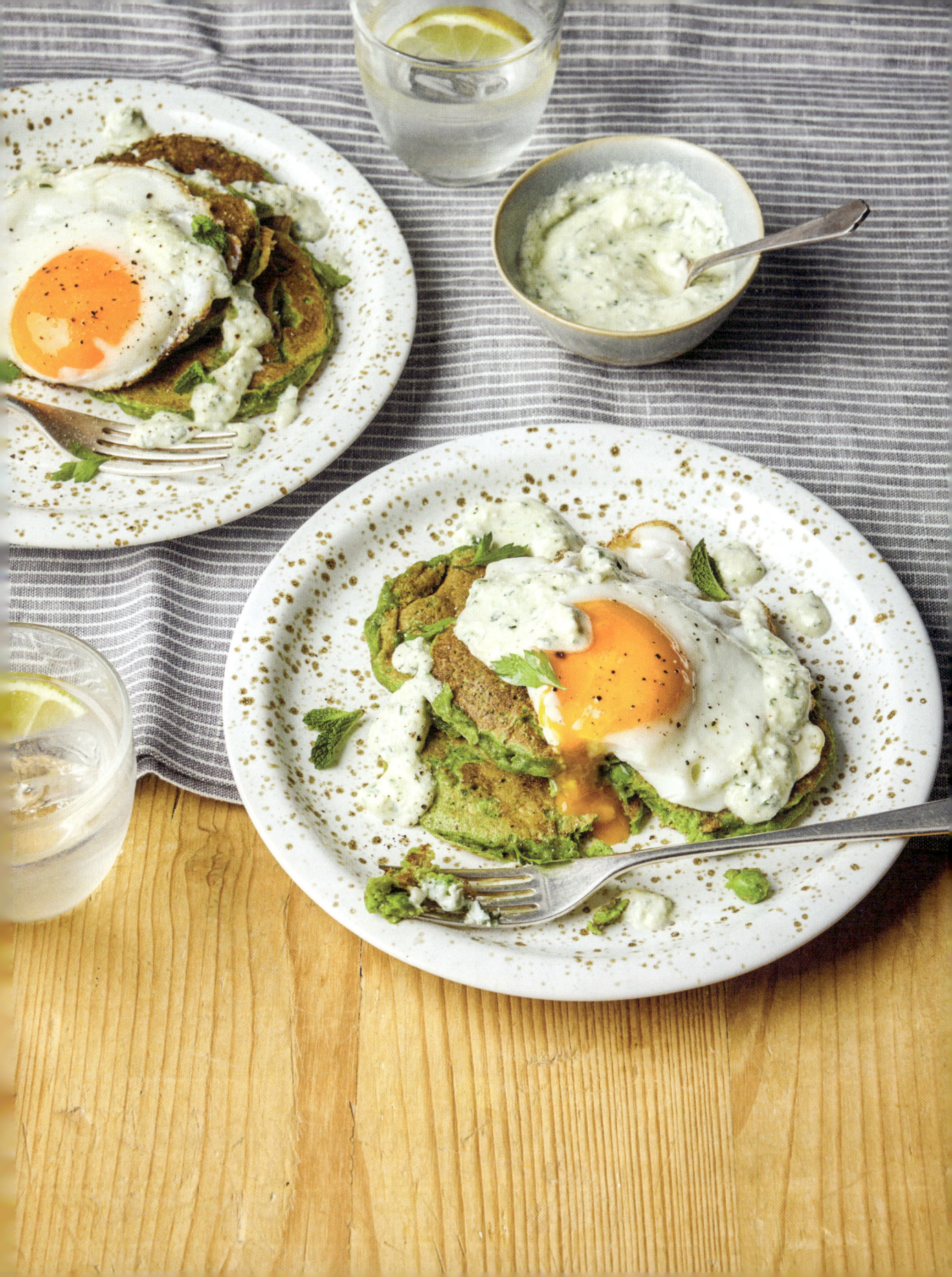

Time is my nemesis, but as a nutritionist and a mother, I've had to adapt to ensure my family always has access to wholesome meals. These are some of my most delicious go-to recipes when I need to get food on the table in a flash but still want to include a nutritional boost.

From twists on comforting classics, like pearl spelt and pea risotto or creamy miso and peanut butter ramen, to fresh and fragrant suppers, like tofu larb or prawn tacos with grapefruit salsa, each dish is packed with gut-loving ingredients, offers alternatives for different dietary requirements, and is quick and simple to prepare.

30-Minute Heroes

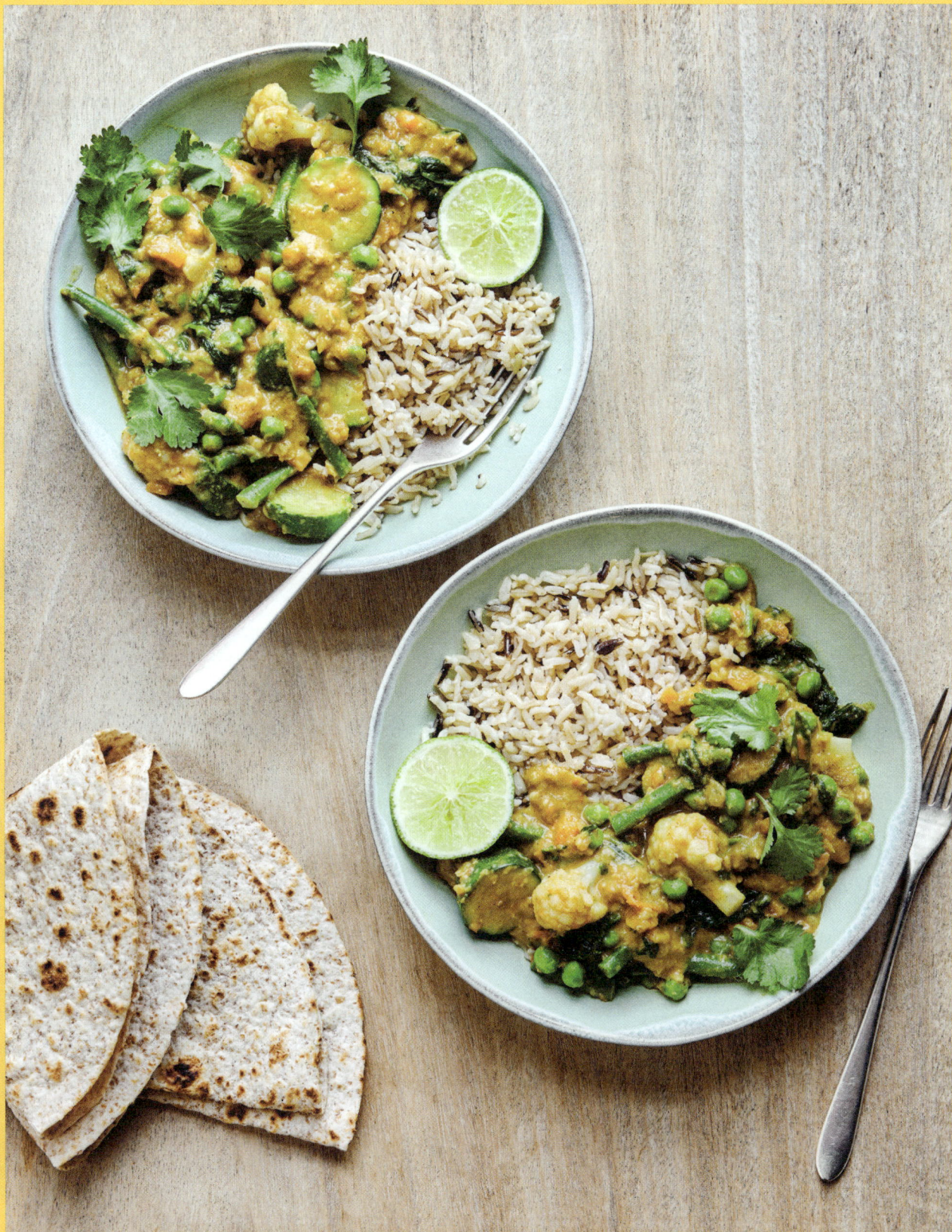

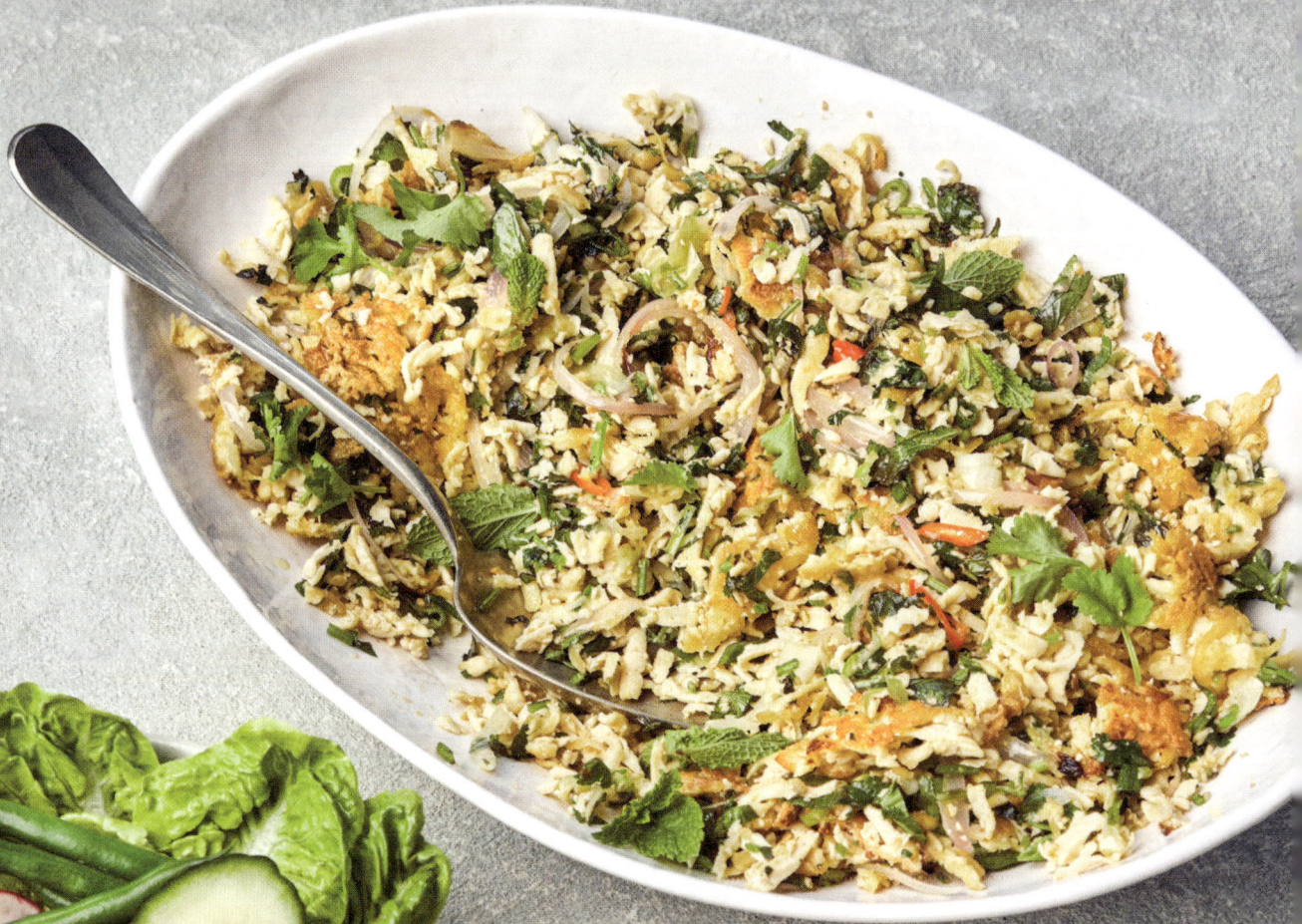

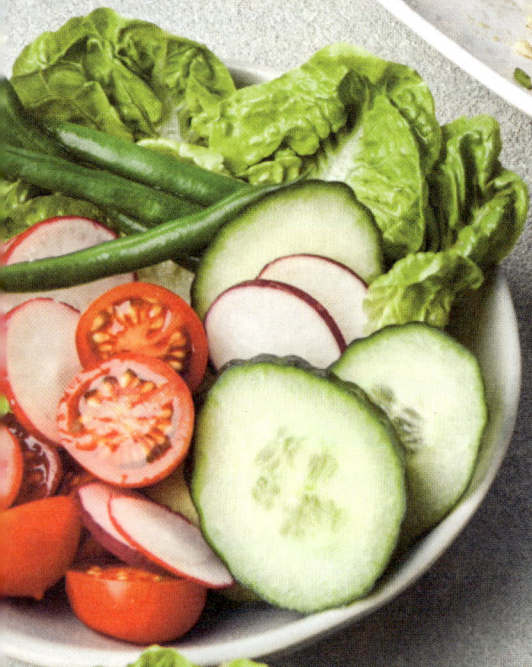

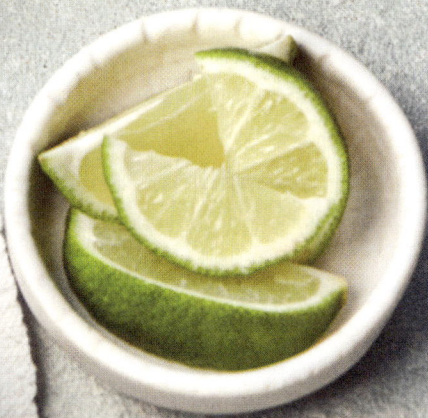

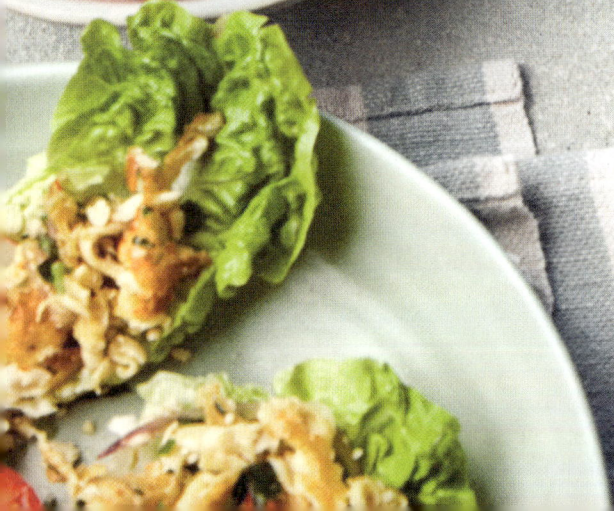

Tofu larb

Serves 4   **Prep** 10 mins   **Cook** 20 minutes

2 tbsp long-grain brown rice

2 tbsp sunflower oil, cold-pressed rapeseed oil, or avocado oil

450g (16oz) firm tofu, patted dry and coarsely grated or finely chopped (or use ground turkey or finely chopped chestnut/brown mushrooms)

2 shallots, finely sliced

½–1 small red bird's eye chilli or ¼ tsp chilli (red pepper) flakes

4 spring (green) onions, finely sliced, white and green parts separated

2–3 tbsp lime juice, plus extra to taste

2 tbsp fish sauce (or use a vegan fish sauce, such as Yondu), plus extra to taste

40g (1½oz) coriander (cilantro), leaves and stems chopped, plus extra to serve

3 mint sprigs, leaves picked and chopped, plus extra to serve

To serve

2 heads of little gem, butterhead or romaine lettuce, leaves separated

½ cucumber, sliced

200g (7oz) green beans, trimmed

Handful of cherry tomatoes, halved

Handful of radishes, sliced

Lime wedges

Tofu is a very underrated ingredient in western cultures, but it's a wonderful source of protein and low in fat. This is a surprisingly filling supper, but you can always cook some extra brown rice to bulk things up if needed. You can make this as mild or as spicy as you like—I tend to add half the chilli at first, adding the other half at the end once I've tasted everything if I feel it needs it.

1. Set a heavy-based frying pan (skillet) over a low–medium heat and toast the brown rice for 4–6 minutes, moving the pan constantly until it's evenly golden-brown. Tip onto a plate and leave to cool for 5 minutes, then transfer to a pestle and mortar or spice grinder and grind to a fine powder. Set aside.

2. Wipe the pan clean, then return it to a medium–high heat and add the oil. Once the oil is shimmering, fry the tofu for 2–3 minutes without stirring it, then stir and continue cooking for another 5 minutes until most of it is golden and crisp. Add half the shallots, the chilli and the spring onion whites and fry for 3–5 minutes before turning off the heat and adding the lime juice, fish sauce, herbs, ground rice, spring onion greens and remaining shallots. Taste and add more chilli, fish sauce and lime juice if needed. It should be quite punchy.

3. Serve everything in the middle of the table for people to help themselves. Spoon some of the warm larb into a lettuce leaf and top with some crunchy vegetables, extra herbs and a squeeze of lime juice.

Note You'll be surprised by just how well the texture of grated or crumbled tofu mimics ground meat, so do give it a go!

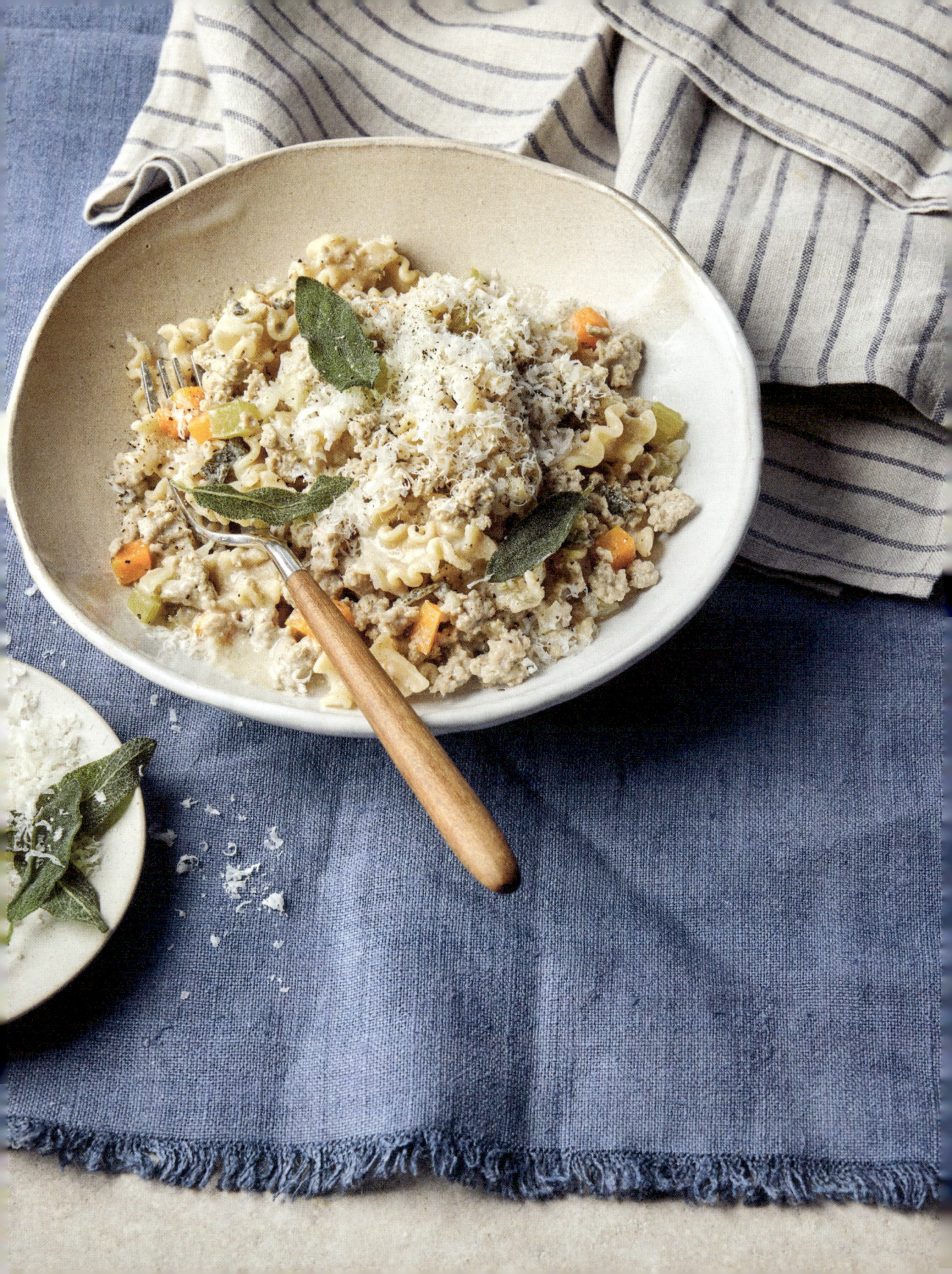

Pork ragu with milk, lemon, and sage

Nutritional info per portion

Fibre 5.3g
Protein 27g
Plant Points 6.75

● **Serves** 6   ● **Prep** 5 mins   ● **Cook** 25 minutes

3 tbsp olive oil

1 large onion, chopped

1 celery stalk, chopped

1 carrot, chopped

2 garlic cloves, chopped

1 bay leaf

500g (18oz) high-quality ground pork

1 tsp fennel seeds

300ml (1¼ cups/10½fl oz) whole milk

3 tbsp white wine vinegar

10 sage leaves, roughly chopped

2 pared strips of lemon peel

A few gratings of nutmeg

500g (18oz) dried wholewheat pasta

40g (1½oz) Parmesan, grated, plus extra to serve

Sea salt and freshly ground black pepper

This is a great example of how to make a meat sauce for pasta without the need of tomatoes and a long cook time—and is a lovely way to bring some variation to your weeknight cooking repertoire. Here milk, lemon and sage are used to create an incredibly delicious, intense sauce.

To make this veggie or vegan, use 250g (9oz) finely chopped cauliflower and 250g (9oz) lentils in place of the pork, use plant-based milk, and use a vegan alternative to Parmesan.

1. Warm the oil in a deep pan set over a medium heat and fry the onion, celery, carrot, and garlic with the bay leaf and a pinch of salt for 10 minutes until softened.

2. Meanwhile, season the pork in a bowl with plenty of salt, pepper, and the fennel seeds. Give it a quick massage to get the seasoning nicely distributed.

3. Turn up the heat under the veg, then add the meat. Fry, stirring, until it's just cooked through, then add the milk, vinegar, sage, lemon peel, nutmeg, and plenty of salt and pepper and leave to simmer for 15–20 minutes (or longer if you have time) until the meat is tender. Taste and adjust the seasoning. Discard the bay leaf and lemon peel.

4. While the sauce is cooking, bring a pan of salted water to the boil and cook the pasta according to the packet instructions until al dente. Drain, reserving a cup of the pasta water, then transfer the drained pasta and Parmesan to the sauce and stir. Add a few splashes of pasta water if it's looking dry, stir well, then transfer to plates and serve with a little extra Parmesan grated over.

Pearl spelt and pea risotto

Nutritional info per portion

Fibre 11g
Protein 14g
Plant Points 5.5

Serves 4   **Prep** 5 mins   **Cook** 30 mins

4 tbsp olive oil, plus extra to serve

1 celery stalk, chopped

2 leeks or 1 large onion, chopped

200g (7oz) pearl spelt or pearl barley

1.25 litres (5 cups/40fl oz) vegetable or chicken stock

325g (11½oz) frozen and defrosted or fresh peas

2 big handfuls of mint leaves, roughly chopped

2 big handfuls of basil leaves, roughly chopped

30g (1oz) Parmesan, grated, plus extra to serve (or use a vegetarian alternative)

Sea salt and freshly ground black pepper

The inspiration for this dish, traditionally called risi bisi, is usually made with a 1:1 ratio of rice to peas, but here I've blended some extra peas to make a delicious herby purée to amp up the pea flavor. Peas are often overlooked when it comes to protein sources, but they are a really nourishing source of nutrition. This is a particularly easy dish as, although it's similar to a risotto, very little stirring is required so you don't need to stand by the stove for a lifetime. You can eat it thick like a risotto, or add a little more liquid (as the Venetians do) and serve it as a thick soup with a spoon. You can also leave the spelt/barley unrinsed for a creamier dish.

1. Set a large pan over a medium heat and add 3 tablespoons of the olive oil. When hot, add the celery and leeks or onion, and a pinch of salt and fry for 10 minutes until softening but not colored.

2. Add the pearl spelt (or barley), stock, and 1 teaspoon of salt, then bring to a simmer and cook for 10 minutes (30 minutes if using barley), ensuring the spelt is always just covered in liquid (add a little water if needed). Add 225g (8oz) of the peas and continue simmering for 10–15 minutes until the spelt (or barley) is tender.

3. Meanwhile, place the remaining 100g (3½oz) of peas, the remaining 1 tablespoon of oil, half the herbs, and the grated Parmesan in a blender with 2 tablespoons of water and blitz to form a bright green purée.

4. Stir the purée into the pan until you have a thick, soupy texture (add a little more water if needed). Season to taste with salt and pepper, stir in the remaining mint and basil, then serve in bowls with plenty of grated Parmesan and a little drizzle of olive oil. This freezes very well.

Note You can top the risotto with any extra burst of flavor; some ricotta, mozzarella, or crumbled walnuts would be great. You can also add extra vegetables while cooking—chopped courgettes (zucchini) and spinach both work well.

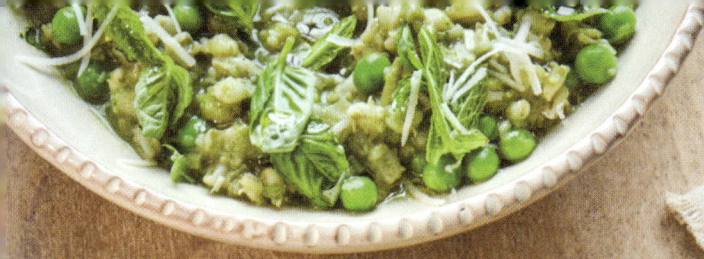

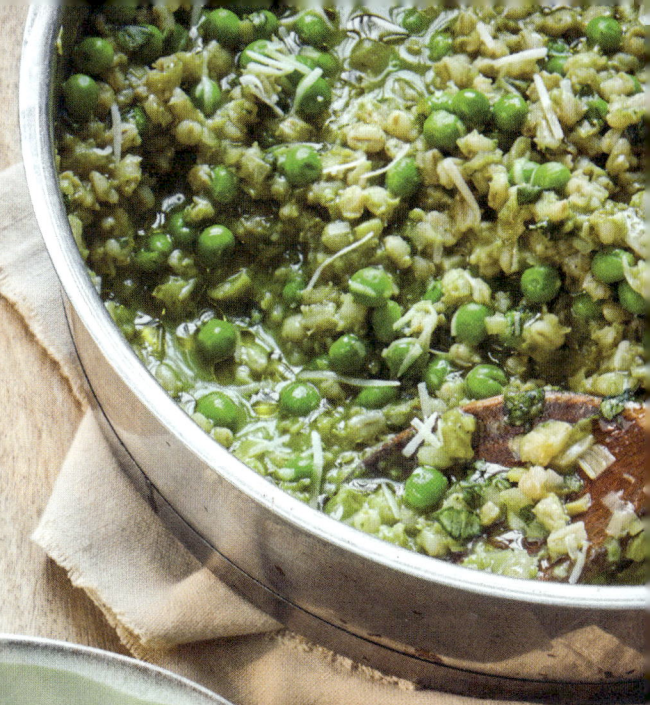

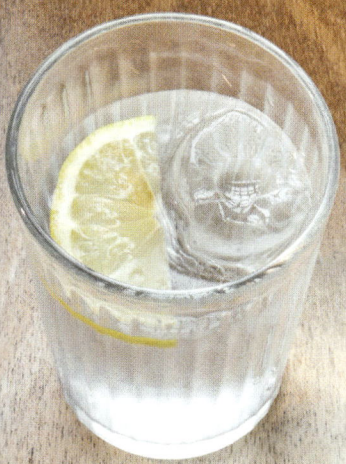

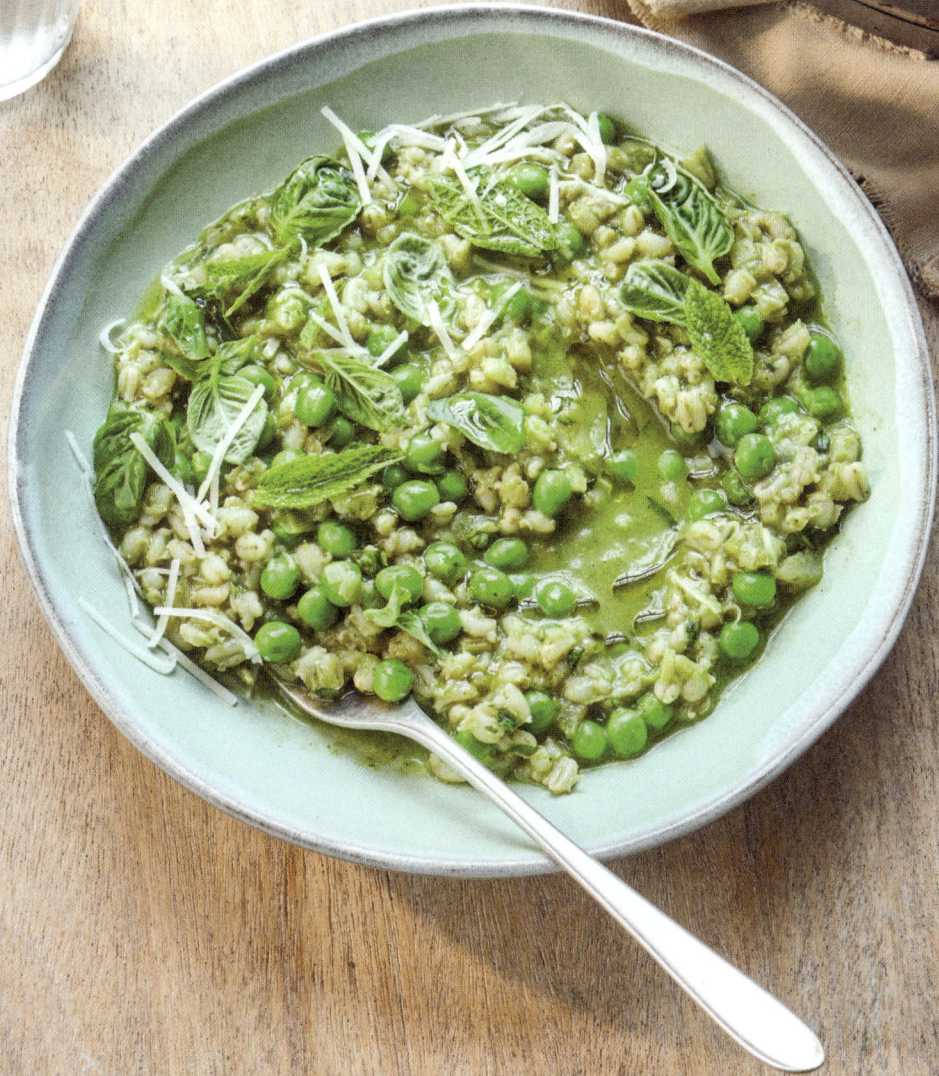

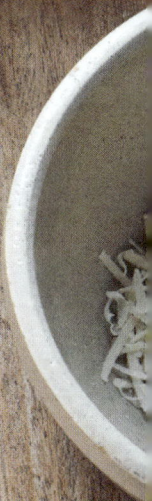

Sweet potato and chicken curry

Nutritional info per portion

Fibre 8.5g
Protein 36g
Plant Points 6.5

Serves 4   **Prep** 5 mins   **Cook** 25 mins

2 tbsp coconut oil

400g (14oz) skinless, boneless chicken thighs or skinless breast, cut into 2cm (1 inch) chunks

1 × 400g (14oz) can coconut milk, creamy top layer and liquid milk separated

300g (10½oz) sweet potato, peeled and cut into 2cm (1 inch) chunks

200g (7oz) carrots, sliced into 1cm (½ inch) rounds

1–2 tbsp fish sauce (optional)

½ tsp brown sugar (optional)

Handful of coriander (cilantro) leaves

Cooked long-grain brown rice or wholewheat noodles, to serve

Lime wedges, to serve

Sea salt and freshly ground black pepper

For the curry paste

2 lemongrass stalks, tough outer layer discarded (see intro) and tender core roughly chopped

1 thumb-sized piece fresh ginger, peeled and chopped

2 garlic cloves, chopped

2 shallots, chopped

2 tbsp curry powder, ideally Madras

Another curry that will delight every member of the family. This has quite a wet sauce, so definitely serve it with either brown rice or noodles (if opting for brown rice, add the tough outer layer of the lemongrass stalk to the water as it cooks, to impart extra flavor and fragrance). You can make this vegan by omitting the fish sauce and substituting the chicken for tofu, celeriac, potato, or cauliflower. Feel free to make extra curry paste and use my ice-cube trick for easy meals in the future (see page 143).

1. First, make the curry paste. Place the lemongrass, ginger, garlic, and shallots in a blender or a food processor and blitz until finely chopped. Add the curry powder and ½ tsp freshly ground black pepper and blitz to a paste (add 2–3 tablespoons of water if it needs a little help breaking down).

2. Warm the coconut oil in a wide pan set over a low–medium heat and add the curry paste. Cook for 3–5 minutes, stirring constantly, until fragrant.

3. Season the chicken pieces with salt and pepper, then add them to the pan and stir fry for 1–2 minutes. Add the liquid from the can of coconut milk (save the thick cream layer for later), the sweet potatoes, carrots, and some salt and pepper. Add enough water to just cover everything (about 120ml/½ cup/4fl oz), then bring to a simmer and cook for 20–25 minutes until the potatoes and carrots are tender. Taste and adjust the seasoning, adding the fish sauce and sugar if you feel it needs it.

4. Just before serving, swirl the reserved coconut cream through the curry and scatter over the coriander leaves. Serve over rice or noodles, with lime wedges on the side for squeezing.

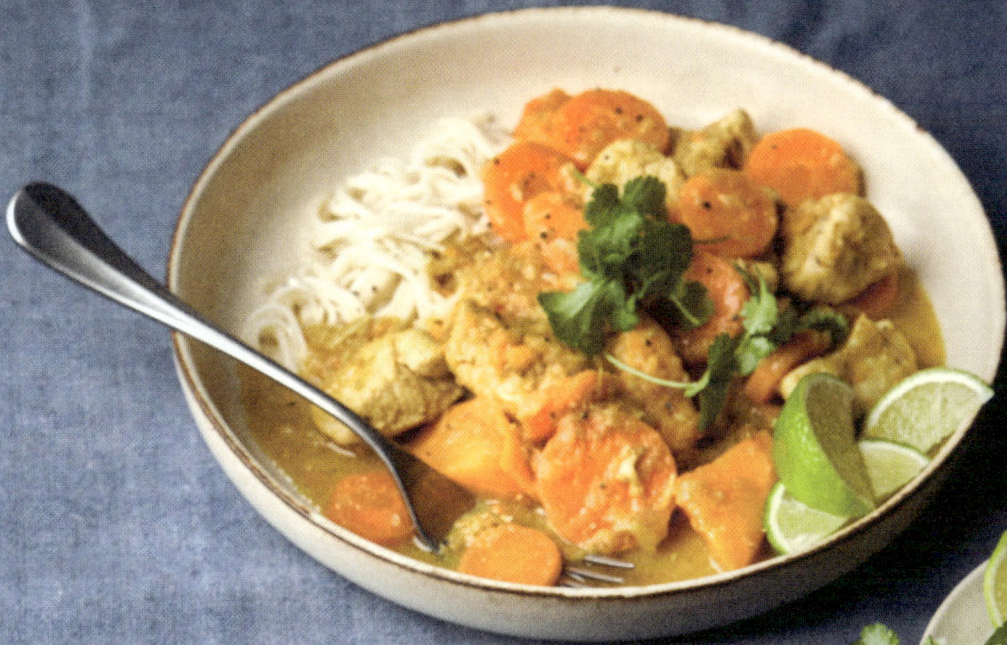

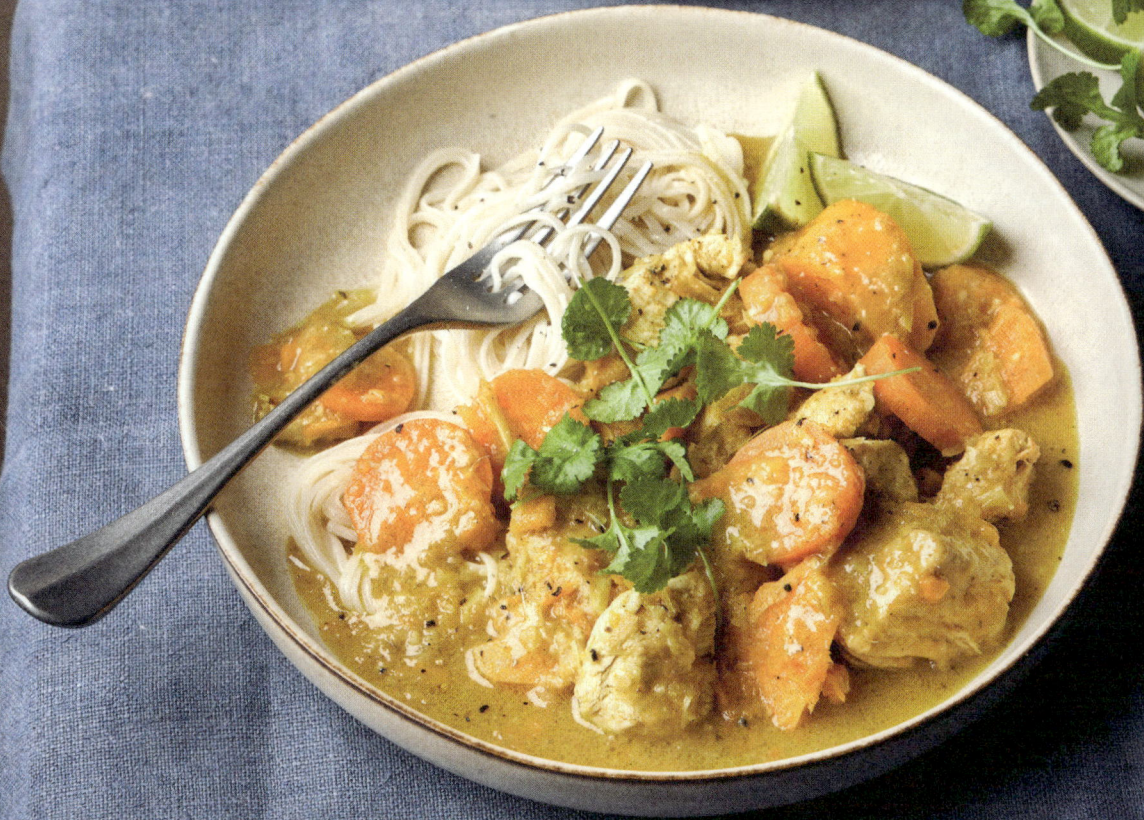

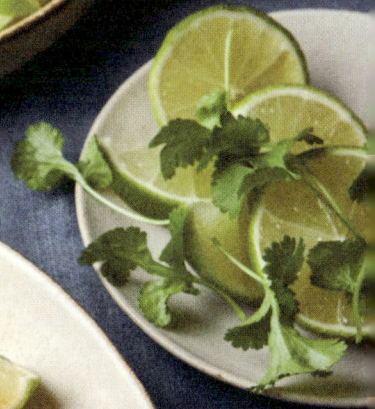

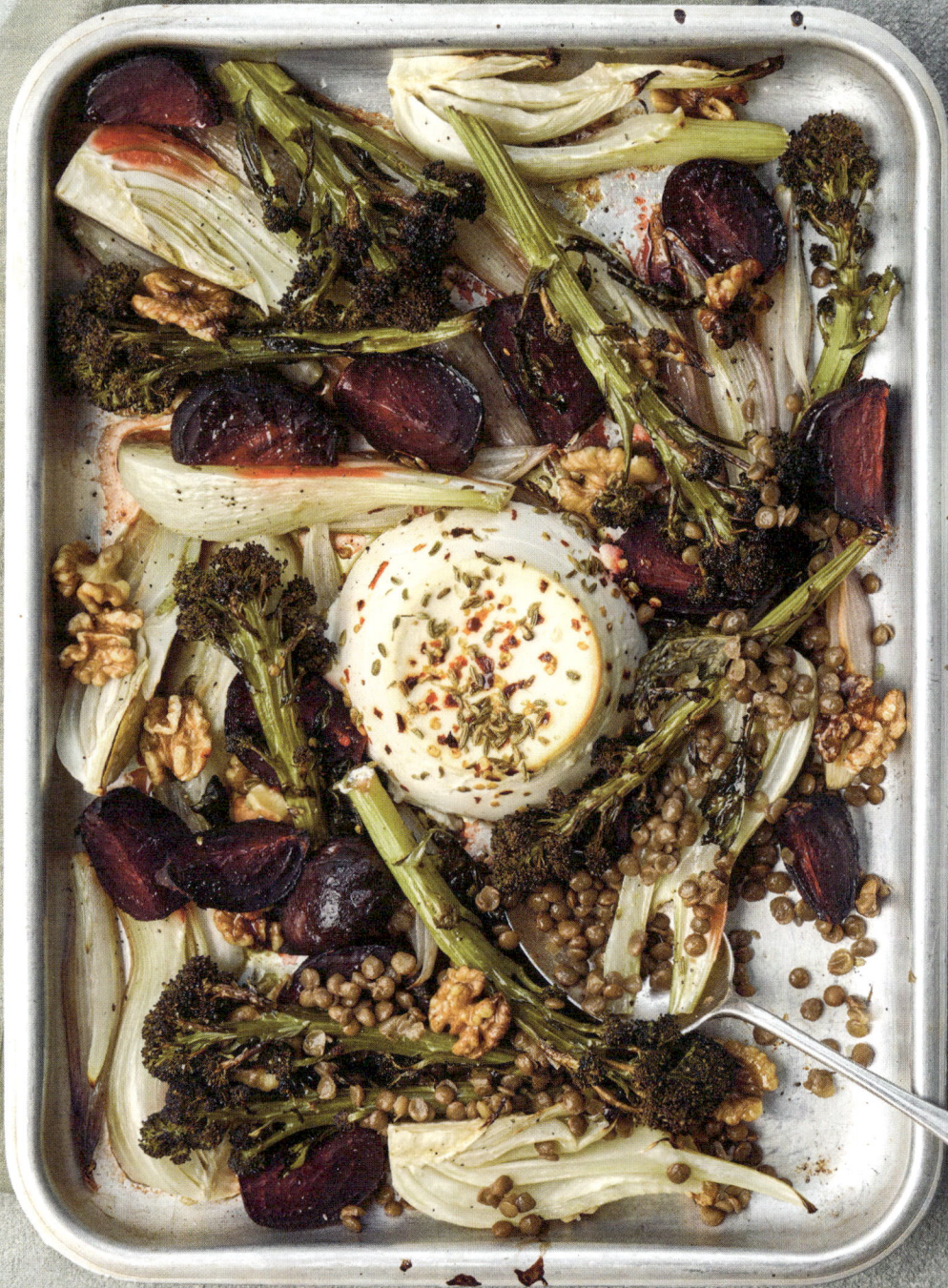

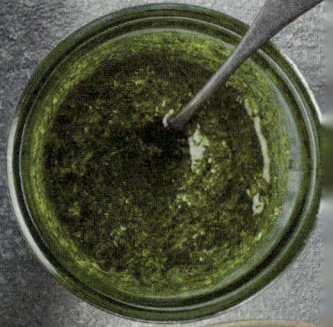

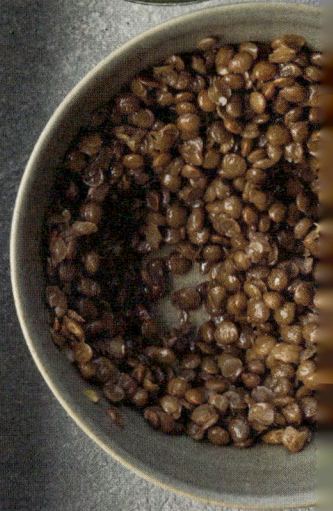

Baked ricotta, beetroot, and walnut traybake

Nutritional info per portion

Fibre 11g
Protein 18g
Plant Points 13.25

Serves 4   Prep 5 mins   Cook 25 mins

1 large or 2 small fennel bulbs, tough outer layer discarded, cut into eighths

4 shallots, quartered

200g (7oz) tenderstem or purple sprouting broccoli (broccolini)

250g (9oz) cooked vac-packed or canned beetroot (beets), quartered

60g (2oz) walnuts

4 tbsp olive oil, plus extra to drizzle

250g (9oz) ricotta

Pinch of dried chilli (red pepper) flakes

½ tsp fennel seeds, roughly crushed

Sea salt and freshly ground black pepper

For the lentils

175g (6¼oz) dried brown or black lentils, rinsed

2 garlic cloves, minced

2 tbsp olive oil

Juice of ½ lemon

For the green sauce

40g (1½oz) parsley, leaves and stalks

5g (¼oz) tarragon leaves

½ garlic clove, peeled

1 tbsp capers in brine, plus 2 tbsp brine from the jar

6 tbsp olive oil

The ultimate easy-peasy dinner to make at the end of a busy day. To make this even more speedy, you can use a couple of cans or pouches of pre-cooked lentils—if so, there's no need to boil them; simply combine with the garlic, olive oil, and lemon. For variation, try swapping the ricotta for some chicken thighs (just be sure to cook them for at least 25–30 minutes). And if you'd like to make this vegan, just omit the ricotta, double the amount of beetroot and broccoli, and sprinkle with toasted seeds before serving.

1. Preheat the oven to 220°C/200°C fan/425°F.

2. Place the lentils, garlic, and a pinch of salt in a saucepan and cover with plenty of boiling water. Set over a medium heat, bring to a simmer, and cook for 20–25 minutes until tender. Once tender, drain into a sieve (strain), then return to the pan. Mix the garlic with the oil, lemon juice, and some salt and pepper in a small bowl, then stir this through the lentils. Place a lid on the pan and set aside.

3. While the lentils are cooking, place the fennel, shallots, broccoli, beetroot, and walnuts in a large baking dish, then drizzle with most of the oil. Toss to coat the vegetables, then make a space in the centre of the tray and turn out the ricotta into the space. Scatter over the chilli flakes and fennel seeds and season with plenty of salt and pepper, then drizzle over the remaining oil. Roast for 25–30 minutes, or until everything is tender and a little crisp at the edges.

1. Meanwhile, place all the ingredients for the green sauce in a blender, along with 1 tablespoon of water, and blitz to a smooth green purée. Season with salt and pepper to taste, then set aside.

2. Stir the lentils through the roasted veg, breaking up the ricotta, then serve up on plates with dollops of the green sauce.

Note You can make part of this in your air fryer too! Preheat your air fryer to 190°C/375°F. Place the fennel, shallots, broccoli, beetroot, and walnuts in your air fryer, then drizzle with most of the oil and toss to coat. Make a space in the centre of the veggies and turn out the ricotta into the space. Scatter over the chilli flakes and fennel seeds and season with plenty of salt and pepper, then drizzle over the remaining oil and air fry for about 15 minutes until the fennel is tender. Depending on the size of your air fryer, you may want to halve the quantities in this recipe, or simply air fry in 2 batches.

Any leftovers are perfect for lunch the next day, you can even stir in some spinach or rocket (arugula) to turn it into a vibrant salad.

Prawn tacos with grapefruit salsa

Serves 4   **Prep** 5 mins   **Cook** 20 mins

For the prawns (shrimp)

250g (9oz) shelled king prawns (jumbo shrimp), defrosted if frozen

¼ tsp ground cumin

¼ tsp chipotle flakes or sweet paprika

Zest of 1 lime

1 tbsp olive oil, cold-pressed rapeseed oil, or avocado oil

For the black beans

2 tbsp olive oil, cold-pressed rapeseed oil, or avocado oil

1 garlic clove, chopped

1 tsp cumin seeds

1 × 400g (14oz) can black beans, drained and rinsed

For the grapefruit salsa

1 pink grapefruit

½ red onion, finely sliced

Juice of ½ lime

½ red chilli, finely chopped

Handful of coriander (cilantro) leaves, chopped

Handful of mint leaves, chopped

1 avocado, peeled, de-stoned and cubed

Sea salt and freshly ground black pepper

To serve

12 small flour or corn tortillas

¼ white cabbage, finely shredded

Lime wedges

Taco night is always a favourite in our house, and they're a wonderful way to add plenty of nutrition and color to your plate. This version is zesty and fresh, with plenty of protein from the black beans and prawns. To make this veggie/vegan, simply use roasted cauliflower or tofu instead of prawns.

1. Begin with the prawns. Combine all the ingredients in a bowl with a pinch of salt and mix well to coat. Set aside to marinate while you prepare the beans and salsa.

2. To make the black beans, warm the oil in a small pan set over a low heat. Add the garlic and gently fry until it begins to color, then add the cumin seeds and toast for 30–60 seconds. Add the black beans, 100ml (scant ½ cup/3½fl oz) water, and plenty of salt and pepper. Roughly crush about half the beans with a fork, then simmer for 15 minutes. Add splashes of water if it begins to look too dry.

3. While the beans are cooking, make the grapefruit salsa. Use a serrated knife to cut away the pith of the grapefruit, then cut the flesh into segments (do this over a bowl to catch the juices). Cut each segment into 1cm (½ inch) pieces, then add these to the bowl of juices along with the onion, lime juice, and a big pinch of salt. Mix really well, then stir through the chilli, herbs, and avocado. Set aside.

4. Place a dry frying pan (skillet) over a high heat and toast the tortillas for about 30 seconds on each side until warm and floppy. Wrap them in a kitchen towel to keep warm.

5. Place the frying pan back over a medium–high heat. When it's super-hot, add the prawns in a single layer (you may have to do this in batches). Cook them for 3–4 minutes, turning halfway, until deep pink.

6. Pile each warm tortilla with some of the black beans, then top with a little cabbage, a few prawns and some salsa. Serve with the lime wedges for squeezing over.

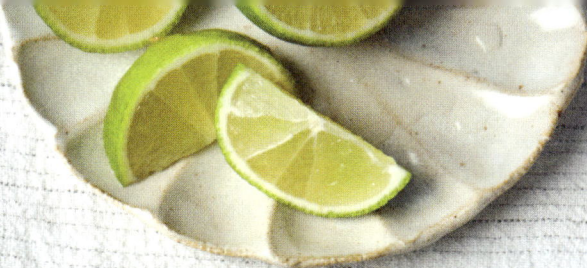

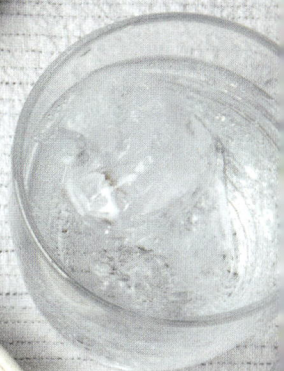

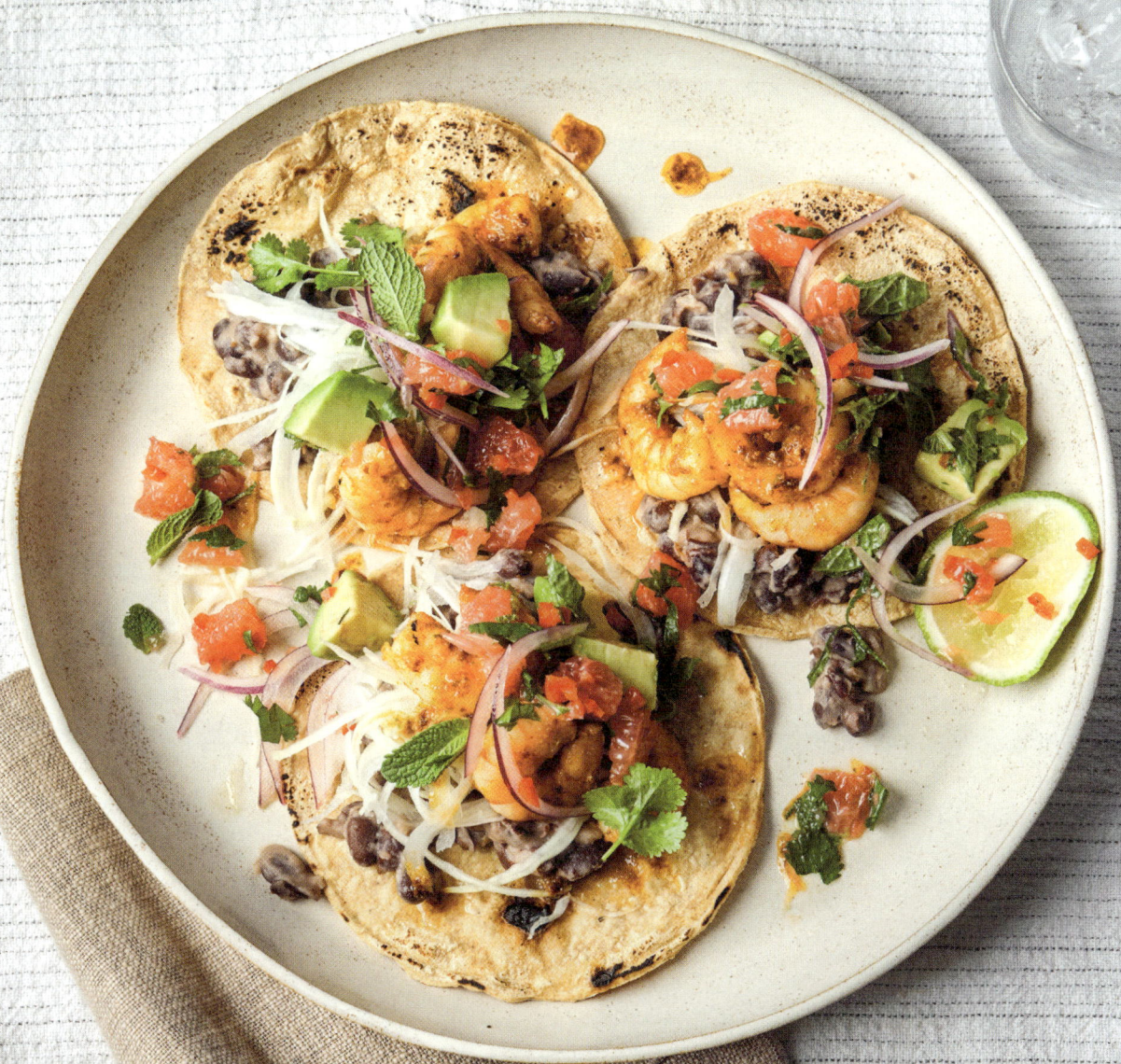

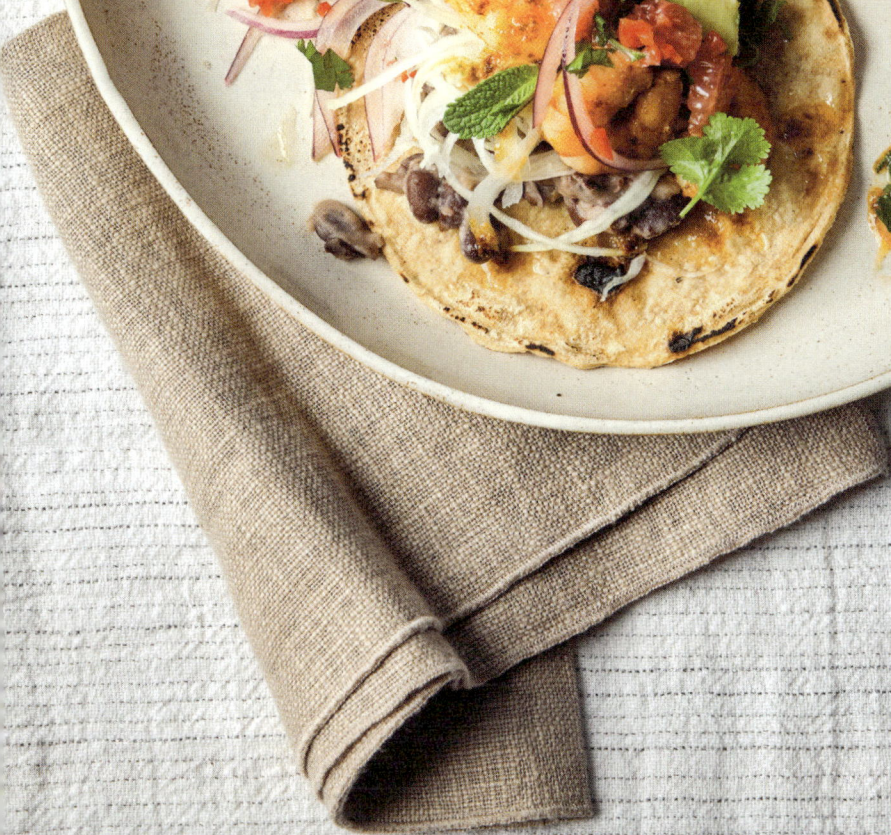

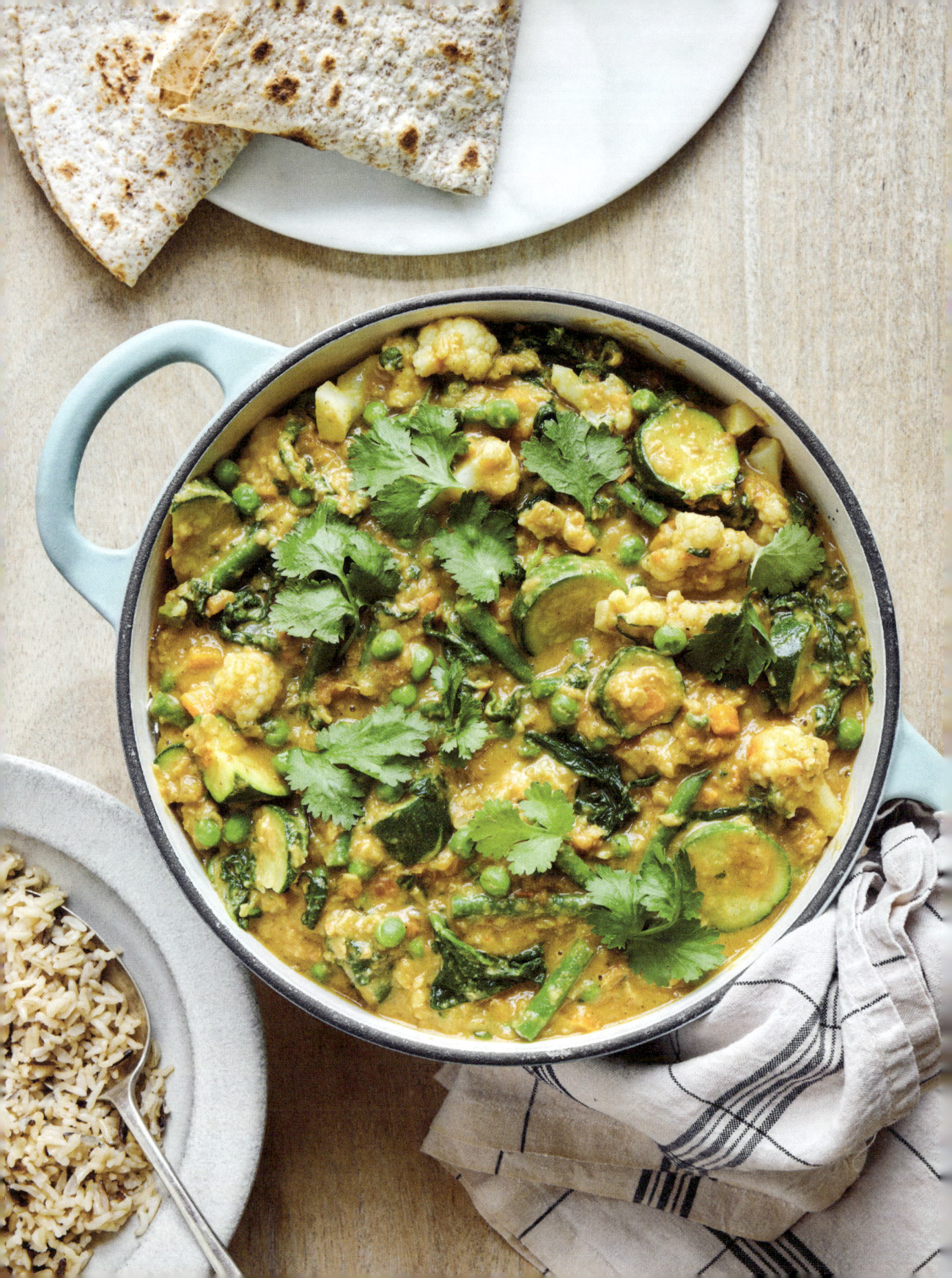

Eight-veg curry

Serves 4–6 (spice paste makes enough for 8–12 portions) **Prep** 5 mins **Cook** 25 mins

½ × 400g (14oz) can plum (Roma) tomatoes

50g (¼ cup/1¾oz) dried red lentils, rinsed

¼ cauliflower, broken into small florets

1 courgette (zucchini), cut into 1cm (½ inch) rounds

100g (3½oz) frozen peas

100g (3½oz) fresh or frozen green beans, trimmed and cut into 2cm (1 inch) lengths

½ × 400g (14oz) can coconut milk

3 tbsp smooth or crunchy peanut or almond butter

100g (3½oz) frozen spinach (or 250g/9oz fresh spinach)

200–300g (7–10½oz) long-grain brown rice

2 handfuls of coriander (cilantro) leaves, chopped

Lime wedges, to serve

Sea salt and freshly ground black pepper

For the spice paste

8 garlic cloves, chopped

2 thumb-sized pieces fresh ginger, peeled and chopped

1–2 red or green chillies, roughly chopped (optional)

2 onions, chopped

4 tbsp olive oil, cold-pressed rapeseed oil, or avocado oil

1 large carrot, chopped

1½ tsp ground cumin

½ tsp ground turmeric

½ tsp ground cinnamon

1 tsp sweet paprika

2 tsp garam masala

2 tsp sea salt

Curries are a great way to pack in as many plant points as possible into one meal. Unlike a curry you might have as part of a takeaway—usually containing lots of cream and sugar—the focus here is to create a balanced meal using whatever you have in your fridge or freezer.

1. First, make the spice paste. Place the garlic, ginger, chillies, and ¼ of the onion in a blender with 2–3 tablespoons of water and blitz to a paste. Set aside.

2. Warm the oil in a large, wide pan set over a medium heat and add the remaining onion and the carrot. Cook, stirring until golden and soft, for 5–7 minutes, then add the paste and continue cooking for another 4–5 minutes until it begins to darken in color and smell fragrant. Add splashes of water if it begins to stick to the pan.

3. Stir in the spices and salt and cook for a further 1 minute, then remove the pan from the heat. Remove half the spice paste from the pan and allow it to cool before evenly spooning it into an ice-cube tray (this will be roughly 150g/⅔ cup/5½oz, which will make 10–12 ice cubes)—see more info about my ice-cube trick in the note below.

4. Set the pan with the remaining spice paste back over a medium heat and add the tomatoes, lentils, and 150ml (⅔ cup/5½fl oz) water. Scrape up any stuck bits on the base of the pan, then simmer for 5 minutes. Add the rest of the vegetables (apart from the spinach), the coconut milk, nut butter, and 200ml (generous ¾ cup/7fl oz) water. Bring back to a simmer and cook for 10–15 minutes until the veg is tender (the cauliflower will probably take the longest) and the lentils are soft and have disappeared into the sauce. Stir in the spinach, allow it a moment to defrost (or wilt) and check the seasoning, adding salt and pepper to taste. If it looks a little wet, simply cook it for a few minutes more.

5. Meanwhile, cook the brown rice according to the packet instructions.

6. Divide the rice and curry between bowls, then scatter over plenty of coriander and serve with lime wedges on the side for squeezing.

Note This recipe is a great example of my ice-cube trick. As we're going to the effort of making a spice paste (albeit a very easy one), I make more than I need and then freeze the excess in ice-cubes trays ready to use in future meals. Once frozen, you can transfer the ice cubes to a labelled sandwich bag and store them in your freezer for easy access. All you have to do is chuck a few ice cubes in a pan set over a low heat and they'll melt in minutes. If you don't fancy using the ice-cube trick in this recipe, just halve the quantities for the spice paste.

Creamy miso and peanut butter ramen

Nutritional info per portion

Fibre 14g
Protein 33g
Plant Points 8

● **Serves** 2   ● **Prep** 2 mins   ● **Cook** 10 mins

125–150g (4½–5½oz) soba or brown rice ramen noodles (or use wholewheat spaghetti)

2 garlic cloves, peeled

1 thumb-sized piece fresh ginger, peeled

4 spring (green) onions, sliced, white and green parts separated

2 tbsp sesame oil

2 tbsp tamari or soy sauce, plus extra to taste

2 tbsp white miso

2 tbsp smooth peanut or almond butter (or use tahini)

600ml (2½ cups/21fl oz) milk of your choice

1 pak choi (bok choy), leaves separated (or use 120g/4oz spinach leaves)

120g (4oz) chestnut (brown) mushrooms, thinly sliced

70g (2½oz) frozen and defrosted or canned sweetcorn

To serve

2 soft-boiled eggs, halved

Chilli oil

A rich but wholesome, vegetable-packed, incredibly speedy meal. You can use any type of mushroom in this, Asian varieties such as shimeji and enoki can be added straight to the broth as specified below, but if you're using button mushrooms or fresh shiitake, you'll want to brown them slightly in a pan first before adding them to the broth.

1. Bring a medium pan of water to the boil and cook the noodles according to packet instructions. Drain and rinse under cold water, then divide between two bowls.

2. Meanwhile, grate the garlic and ginger into a medium saucepan and throw in the spring onion whites. Drizzle in the oil, then place over a low–medium heat and gently fry for 3–4 minutes until fragrant. Add the tamari, reduce for 15 seconds, then add the miso and nut butter and stir to make a paste.

3. Slowly whisk in the milk in a steady stream, then bring to a simmer and add the pak choi and mushrooms, pushing them under the surface of the broth. Simmer for 3–4 minutes (less if using spinach), then add the corn and cook for 1 minute more to warm through.

4. Pour the broth over the noodles, distributing the mushrooms, corn and pak choi evenly between the bowls. Top each bowl of ramen with an egg and the spring onion greens, then drizzle with a little chilli oil and extra tamari, if you like.

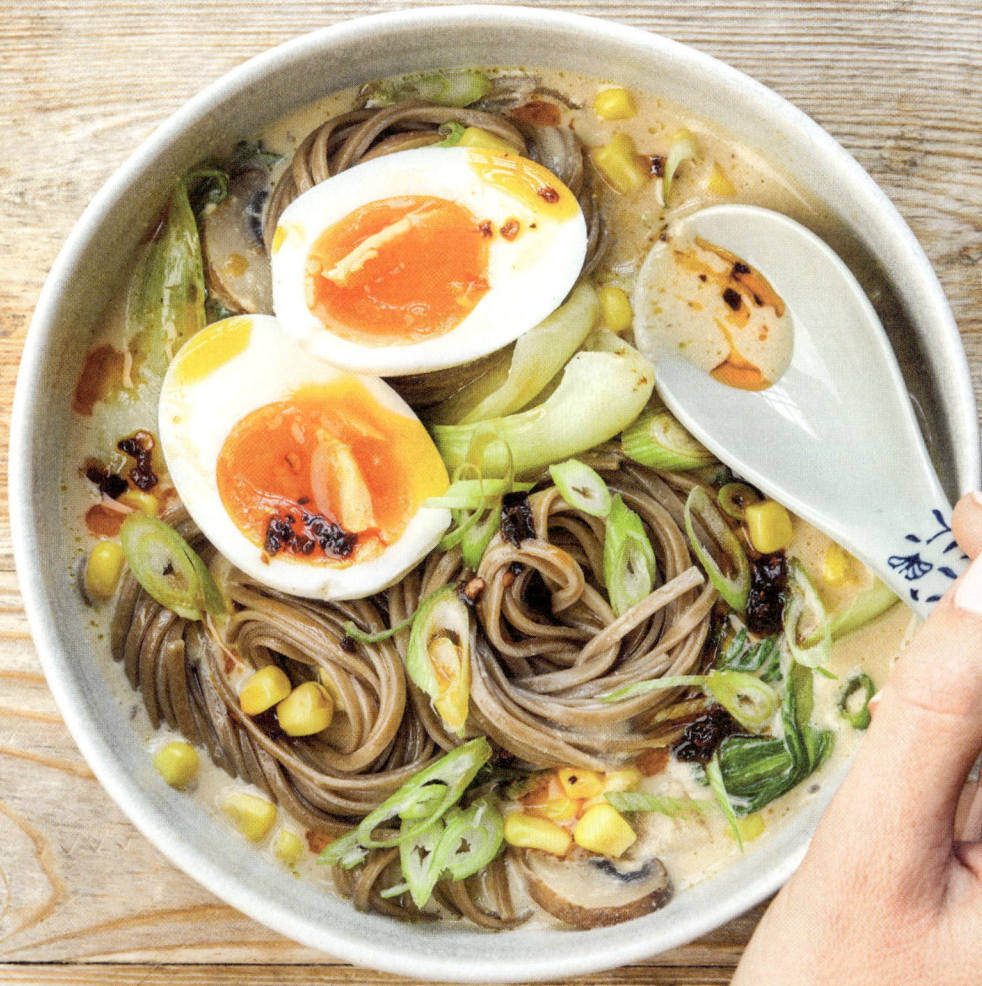

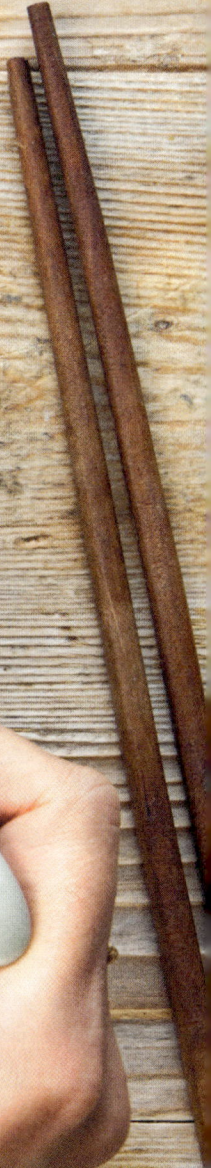

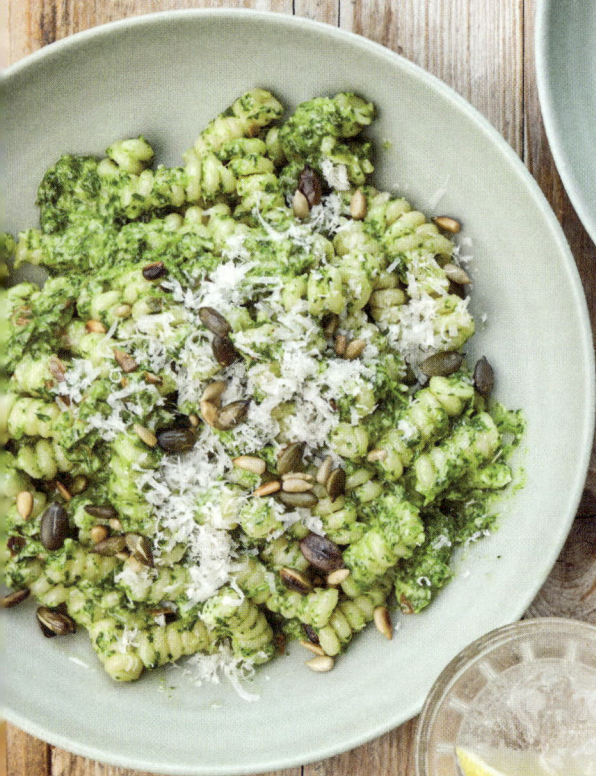

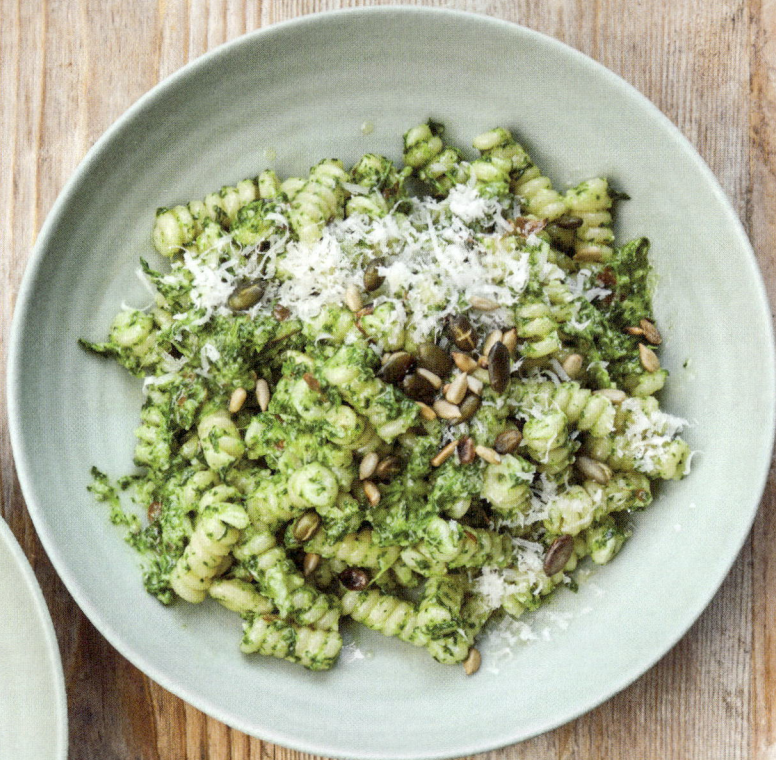

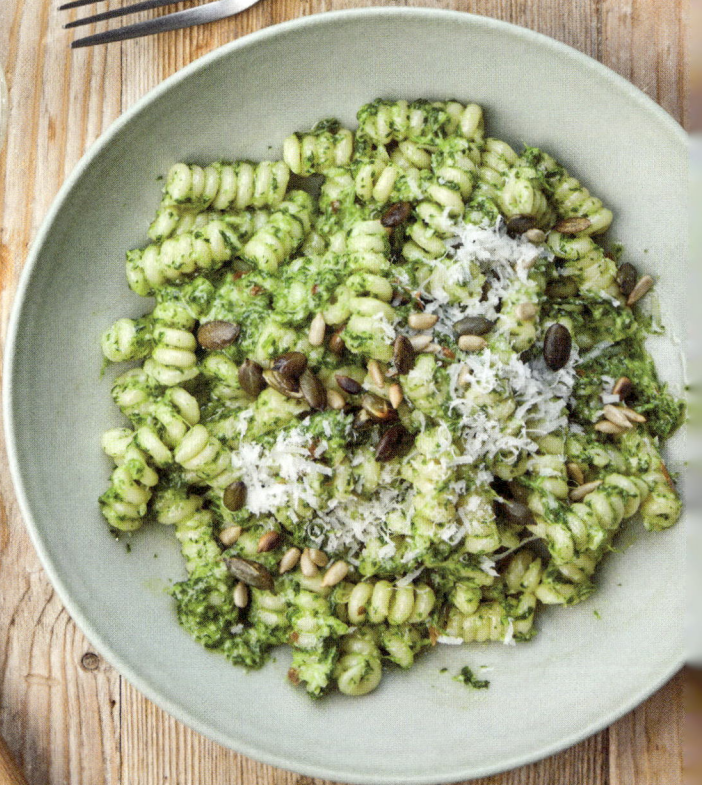

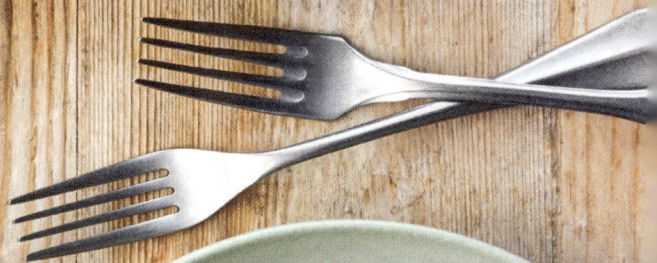

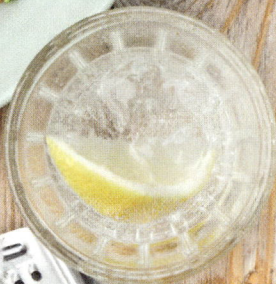

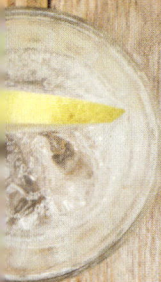

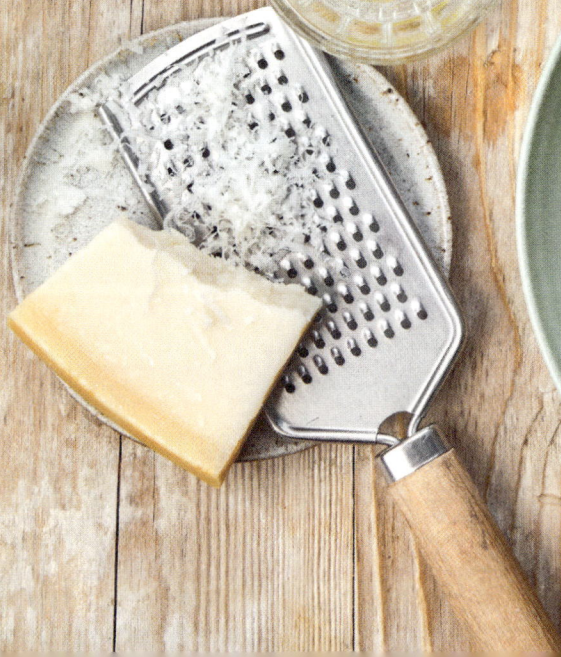

Salad-bag pasta

Nutritional info per portion

Fibre 7.8g
Protein 20g
Plant Points 6.5

Serves 4   **Prep** 2 mins   **Cook** 15 mins

500g (18oz) fusilli, farfalle, or penne

2 garlic cloves, peeled

60g (2oz) whole almonds

250g (9oz) watercress, spinach and/or rocket (arugula) (or use cavolo nero/Tuscan kale or savoy/Napa cabbage, stems removed)

125g (½ cup/4½oz) extra-virgin olive oil, plus extra for drizzling

4 tbsp grated Parmesan (or use vegan alternative), plus extra to serve

3 tbsp toasted pumpkin seeds

3 tbsp toasted sunflower seeds

Sea salt and freshly ground black pepper

This is the quickest pasta ever, with the sauce taking less time to make than the pasta takes to cook! It can be made with a variety of leafy greens for maximum iron and there is absolutely zero skill required. Throwing the almonds into the water might seem a little crazy, but it softens them up and adds body to the sauce. You can slip their skins off after boiling if you prefer, but it's not essential. To make this extra creamy, try stirring in a couple of tablespoons of ricotta before serving. This is also a great recipe to use that special olive oil you've been saving, as you can really taste it.

1. Bring a big pan of salted water to the boil and cook the pasta according to the packet instructions. Scoop the pasta into a colander using a slotted spoon and return the pan to the boil.

2. Add the garlic and almonds to the water and simmer for 2–3 minutes until the garlic is just tender, then add the leaves. Push the leaves under the water so they're just submerged, then drain into a sieve (strainer). Transfer the wilted leaves, garlic, and almonds to a blender or food processor (you can also use an electric hand-held blender), add the olive oil and Parmesan, then blitz to a bright green purée. Season to taste with salt and pepper.

3. Add the sauce back the pan and set over a low heat, then stir in the cooked pasta to ensure everything is hot.

4. Transfer the pasta to bowls, sprinkle over a little extra Parmesan, and the toasted seeds, then drizzle with a little extra oil before serving.

Perhaps the most important meals to get right are the ones you feed your family. Soon, these dishes will become nostalgic food memories, regardless of whether they are remembered fondly or not so fondly! This section is packed with crowd-pleasing recipes—all with added plant points and nutritional balance—that will always justify a second helping!

It's impossible to cook fresh meals every single day for 365 days a year, especially with a busy family life, so setting realistic goals for yourself is essential. Batch cooking and making use of your freezer are key to maintaining a lifestyle that's lower in UPFs – and the recipes in this section cater to this streamlined method of cooking.

Family favourites

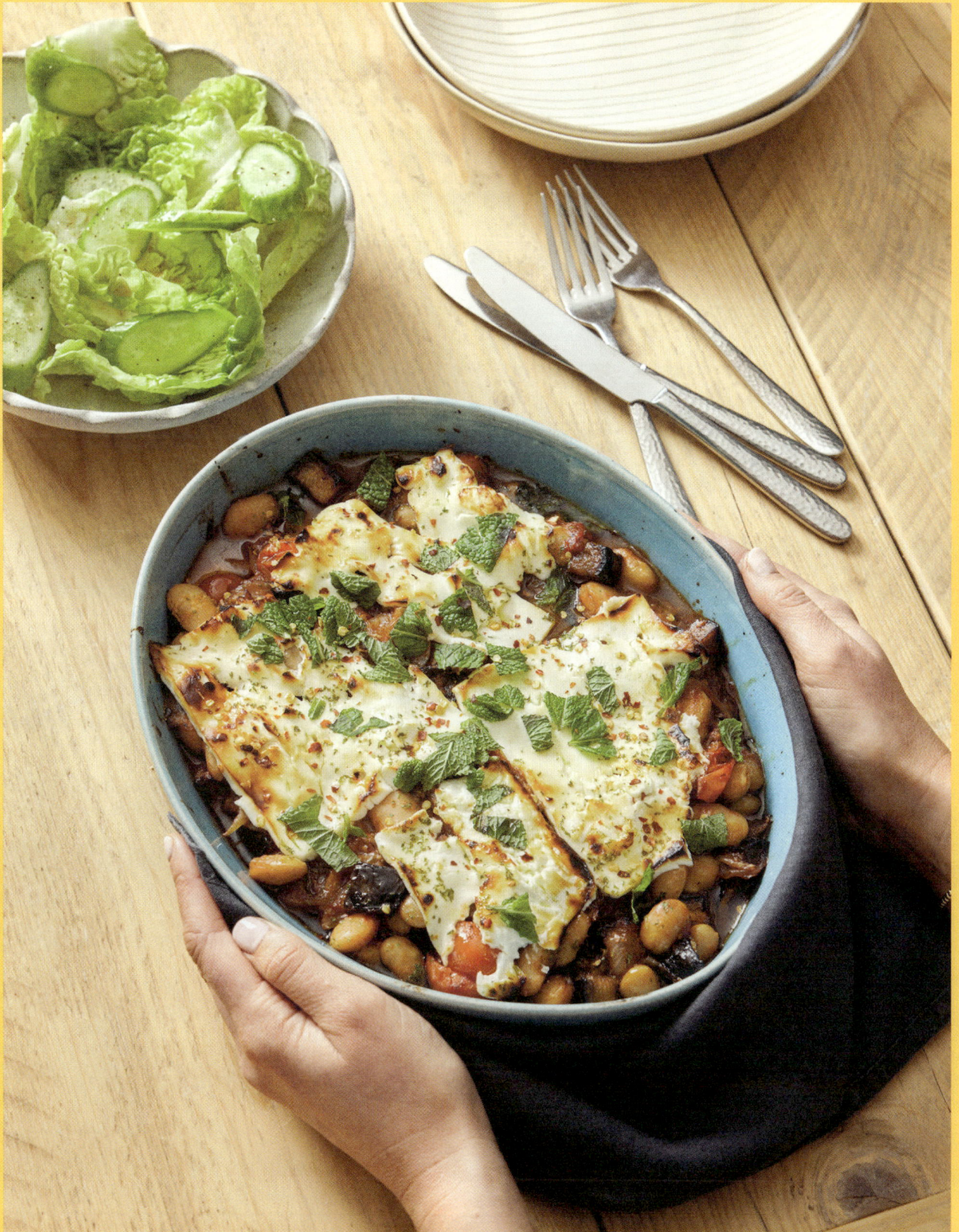

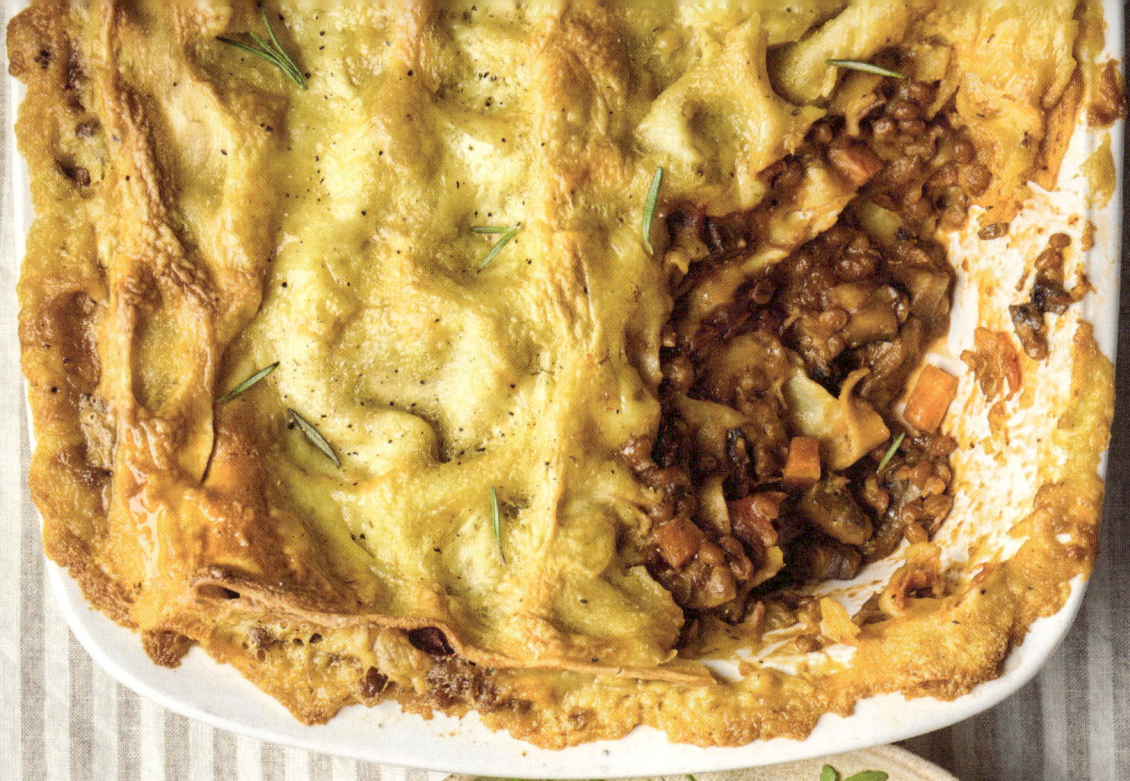

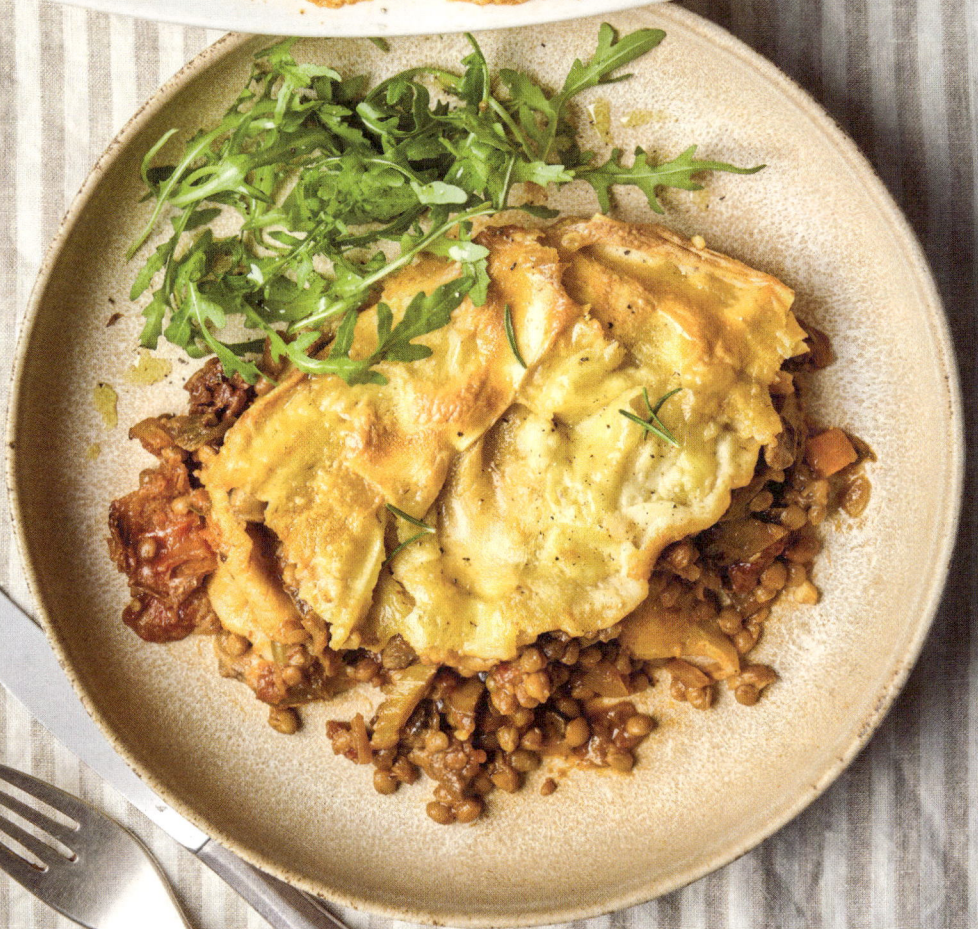

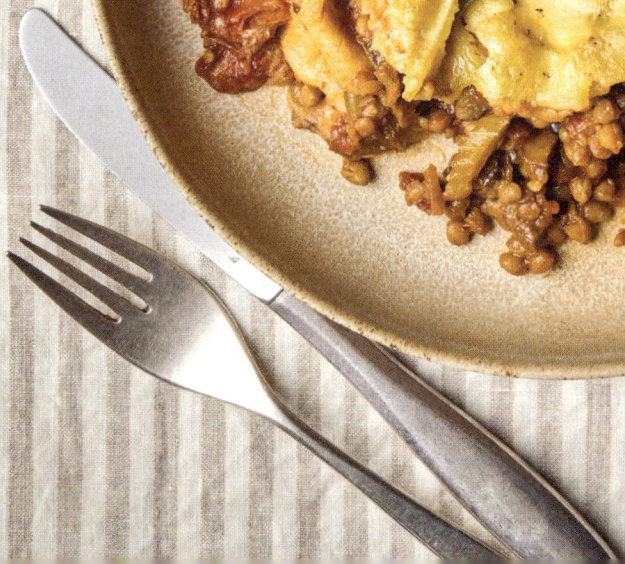

Veggie-loaded lasagna

Nutritional info per portion

Fibre 12g
Protein 17g
Plant Points 9.5

Serves 6   **Prep** 10 mins   **Cook** 1 hour 30 mins

3 tbsp olive oil

300g (10½oz) chestnut (brown) mushrooms, roughly chopped

4 tbsp tamari or soy sauce

1 onion, chopped

2 celery stalks, chopped

2 carrots, chopped

3 garlic cloves, chopped

1 tbsp finely chopped rosemary

1 bay leaf

20g (¾oz) dried porcini soaked in 250ml (1 cup/ 9fl oz) boiling water for 15 minutes (or use 250ml/1 cup/9fl oz mushroom stock)

1 × 400g (14oz) can chopped tomatoes or passata

2 × 400g (14oz) cans brown or green lentils

90g (3oz) sun-dried tomatoes, chopped, plus 3 tbsp oil from the jar

250g (9oz) lasagna sheets (ensure egg-free if vegan)

Sea salt and freshly ground black pepper

For the bechamel

65g (4½ tbsp/2¼oz) butter (or use 6½ tbsp olive oil)

60g (scant ½ cup/2oz) all-purpose flour

750ml (3¼ cups/26fl oz) milk of your choice

A few gratings of nutmeg

Just like the curry over on page 143, this lasagna is such an easy way to pack plenty of plants onto your plate and, despite it being meat-free, the lentils still provide lots of protein and iron when combined with the tomatoes. The sauce also works perfectly served with spaghetti for a veggie or vegan Bolognese, so why not double up on ingredients and pop half the sauce in the freezer for future easy suppers?

1. Warm 2 tablespoons of the oil in a large deep pan set over a medium heat, then add the mushrooms. Cook undisturbed for 5 minutes, then begin stirring, cooking for a further 2–3 minutes, until dark and reduced in volume. Stir in half the tamari and allow it to reduce.

2. Add the remaining tablespoon of oil, then add the onion, celery, carrots, garlic, rosemary, bay leaf, and a big pinch of salt. Fry gently for 10 minutes, then chop the porcini and add it to the pan along with the soaking water. Add the tomatoes, lentils, sun-dried tomatoes and their oil, the remaining tamari, and plenty of salt and pepper, then stir well. Add just enough water to almost cover (about 100ml/⅓ cup/3½fl oz), then bring to a simmer and cook for 20–25 minutes until reduced and delicious.

3. Preheat the oven to 180°C/160°C fan/350°F.

4. While the lentil ragu is simmering, prepare the bechamel. Gently warm the butter in a medium saucepan set over a low heat and stir in the flour until you have a paste. Keep stirring for 2 minutes, then very slowly start adding the milk, whisking constantly. Once all the milk is incorporated, simmer for 5 minutes, or until it thickens, then season generously with salt and pepper and a little nutmeg. Remove from the heat.

5. Spread one third of the lentil ragu over the base of a baking dish. Cover with a layer of lasagna sheets, snapping them to fit if needed, then top with one quarter of the bechamel. Repeat the layers two more times, finishing by topping the lasagna with all the remaining bechamel. Drizzle with a little olive oil, then place in the oven for 45 minutes–1 hour until bubbling, browned, and crisp on top.

Triple-protein dal

Serves 4–6   **Prep** 5 mins   **Cook** 35 mins

3 tbsp olive oil, cold-pressed rapeseed oil, or avocado oil

2 onions, chopped

4 garlic cloves, minced

1 green chilli, chopped, or ¼ tsp dried chilli (red pepper) flakes

1 thumb-sized piece fresh ginger, peeled and grated

1 tsp ground turmeric

1½ tsp ground coriander

1½ tsp ground cumin

3 medium tomatoes or 4 plum tomatoes from a can, chopped

250g (1½ cups/9oz) dried red lentils, rinsed

1 × 400g (14oz) can green or brown lentils, drained and rinsed

150g (5½oz) frozen peas

1 × 400g (14oz) can coconut milk

2 big handfuls of coriander (cilantro) leaves, roughly chopped

Yogurt flatbreads, to serve (page 179)

Cooked long-grain brown rice, to serve (optional)

Sea salt and freshly ground black pepper

For the cucumber raita

½ garlic clove, peeled

¼ cucumber

½ tsp ground coriander

200g (1 cup/7oz) skyr, Greek yogurt or coconut yogurt

This is the ultimate comforting supper, packed with protein, fibre, and iron thanks to the peas and red and green lentils—you can also make the cucumber raita with skyr for a quadruple protein hit!

1. Warm the oil in a large pan set over a medium heat and fry the onions with a pinch of salt for 8–10 minutes until softened. Add the garlic, chilli, ginger, and spices, and cook for another 2–3 minutes, stirring constantly, until fragrant.

2. Add the tomatoes, red lentils, and 700ml (3 cups/25fl oz) water. Allow to simmer for a further 20–25 minutes, until the lentils are tender.

3. Meanwhile, grate the garlic and cucumber for the raita into a small bowl, stir in the ground coriander and yogurt, then lightly season with salt and pepper. Set aside.

4. Once the red lentils are soft and falling apart, add the canned lentils, peas, and coconut milk to the pan. Bring to a simmer, then cook for a further 5 minutes. Taste and adjust the seasoning to your liking, then spoon into bowls. Serve with plenty of coriander, dollops of the cucumber raita, flatbreads, and brown rice, if you like.

Note Try blending any leftovers with a little hot vegetable stock to create a rich and comforting soup.

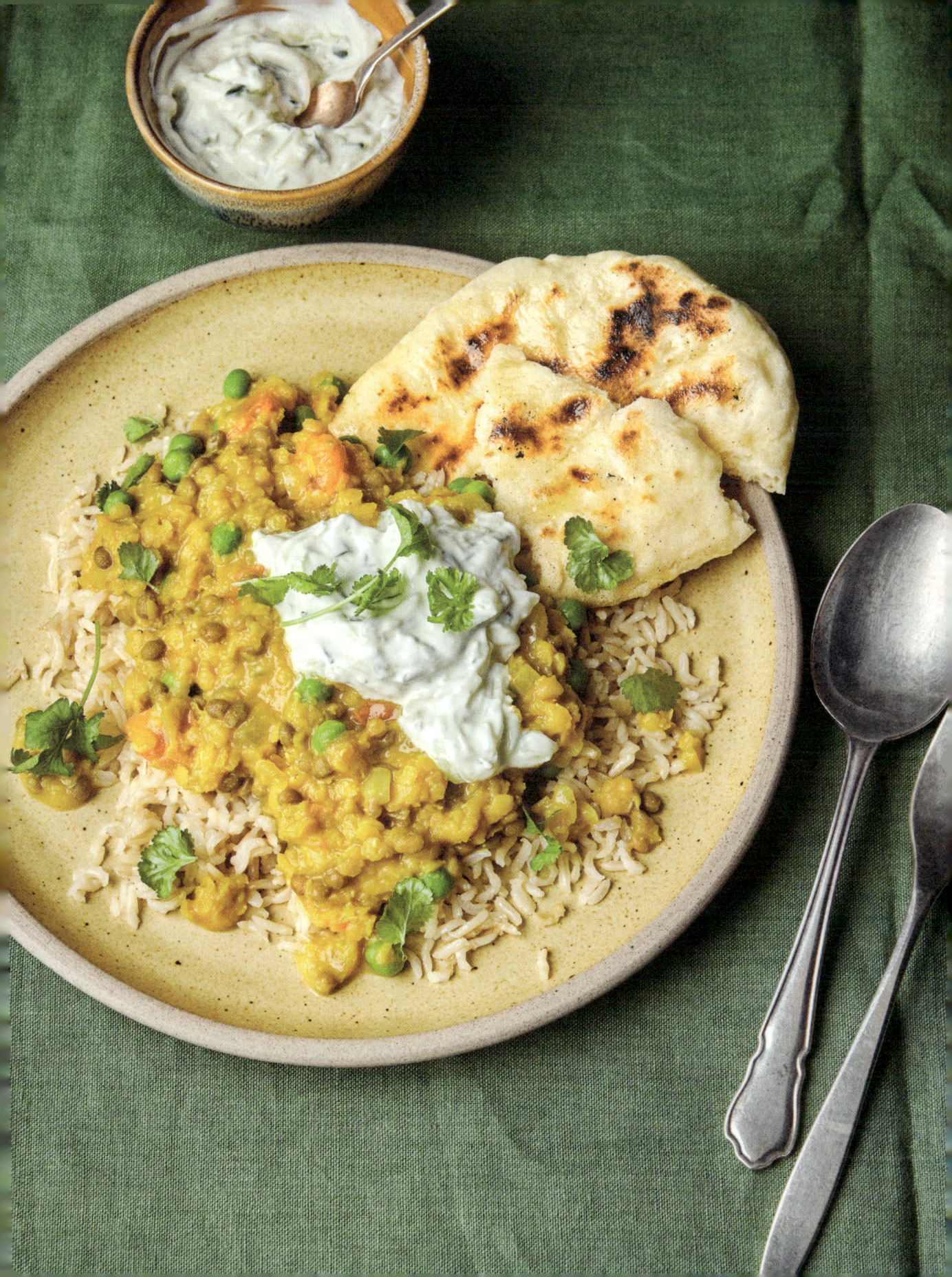

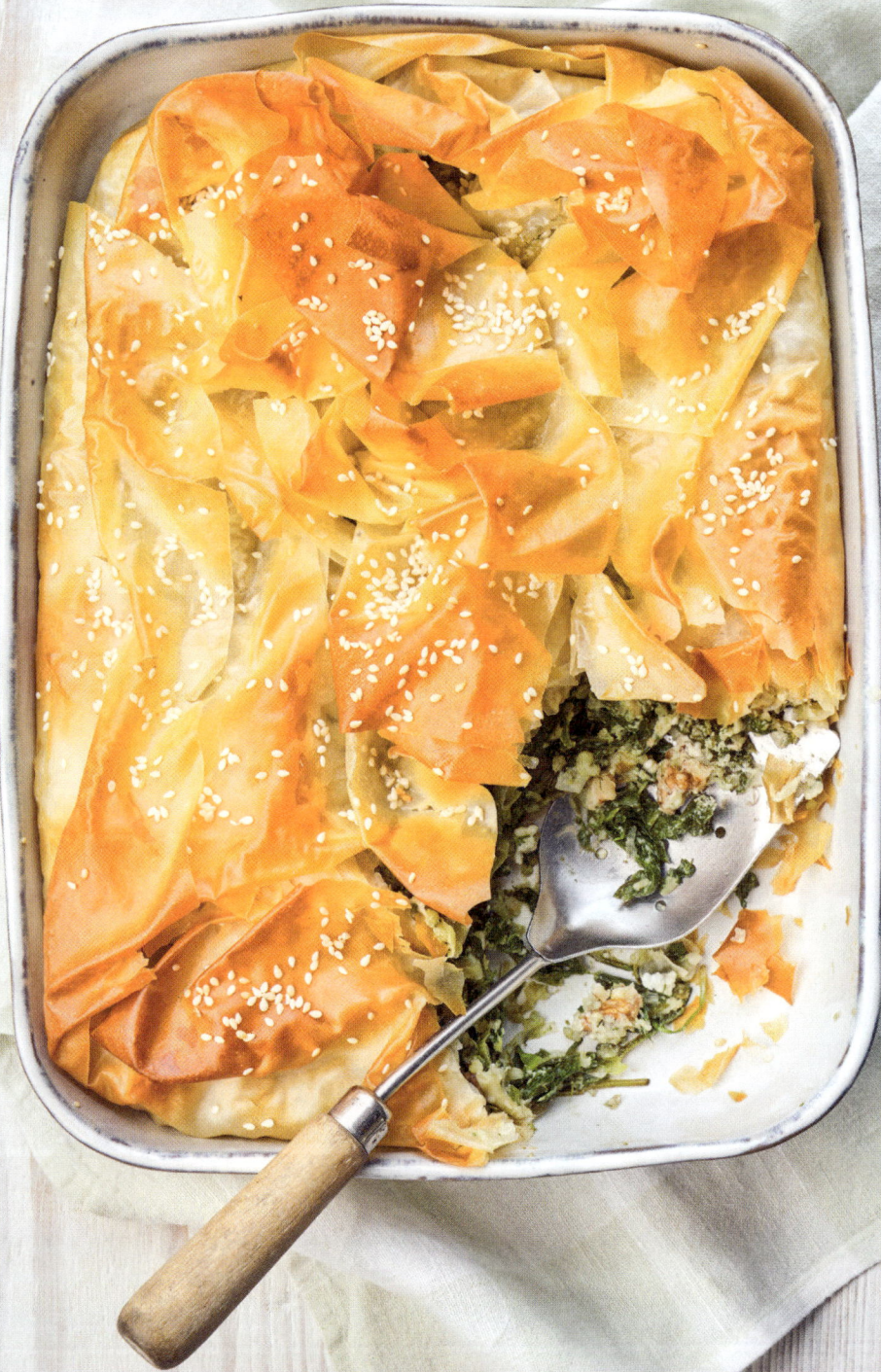

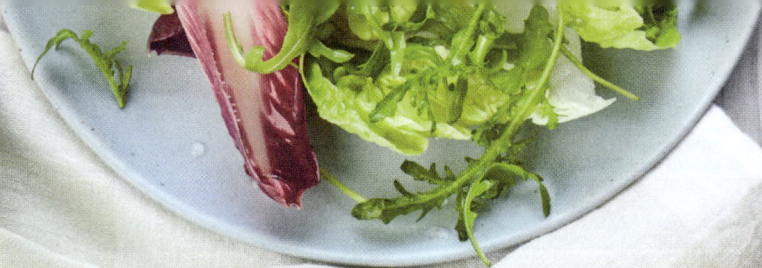

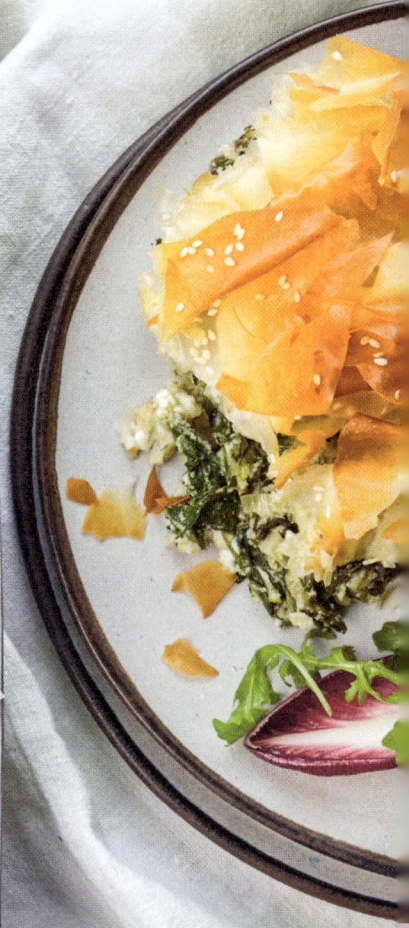

Spanakopita pie

Nutritional info per portion

Fibre 4.4g
Protein 28g
Plant Points 7.75

Serves 4–6　　**Prep** 15 mins　　**Cook** 50 mins

3 tbsp olive oil, plus extra for drizzling and brushing

1 large leek, tough outer leaves discarded, finely sliced

600g (21oz) spinach leaves

60g (2oz) rocket (arugula)

20g (2oz) dill, leaves and stalks chopped

15g (½oz) mint leaves, chopped

4 spring (green) onions, finely sliced

50g (1¾oz) walnuts, finely chopped

50g (1¾oz) bulgar wheat, rinsed

200g (7oz) feta, crumbled

200g (7oz) cottage cheese or ricotta

3 eggs, beaten

7 sheets filo (phyllo) pastry (about 1 × 270g/9½oz packet)

2 tsp black and/or white sesame seeds

My husband is from a Mediterranean family and this dish is often served at family get-togethers. Fun and delicious, my take on it uses one of my favourite ingredients— cottage cheese! You can of course use frozen spinach here—just allow it to defrost first then squeeze out the excess water before adding it to the leek. To make this vegan, omit both cheeses and replace with two cans of drained cooked lentils.

1. Preheat the oven to 180°C/160°C fan/350°F.

2. Warm the olive oil in a deep pan set over a medium heat and fry the leek for 5–7 minutes until beginning to soften. Transfer to a large mixing bowl.

3. While the leek cooks, pile all the spinach into a sieve (strainer), rinse it under cold water, then sprinkle with 1 heaped teaspoon of salt. Vigorously massage, squeezing and crushing it with your hands until it wilts and you have a green mulch. Using your hands, squeeze out as much liquid as possible, then add it to the bowl with the leek.

4. Add the rocket, herbs, spring onions, walnuts, bulgar, feta, and cottage cheese to the bowl, then season lightly with salt and generously with black pepper. Pour over the eggs and mix very thoroughly (your hands are the best tool for this!).

5. Drizzle some oil over the base of a medium baking dish (about 25 × 30cm/ 10 × 12 inches) then add a sheet of filo pastry. Brush the pastry with a little more oil, then layer on another sheet of filo pastry, this time with a little overhang. Repeat with 4 more sheets of filo pastry, brushing with oil between each one and layering so that you have slight overhang all around the dish.

6. Spoon the spinach and cheese mixture into the dish, smooth the top, then fold in the overhanging pastry, gently scrunching it as you do so. Scrunch the final sheet of pastry, then place it on top to cover the filling. Drizzle with a little more oil, sprinkle over the sesame seeds, then bake for 45–50 minutes until the top is crisp and golden. If it colors too quickly, reduce the oven temperature slightly.

7. Allow to cool and firm up for 15 minutes, then serve. It's also delicious at room temperature—slice and wrap for a packed lunch or to take on picnics.

Note You can also cook this in your air fryer! Line your air fryer basket with baking paper (parchment paper), then grease the paper with oil. Build the pie directly in the air fryer basket, following the instructions in steps 5–6, then air fry at 180°C/350°F for 30 minutes. Allow to cool in the air fryer basket for 15 minutes before lifting out using the paper.

Seeded wholemeal fishcakes

Nutritional info per portion

Fibre 12g
Protein 54g
Plant Points 10.5

Serves 4 (makes 8) **Prep** 10 mins **Cook** 30 mins

400g (14oz) floury potatoes such as Maris Piper or Yukon Gold, peeled and cut into 2cm (1 inch) chunks

250g (9oz) skinless white fish, such as haddock, cod, coley, or hake (a mix of smoked and unsmoked is nice), roughly chopped

15g (½oz) parsley, leaves and stalks finely chopped

2 tbsp chopped chives

3 spring (green) onions, finely chopped

1½ tbsp capers, roughly chopped

1 heaped tsp Dijon mustard

Zest of 1 lemon

1 egg, beaten

3 tbsp olive oil, cold-pressed rapeseed oil, or avocado oil

Sea salt and freshly ground black pepper

Tartare sauce (page 208), to serve

For the coating

40g (1½oz) spelt or wholemeal (whole wheat) flour, plus extra for dusting

1 egg

1 tbsp milk

70g (2½oz) fresh wholemeal breadcrumbs

4 tbsp white and/or black sesame seeds

1 tsp chia seeds

1 tsp flaxseeds

Fishcakes are such a convenient supper, but I much prefer making my own so that I know exactly what goes into them. It also means I can add some extra goodness to the coating too, in the form of plenty of seeds. These freeze well, so feel free to double the quantities to make extras. Simply freeze on a tray once coated, then transfer to a labelled sandwich bag and store in the freezer. Allow to defrost fully in the fridge before cooking as below.

1. Preheat the oven to 200°C/180°C fan/400°F.

2. Put the potatoes in a large pan of salted water and bring to the boil. Cook for 10–12 minutes until tender, then drain into a colander and allow to steam dry. Tip into a mixing bowl and use a potato masher to crush them (a few lumps are nice).

3. Meanwhile, place the fish in a food processor with the parsley, chives, spring onions, capers, mustard, lemon zest, and egg. Season well with salt and pepper and pulse until combined but still textured.

4. Tip the fish mixture into the bowl with the potatoes and gently mix. Dust your hands with flour, then shape the mixture into 8 even patties, about 3cm (1¼ inches) thick.

5. To prepare the coating, mix the flour with plenty of salt and pepper then spread it out on a plate; beat the egg with the milk in a shallow bowl; then toss the breadcrumbs and seeds on another plate.

6. Coat each fishcake in the flour, then the egg, and finally the seeded breadcrumbs, pressing them lightly to help them stick.

7. Drizzle about half the oil into a medium baking dish and arrange the fishcakes on top, making sure they have a little space between them. Drizzle over the remaining oil and place in the oven for 20–25 minutes, turning them over after 15 minutes, until golden and crisp.

8. Slice your zested lemon into wedges, then serve alongside the fishcakes for squeezing. These are best served with tartare sauce and a green salad.

Note You can also cook the fishcakes in your air fryer! Heat the air fryer to 200°C/400°F and air fry for 10–12 minutes, carefully flipping halfway.

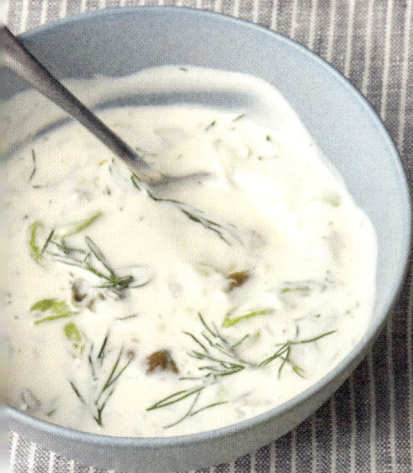

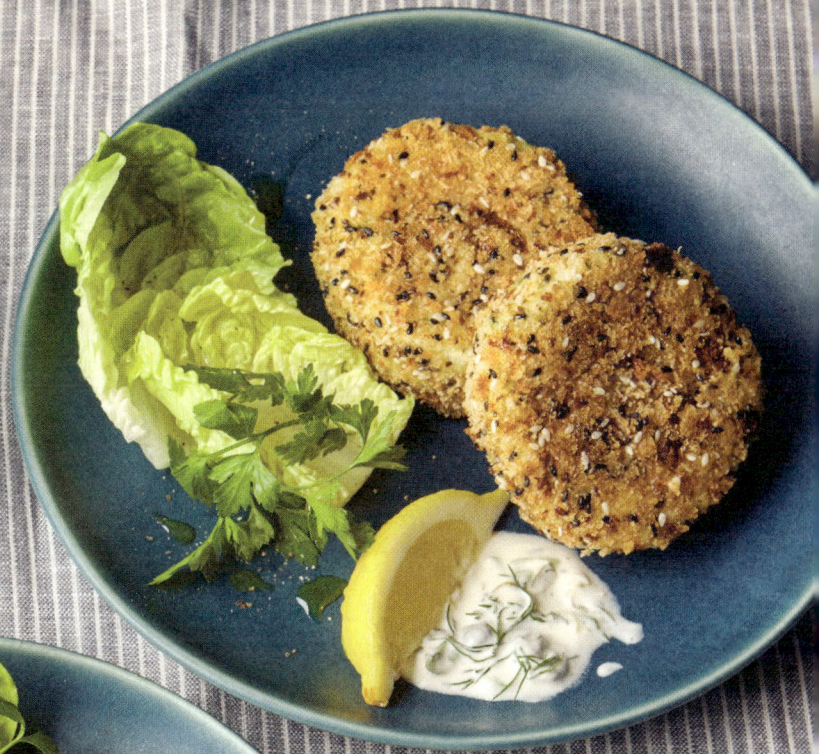

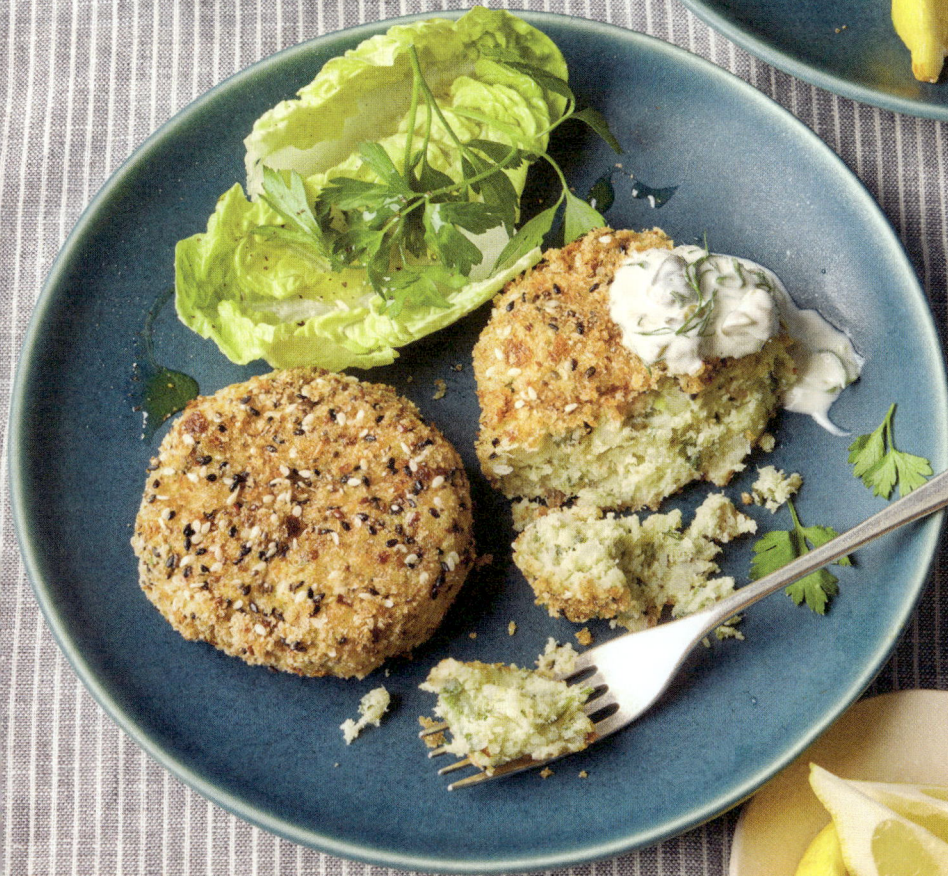

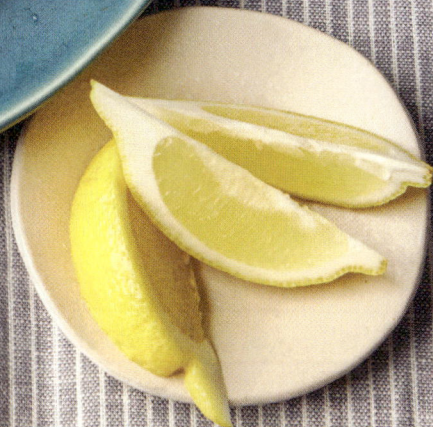

Aubergine, tomato, and butter bean stew with baked feta

Serves 4   **Prep** 5 mins   **Cook** 55 mins

450g (16oz) aubergine (eggplant), cut into 2cm (1 inch) chunks

6 tbsp olive oil, plus extra for drizzling

2 small onions, sliced

4 garlic cloves, chopped

1 × 400g (14oz) can cherry tomatoes or chopped tomatoes

3 tbsp honey or maple syrup

2 × 400g (14oz) cans butter (lima) beans, drained and rinsed

1 tsp sweet paprika

1 tsp ground coriander

½ tsp ground cinnamon

1 tsp pul biber, Aleppo pepper, or a pinch of dried chilli (red pepper) flakes, plus extra to serve

2 tsp dried oregano, plus extra for sprinkling

200g (7oz) feta, sliced into thirds

Handful of mint leaves, roughly chopped

Sea salt and freshly ground black pepper

Salty and sweet, this recipe is based on the Greek dish plaki, a traditional butter bean, tomato, and olive oil stew. I've added aubergine for extra plant points, and feta to add protein and make it into a complete meal. I also like to serve it with a green salad on the side. To make this vegan, simply use maple syrup instead of honey and use a vegan alternative to feta.

1. Preheat the oven to 220°C/200°C fan/425°F.

2. Place the aubergine in a large baking dish, toss with half the oil, and season generously with salt and pepper. Roast for 25–30 minutes, stirring after 15 minutes, until tender and charred on the edges.

3. Meanwhile, warm the remaining oil in a wide pan set over a medium heat and fry the onions with a big pinch of salt for 12–15 minutes until soft and caramelized. Add the garlic and cook for another 2–3 minutes until fragrant, then add the tomatoes, 1 tablespoon of the honey, the butter beans, spices, dried oregano, and some salt and pepper. Bring to a simmer while you wait for the aubergine to finish cooking.

4. Once the aubergine is tender, pour over the butter bean mixture, add 250ml (1 cup/9fl oz) water to the baking dish, and stir well. Return the dish to the oven for a further 15–20 minutes until the sauce has reduced and is beginning to color on top.

5. Change the oven setting to grill (broil), then lay the feta pieces (don't worry if they break up a bit) on top of the beans. Drizzle over the remaining two tablespoons of honey and a little extra olive oil, sprinkle over some extra dried oregano, then place under the grill for 4–5 minutes, watching it carefully, until the feta darkens in places.

6. Scatter over the mint and sprinkle with a little extra pul biber before serving with a green salad.

Note Any leftovers are perfect for lunch the next day, you can even stir in some spinach or rocket (arugula) to turn it into a vibrant salad.

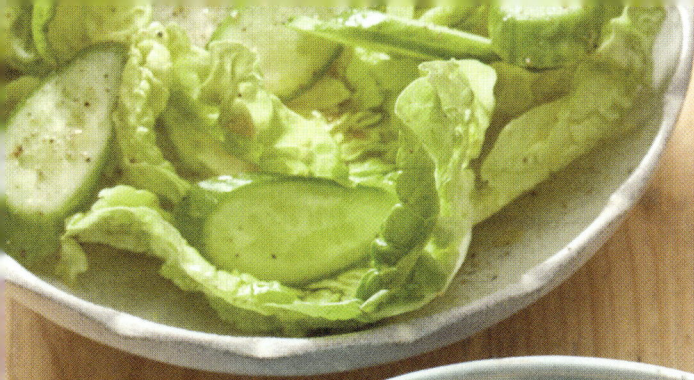

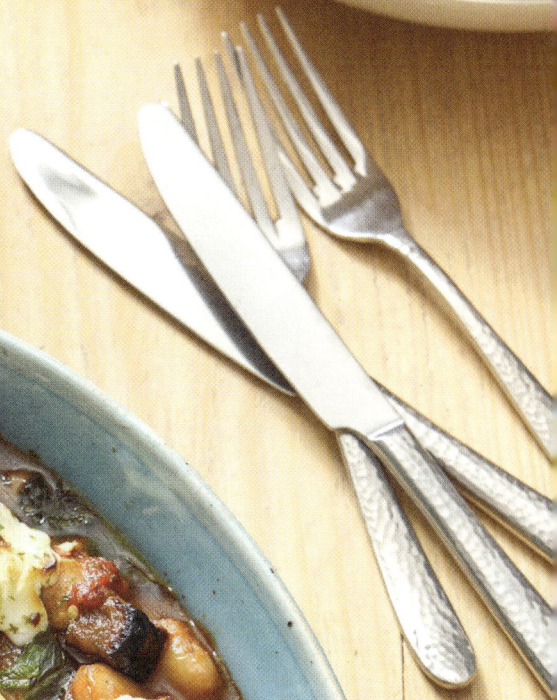

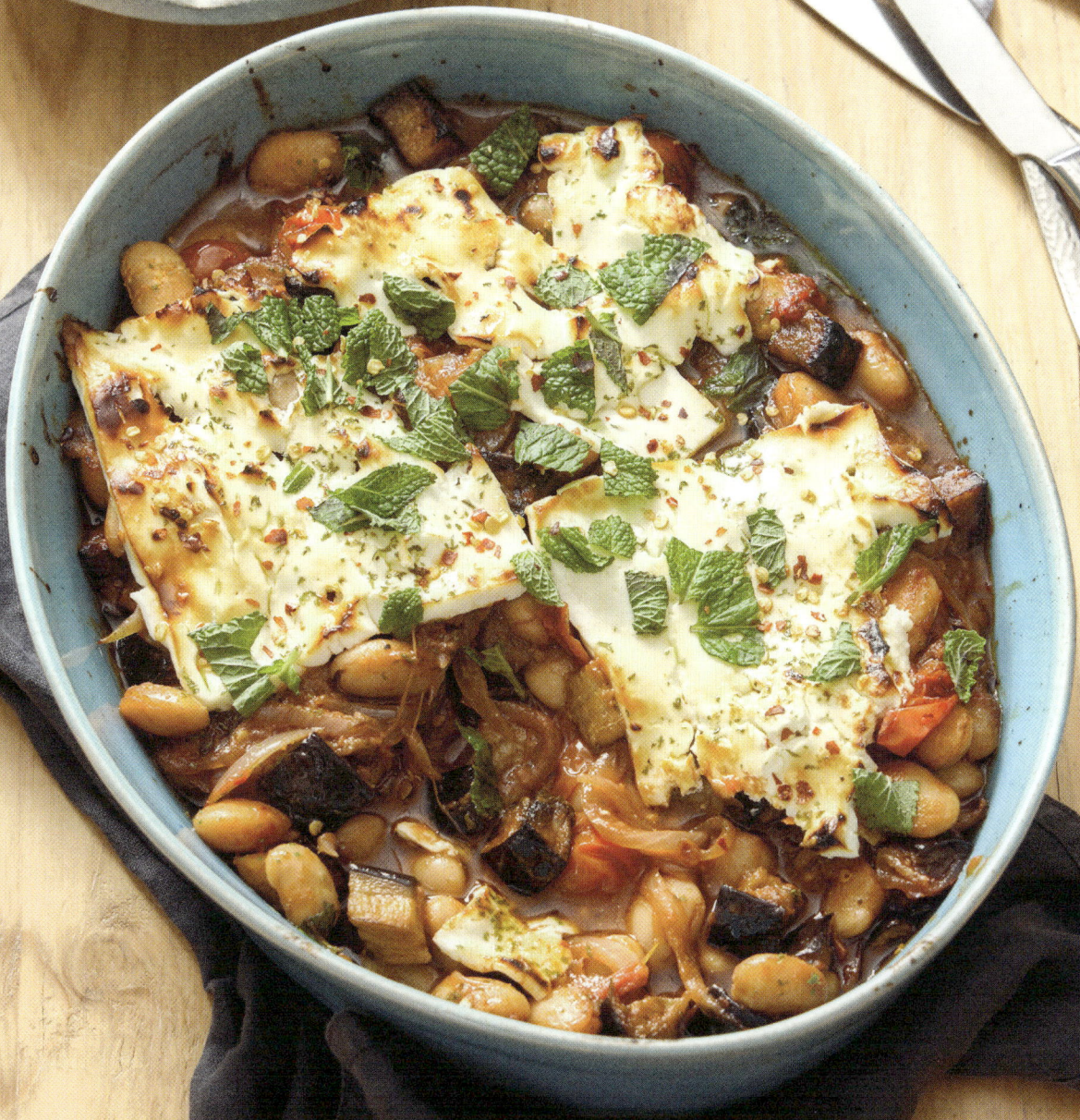

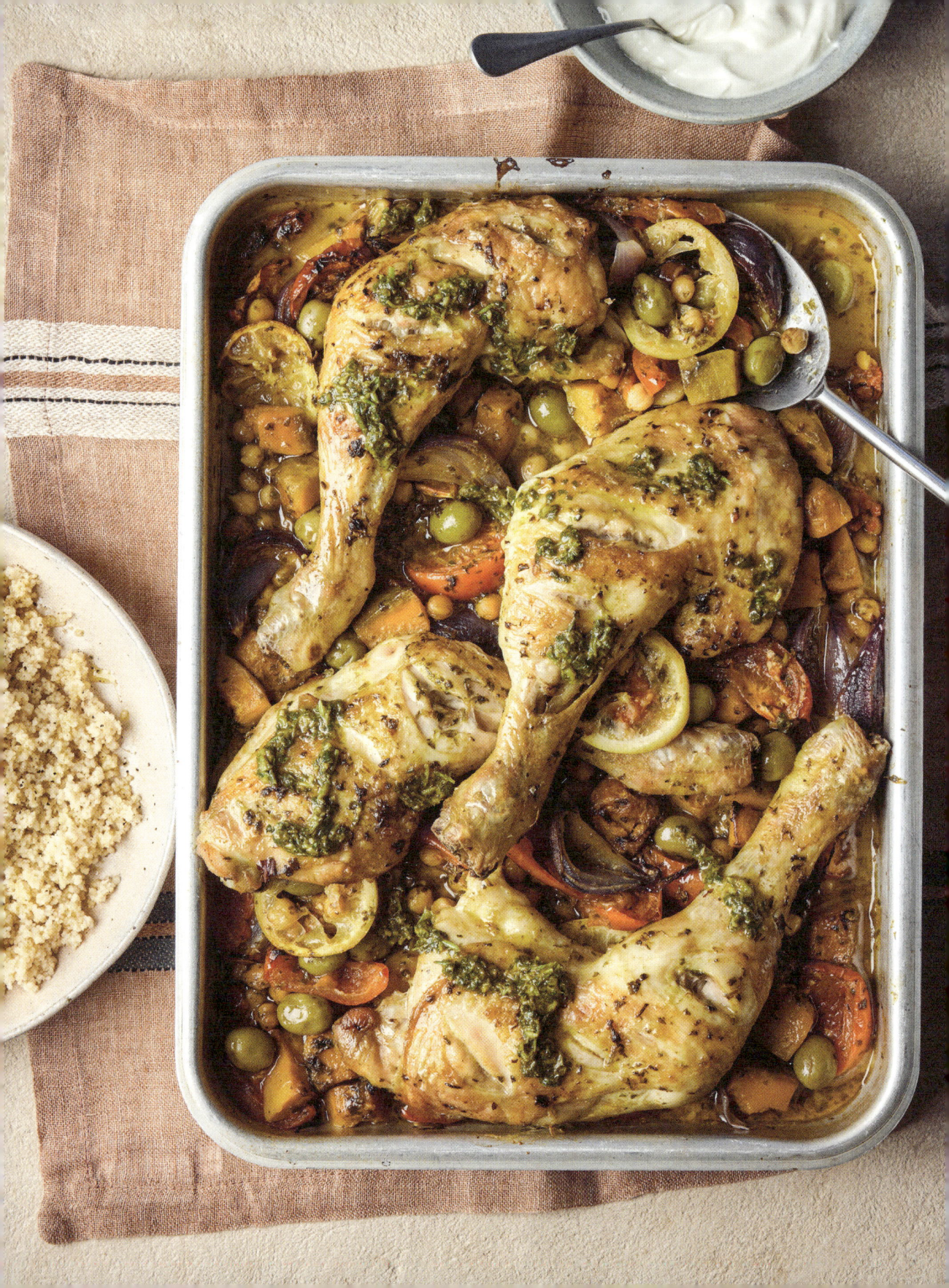

Chicken, pumpkin, and chickpea traybake

Nutritional info per portion

Fibre 14g
Protein 16g
Plant Points 9.5

Serves 4   **Prep** 10 mins   **Cook** 35 mins

4 chicken legs

2 small red onions, each cut into 8 wedges

400g (14oz) acorn or kabocha pumpkin/squash, peeled and cut into 2cm (1 inch) chunks

1 × 400g (14oz) can chickpeas, drained and rinsed

4 medium tomatoes, each cut into 8 wedges

1 small lemon, finely sliced

Drizzle of olive oil

80g (2¾oz) pitted green olives

Sea salt and freshly ground black pepper

For the chermoula

30g (1oz) coriander (cilantro), roughly chopped

15g (½oz) parsley, roughly chopped

2 garlic cloves, chopped

½ tsp ground cumin

½ tsp ground coriander

¼ tsp ground turmeric

1 tsp sweet paprika

¼ tsp dried chilli (red pepper) flakes, plus extra to serve

Juice of 1 small lemon

4 tbsp olive oil, plus extra to drizzle

To serve

Cooked wholegrain couscous

Greek yogurt or coconut yogurt

This is a speedy and delicious recipe for autumn and winter when you fancy something comforting but still nutritious. To make it vegan, simply omit the chicken and increase the amount of onion, pumpkin, and chickpeas. You could also add other vegetables—aubergines (eggplants) halved lengthways make a really great veggie centrepiece.

1. Preheat the oven to 200°C/180°C fan/400°F.

2. First, make the chermoula. Place all the ingredients in a blender or food processor along with ½ teaspoon of salt, a few grindings of black pepper, and 1 tablespoon of water. Blitz to a smooth paste, then transfer 4 tablespoons of the chermoula to a large bowl.

3. Use a sharp knife to make 4 slits in each of the chicken legs, then add these to the large bowl too, along with all the other ingredients (apart from the olives). Use your hands to toss everything well, ensuring the chicken gets plenty of chermoula rubbed into the slits.

4. Tip everything into a large baking dish, then arrange so the vegetables are in a single layer with the chicken sitting on top. Drizzle with a little oil and sprinkle some salt on the chicken, then place in the oven for 25 minutes.

5. Stir the vegetables, add the olives, and return to the oven for a further 10–15 minutes until the chicken is cooked though (cut into the middle of the largest piece to check) and the vegetables are tender and colored at the edges.

6. To serve, spoon onto plates along with some couscous, drizzle with the leftover chermoula and some yogurt, then sprinkle with extra chilli flakes, if you like.

Note You can also make this in your air fryer! Preheat your air fryer to 200°C/400°F. Follow the recipe above, but when you get to step 4, arrange everything in your air fryer basket, ensuring the chicken legs sit on top of the veggies and do no overlap. Depending on the size of your air fryer, you may want to halve the quantities in this recipe, or simply air fry in 2 batches. Air fry for 20 minutes, then flip the chicken legs and air fry for a further 10–12 minutes.

Any leftovers are perfect for lunch the next day; you can even shred the chicken (remove the bones) and stir in some spinach to turn it into a vibrant salad.

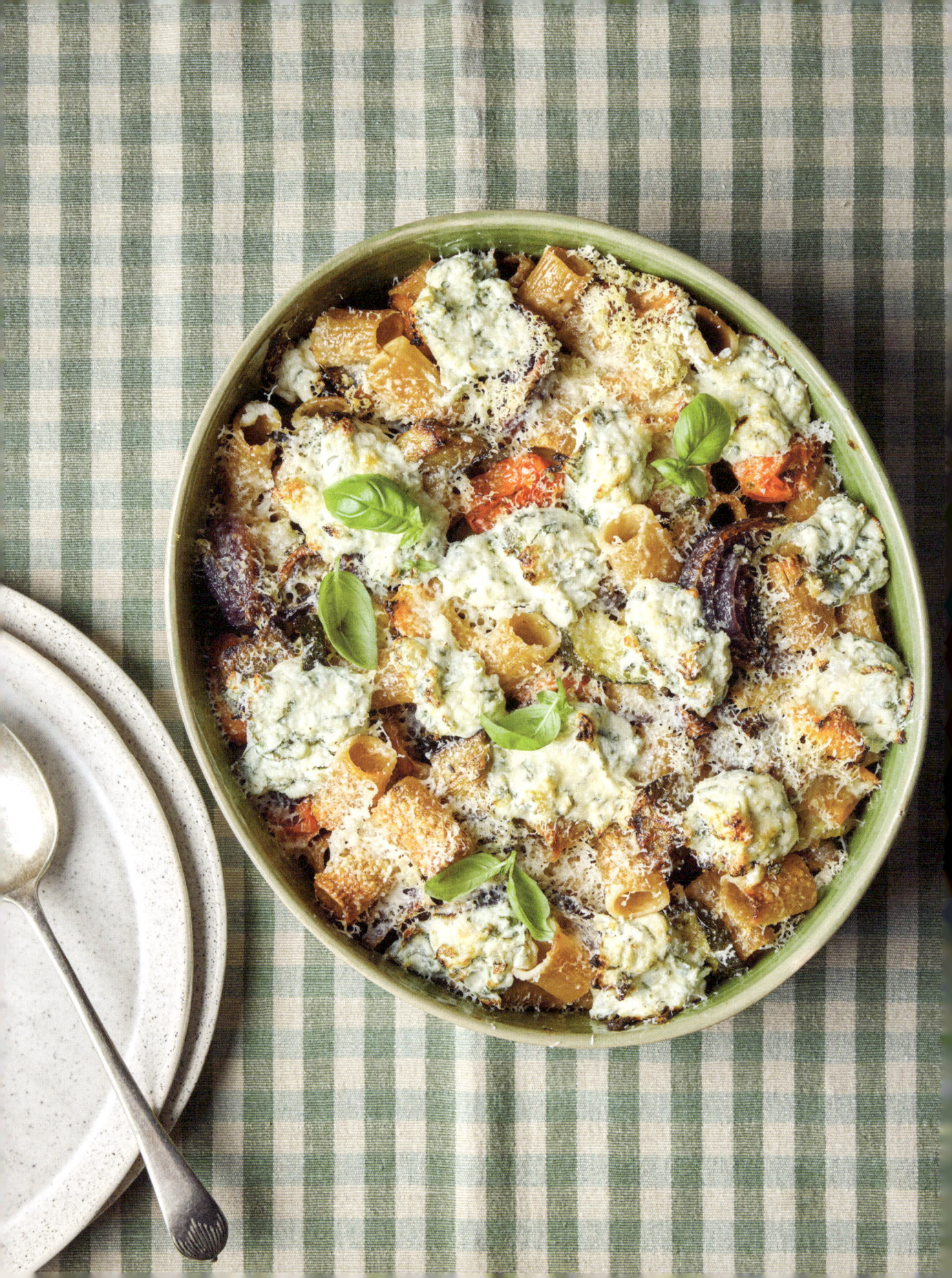

Veg-heavy pasta bake

Nutritional info per portion

Fibre 7.3g
Protein 17g
Plant Points 7.25

Serves 4   **Prep** 10 mins   **Cook** 50 mins

1 medium aubergine (eggplant), cut into 2cm (1 inch) chunks

1 red, orange, or yellow (bell) pepper, deseeded and cut into 2cm (1 inch) chunks

350g (12½oz) cherry tomatoes (or use a 400g/14oz can cherry tomatoes, rinsed)

1 courgette (zucchini), sliced into 2cm (1 inch) half-moons

2 small red onions, sliced into 2cm (1 inch) wedges

6 garlic cloves, halved lengthways

3½ tbsp olive oil, plus extra to drizzle

2 tsp dried oregano

250g (9oz) wholewheat penne, rigatoni or conchiglie

175g (6¼oz) ricotta (or use cashew cream)

2 big handfuls of basil leaves, finely chopped

75g (2¾oz) Parmesan, grated (or use vegan alternative)

Sea salt and freshly ground black pepper

It just makes sense to bulk out a firm family favourite with as much goodness as possible. Whenever I cook a recipe like this for my children, my goal is to pack as many nutritional benefits into it as possible without compromising on the taste (and I think it actually tastes better with all the added veggies!). This is a great recipe for prepping ahead—make it at the weekend and store it covered in the fridge for a couple of days before cooking, or once cooked, simply portion and freeze it ready for those nights when you don't have time to cook from scratch.

1. Preheat the oven to 220°C/200°C fan/425°F and line a large baking sheet with baking paper (parchment paper).

2. Scatter all the vegetables on the baking sheet, drizzle with the oil, sprinkle with the oregano, and season with plenty of salt and pepper. Use your hands to toss everything together so each piece is coated, then roast for 30–40 minutes, giving everything a stir after 20 minutes, until the veg is tender and a little charred.

3. Meanwhile, bring a pan of salted water to the boil and cook the pasta according to the packet instructions until al dente. Drain, keeping a cup of the cooking water, then rinse the pasta under cold water to prevent it sticking. Set aside.

4. In a small bowl, combine the ricotta, chopped basil, and half the Parmesan and season with salt and pepper. Set aside.

5. Once the vegetables are cooked, transfer them to a large baking dish. Add about 125ml (½ cup/4fl oz) of the pasta cooking water, then tip in the pasta and gently stir to combine everything. Dollop over the ricotta in heaped teaspoons, pushing it down a little as you do so.

6. Sprinkle over the remaining Parmesan, drizzle with a little extra oil, then place in the oven for 20–25 minutes until bubbling. Serve with a green salad.

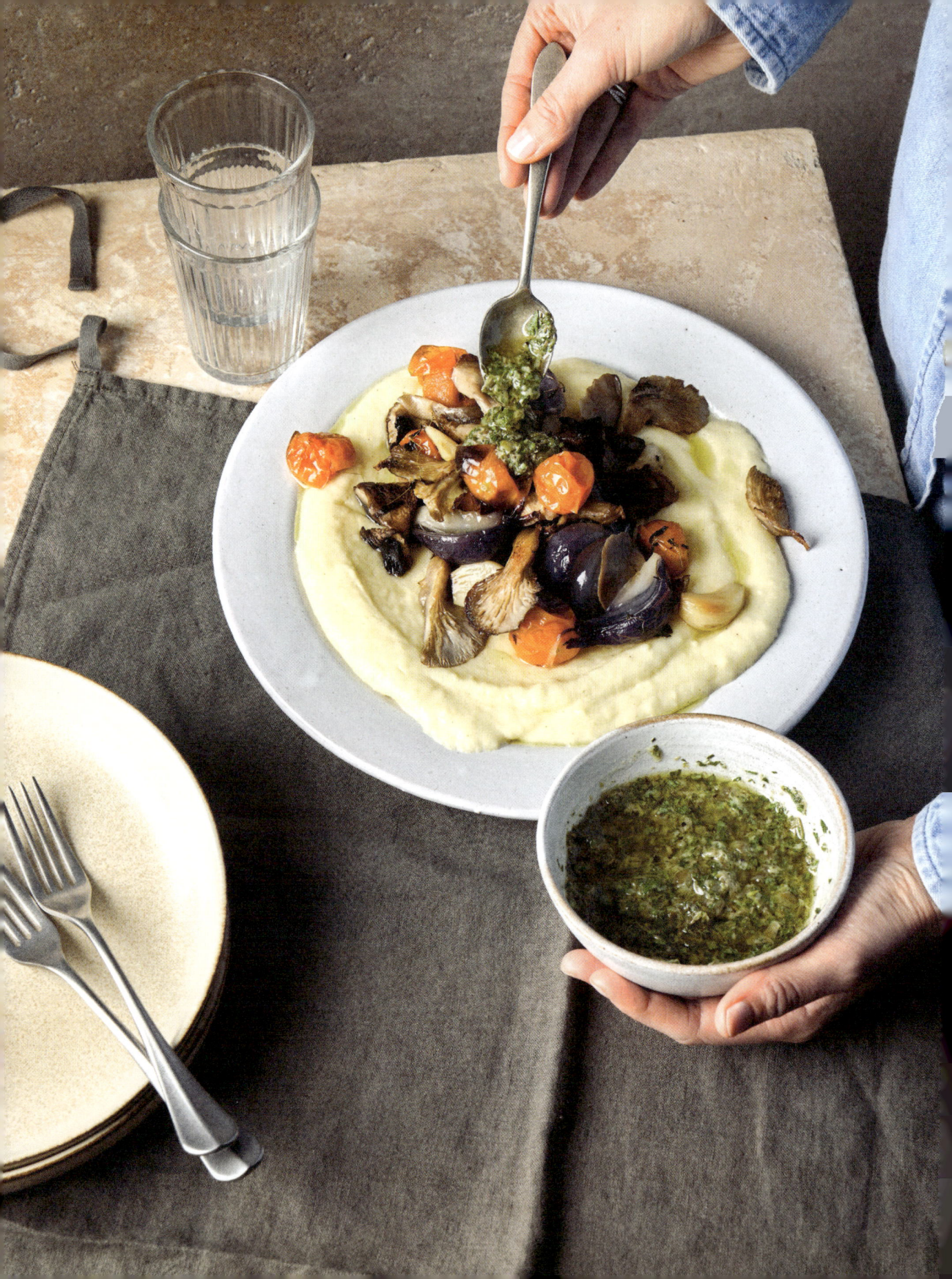

Roast mushrooms with polenta and salsa verde

Nutritional info per portion

Fibre 7.8g
Protein 17g
Plant Points 8.25

Serves 4   **Prep** 10 mins   **Cook** 30 mins

2 small red onions, each cut into 8 wedges

6 garlic cloves, unpeeled

300g (10½oz) portobello mushrooms (about 4 mushrooms), cut into 3cm (¼ inch) pieces

300g (10½oz) oyster or chestnut (brown) mushrooms, torn or cut into 3cm (¼ inch) pieces

250g (9oz) cherry tomatoes, pierced with the tip of a knife

1 tbsp thyme leaves

3 tbsp olive oil

Sea salt and freshly ground black pepper

For the polenta

250g (scant 1¾ cups/9oz) quick-cook polenta (cornmeal)

50g (3½ tbsp/1¾oz) butter (or use 5 tbsp extra-virgin olive oil)

75g (2¾oz) Parmesan (or use vegan alternative), grated, plus extra to serve

For the salsa verde

1 small garlic clove, grated

1½ tbsp capers, chopped

40g (1½oz) parsley leaves, finely chopped

1½ tsp Dijon mustard

Zest and juice of 1 small lemon

5 tbsp extra-virgin olive oil

We should all be eating more mushrooms—they are full of flavor and texture and are a great source of vitamin D. This is a complete meal as is, but it's also wonderful served alongside a roast chicken or a pork roast as an alternative take on a Sunday dinner. I like to add some toasted nuts or seeds when I want a protein boost.

1. Preheat the oven to 220°C/200°C fan/425°F and line your largest baking sheet with baking paper (parchment paper).

2. Spread out the onions and garlic on the baking sheet, then top with the mushrooms and tomatoes, ensuring they're evenly spaced. Sprinkle over the thyme, drizzle with the oil, and season with plenty of salt and pepper. Place in the oven for 30 minutes, tossing halfway, until the mushrooms are golden and crisp on the edges but still tender inside.

3. Meanwhile, place the polenta in a medium saucepan along with 1 teaspoon salt and 1.2 litres (5 cups/40fl oz) cold water, and whisk to combine. Set over a medium heat and bring to the boil. As soon as it starts simmering, whisk continuously for about 6–8 minutes until smooth and thickened, turning down the heat if the polenta begins to spit. Stir in the butter and Parmesan, then remove from the heat and keep warm while you finish off everything else.

4. To make the salsa verde, combine all the ingredients in a small bowl with ½ tablespoon of cold water and season with a little salt and pepper.

5. To serve, spoon the polenta onto a big serving dish or individual plates and sit the mushrooms, onions, and tomatoes on top (peel the garlic and add it to the plates too). Spoon over some salsa verde and scatter with a little extra Parmesan.

Note You can also cook the onions, mushrooms and tomatoes in your air fryer! Heat the air fryer to 200°C/400°F and air fry for 10–12 minutes, tossing halfway.

Chicken, date, and almond pilaf

Serves 4

Prep 5 mins (plus 1 hour soaking)

Cook 1 hour

2 tbsp olive oil, cold-pressed rapeseed oil, or avocado oil

400g (14oz) skinless, boneless chicken thighs or skinless breast, cut into 3cm (1¼ inch) chunks

1½ tbsp butter (or use extra-virgin olive oil)

40g (1½oz) blanched almonds, each roughly chopped into 2–3 pieces

1 large onion, thinly sliced

1 tsp ground allspice

½ tsp freshly ground black pepper

1 cinnamon stick or ½ tsp ground cinnamon

40g (1½oz) pitted dates, quartered (or 50g/1¾oz sour cherries, halved)

250g (9oz) long-grain brown rice, soaked in water for 1 hour

Pinch of saffron (optional)

Handful of parsley leaves, roughly chopped

Handful of dill, roughly chopped

Seeds from ¼ pomegranate

¼ tsp dried chilli (red pepper) flakes (optional)

Greek yogurt or coconut yogurt, to serve

Sea salt and freshly ground black pepper

Everyone needs a delicious rice dish in their repertoire and this pilaf is fresh, fragrant, and super easy to pull together. Combining dates (nature's toffee!) with nutty almonds is a combination you really can't go wrong with. To make this vegan, substitute the chicken for the same weight of quartered and roasted cauliflower.

1. Warm 1 tablespoon of the oil in a large, lidded pan set over a medium–high heat. Season the chicken pieces with salt and pepper, then arrange them in a single layer in the pan. Cook uncovered and undisturbed, for 3–4 minutes, then turn and cook for another 2–3 minutes until golden on both sides and cooked through. Remove to a plate and set aside.

2. Add the remaining oil and the butter and almonds to the same pan. Cook, stirring, for 2–3 minutes until the almonds get a bit of color, then turn the heat down to medium and add the onion, allspice, black pepper, and cinnamon. Scrape up any stuck bits of chicken from the base of the pan, then fry the onions for 10 minutes, stirring occasionally, until they're soft and a little colored.

3. Stir the dates into the pan, then drain the rice and add it to the pan too along with the saffron (if using). Season with 1 teaspoon of salt, then pour over boiling water from a kettle so the water comes roughly 3cm (1¼ inches) above the rice. Stir gently, then cover the pan with the lid. Turn the heat up to high and cook for 7 minutes, before turning the heat down to low and cooking for a further 20 minutes. Check that the rice is just cooked before turning off the heat.

4. Working quickly so not too much heat escapes, remove the lid, scatter over the chicken, gently push it under the rice, then pop the lid back on. Leave to rest for 10 minutes.

5. Remove the lid, fluff the rice up with a fork and stir through the herbs. Top with the pomegranate seeds and chilli flakes (if using), then serve the pilaf in bowls with dollops of yogurt.

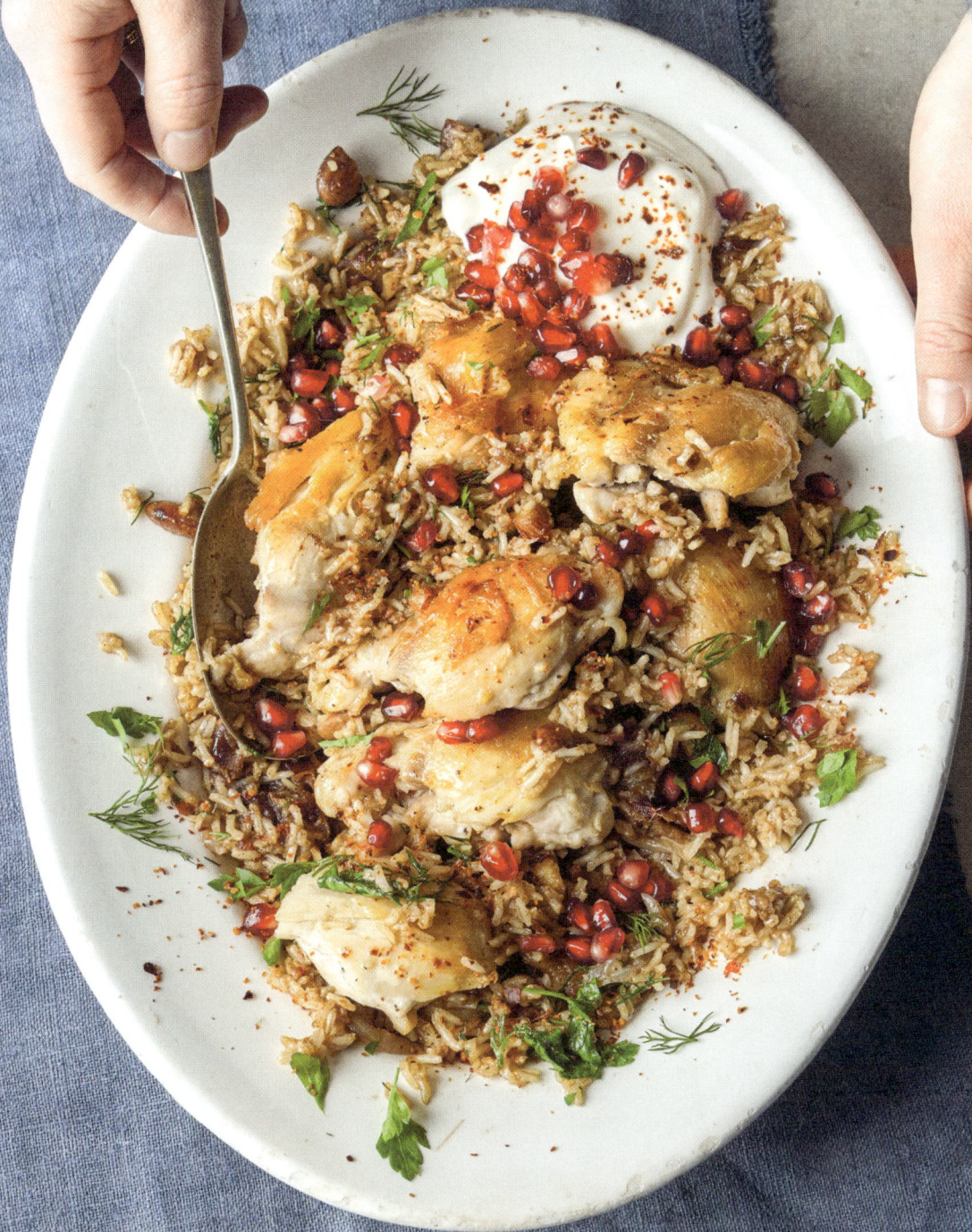

Fish sticks, chips, and peas

Nutritional info per portion

Fibre 11g
Protein 42g
Plant Points 8.5

Serves 4   **Prep** 10 mins   **Cook** 30 mins

500g (18oz) small sweet potatoes, scrubbed then quartered lengthways

5–6 tbsp olive oil, cold-pressed rapeseed oil, or avocado oil

500g (18oz) skinless white fish such as haddock, cod, coley, or hake, sliced into 2cm (1 inch) strips

Tartare sauce (page 208), to serve

Sea salt and freshly ground black pepper

For the coating

50g (6 tbsp/1¾oz) spelt or wholemeal (whole wheat) flour

½ tsp sweet paprika

2 eggs

1 tbsp milk

120g (4oz) fresh wholemeal (whole wheat) breadcrumbs

For the mushy peas

400g (14oz) frozen peas

20g (1½ tbsp/¾oz) butter

Zest of 1 lemon

Small handful of mint leaves, finely chopped

2 tbsp Greek yogurt

Who doesn't love fish sticks? Instead of grabbing a box from the freezer aisle, try this homemade version instead. I promise they'll taste a million times better, plus you'll know exactly what's gone into them. If you get the potatoes in the oven while you're preparing the fish sticks, you should find that everything is ready at the same time. To make them vegan simply swap the fish for tofu to create tofu fingers.

1. Preheat the oven to 220°C/200°C fan/425°F.

2. Toss the sweet potato quarters in half the oil on a baking sheet, then season with salt and pepper. Roast in the oven for 30 minutes until tender and golden.

3. Meanwhile, prepare the coating for the fish sticks. Mix the flour with the paprika (if using) and plenty of salt and pepper, then spread out on a plate; beat the eggs with the milk in a shallow bowl; then spread out the breadcrumbs on another plate.

4. Line a separate large baking sheet with baking paper (parchment paper) and drizzle it with the remaining oil.

5. One by one, lightly coat the fish pieces in the flour mixture, then gently dip into the egg, then roll in the breadcrumbs, pressing them lightly to help them stick. Place the fish sticks on the lined baking sheet and gently turn them in the oil so they get very lightly coated (add more oil if needed). Place in the oven for 20 minutes until golden and crisp.

6. While everything is in the oven, simmer the peas in a pan of salted boiling water for 5–6 minutes until completely tender. Drain, transfer to a bowl with the butter and lemon zest, then use a potato masher or an electric hand-held blender to roughly mash. Add the mint and yogurt, season with a little salt and pepper, and stir well.

7. Serve up the fish sticks and sweet potato chips (fries) with the mushy peas and some tartare sauce on the side.

Note You can also make this in your air fryer (although it's best if you have a two-drawer air fryer so the fish sticks and fries are ready at the same time). Fish sticks: air fry at 180°C/350°F for 8–10 minutes. Fries: air fry at 190°C/375°F for 20 minutes, shaking every 5 minutes.

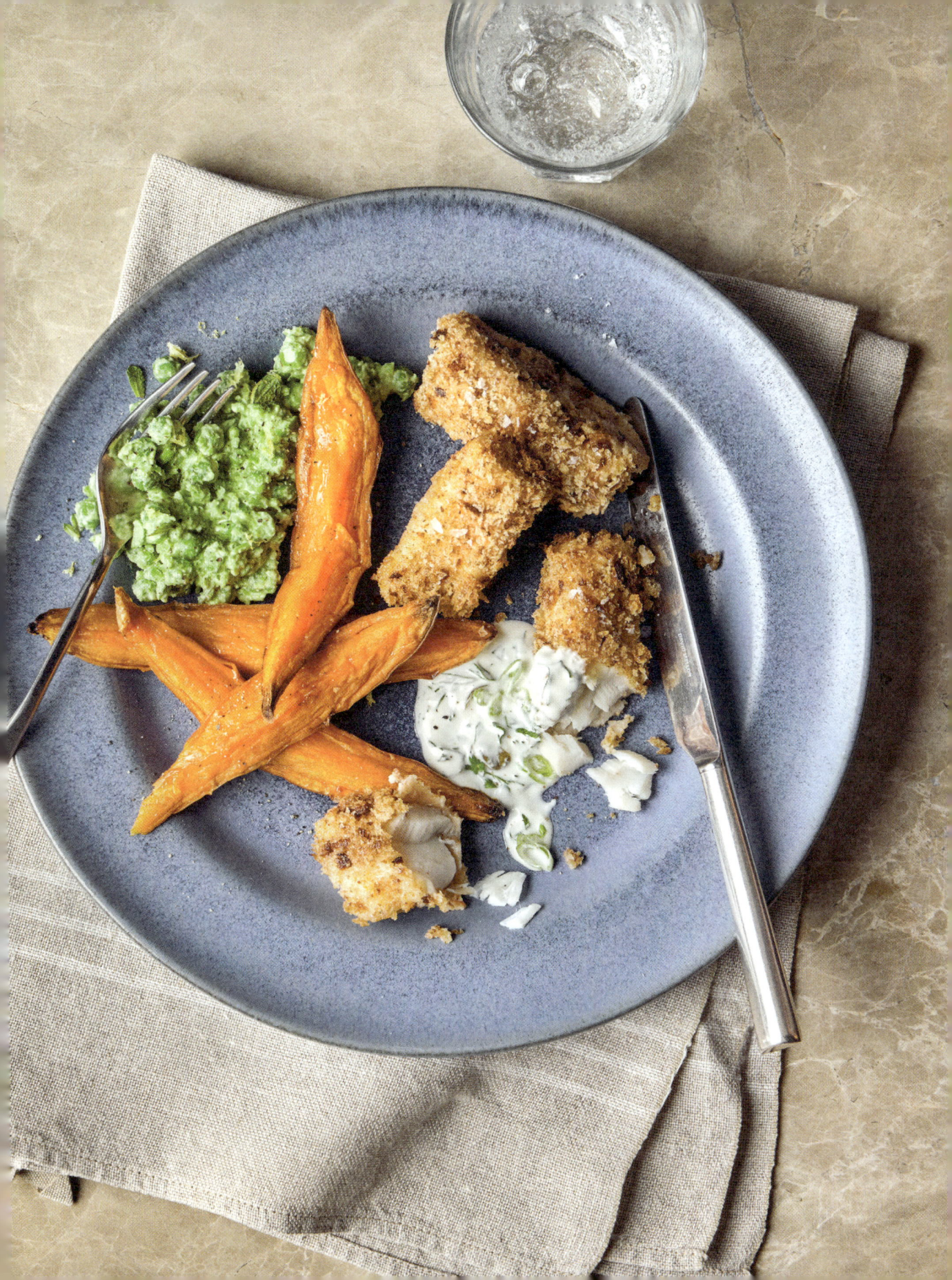

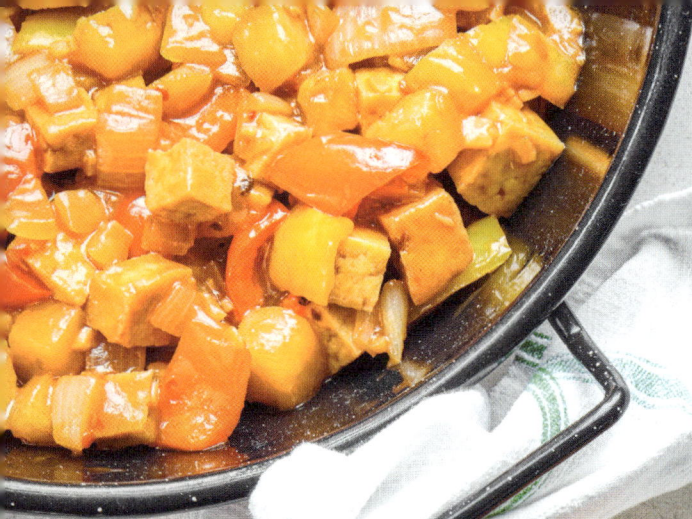

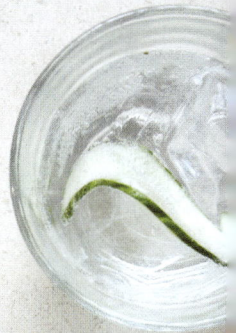

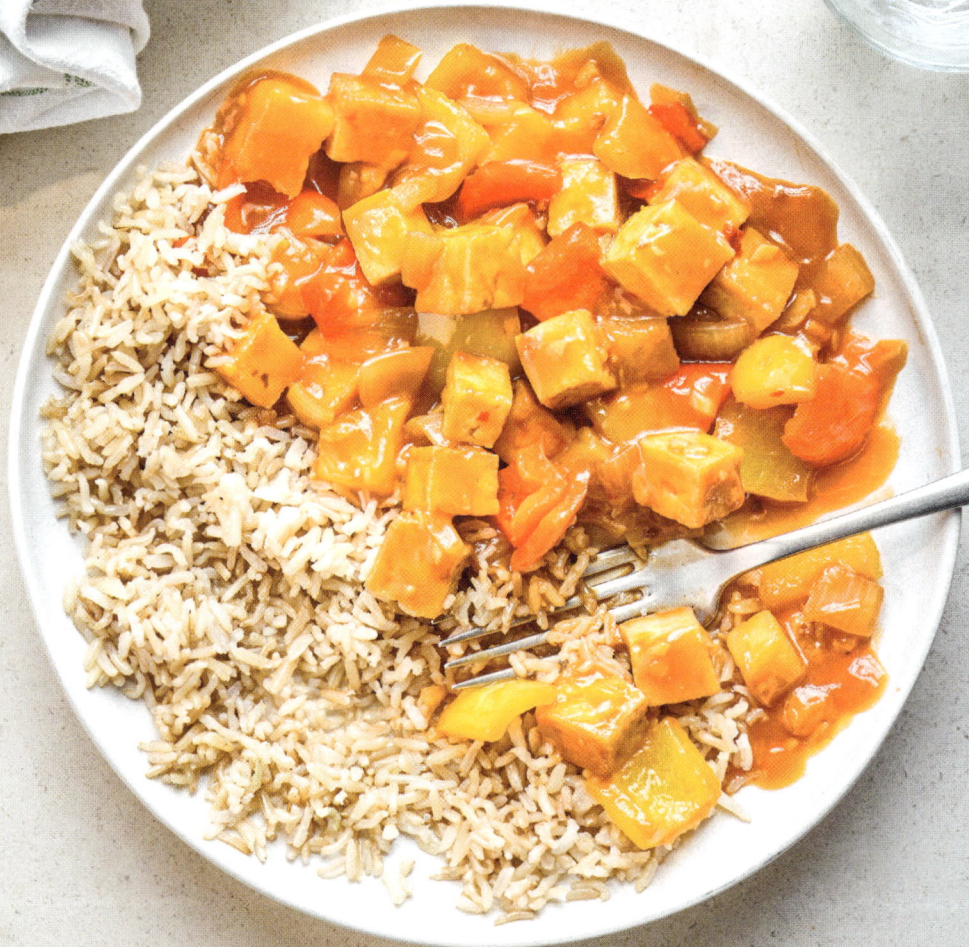

Sweet and sour sticky tofu

Nutritional info per portion

Fibre 8.2g
Protein 23g
Plant Points 7.25

● **Serves** 4   ● **Prep** 15 mins   ● **Cook** 20 mins

4 tbsp olive oil, cold-pressed rapeseed oil, or avocado oil

1 × 450g (16oz) block of firm tofu, patted dry with paper towel and cut into 2cm (1 inch) chunks

2 onions, chopped into 1cm (½in) chunks

1 red (bell) pepper, deseeded and chopped into 2cm (1 inch) chunks

1 yellow (bell) pepper, deseeded and chopped into 2cm (1 inch) chunks

2 large garlic cloves, grated

1 thumb-sized piece fresh ginger, grated

300g (10½oz) fresh pineapple, chopped into 2cm (1 inch) chunks

¼–½ tsp dried chilli (red pepper) flakes (optional)

1 tsp garlic powder (optional)

Cooked long-grain brown rice, to serve

For the sauce

½ tbsp cornflour (cornstarch)

4 tbsp rice wine vinegar

4 tbsp light soy sauce

4 tbsp maple syrup

4 tbsp tomato ketchup (see page 206 for homemade)

A take-out classic and one of my firm favourites, the sweet and sour flavors of this dish are hard to beat—luckily for you, it can be recreated at home in a much healthier manner than the one you order from your local take-out place. This recipe contains loads of nutrients from a variety of plants and a nice boost of protein from the tofu (but feel free to substitute the tofu with the same quantity of chicken or prawns/shrimp). I promise, you may think twice before ordering it once you've tried this recipe!

1. First, prepare the sauce. In a small bowl, whisk the cornflour into 1 tablespoon of the vinegar until smooth. Now add the remaining sauce ingredients, whisk well, then pour in 100ml (scant ½ cup/3½fl oz) water. Whisk again and set aside.

2. Add half the oil to a non-stick pan set over a medium heat. When hot, add the tofu in a single layer and fry for 6–8 minutes, turning regularly, until golden on all sides. Transfer the tofu to a plate.

3. Place the pan back over a medium heat and add the remaining oil along with the onions and both peppers and fry for 5–6 minutes until softened and browning on the edges. Add the garlic and ginger and fry for 2–3 minutes until fragrant, then stir through the pineapple, chilli flakes, and garlic powder (if using).

4. Give the sauce a quick stir, then pour it into the pan and bring to a vigorous simmer. Simmer for 4–5 minutes, stirring slowly, until it begins to thicken and any cornflour taste has disappeared (add a splash of water if you'd like the sauce a little looser). Add the tofu back to the pan and stir to coat it in the sauce, then serve with brown rice. This freezes well in an airtight container for up to 3 months.

Note Opt for a calcium-set tofu for an added boost of calcium.

Snacks are an incredibly important part of our diet, providing us with an energy boost and an opportunity to add further nourishment to our bodies. They are often seen as inherently "bad", but this couldn't be further from the truth if you're making good food choices (like opting for a piece of fruit or one of the nutrient-dense recipes in this section). The problem lies in the UPF snack foods that we all know and can't help but love, which are designed to be hyper-palatable. Here you'll find healthier versions for all your favourites, to help satisfy those hunger cravings while doing you good.

In some cases, utilizing good-quality processed products can be convenient and still better for you than purchasing UPF items. Turn to page 87 to understand why I use store-bought tortilla wraps when making my tortilla chips (page 176).

Snacks and dips

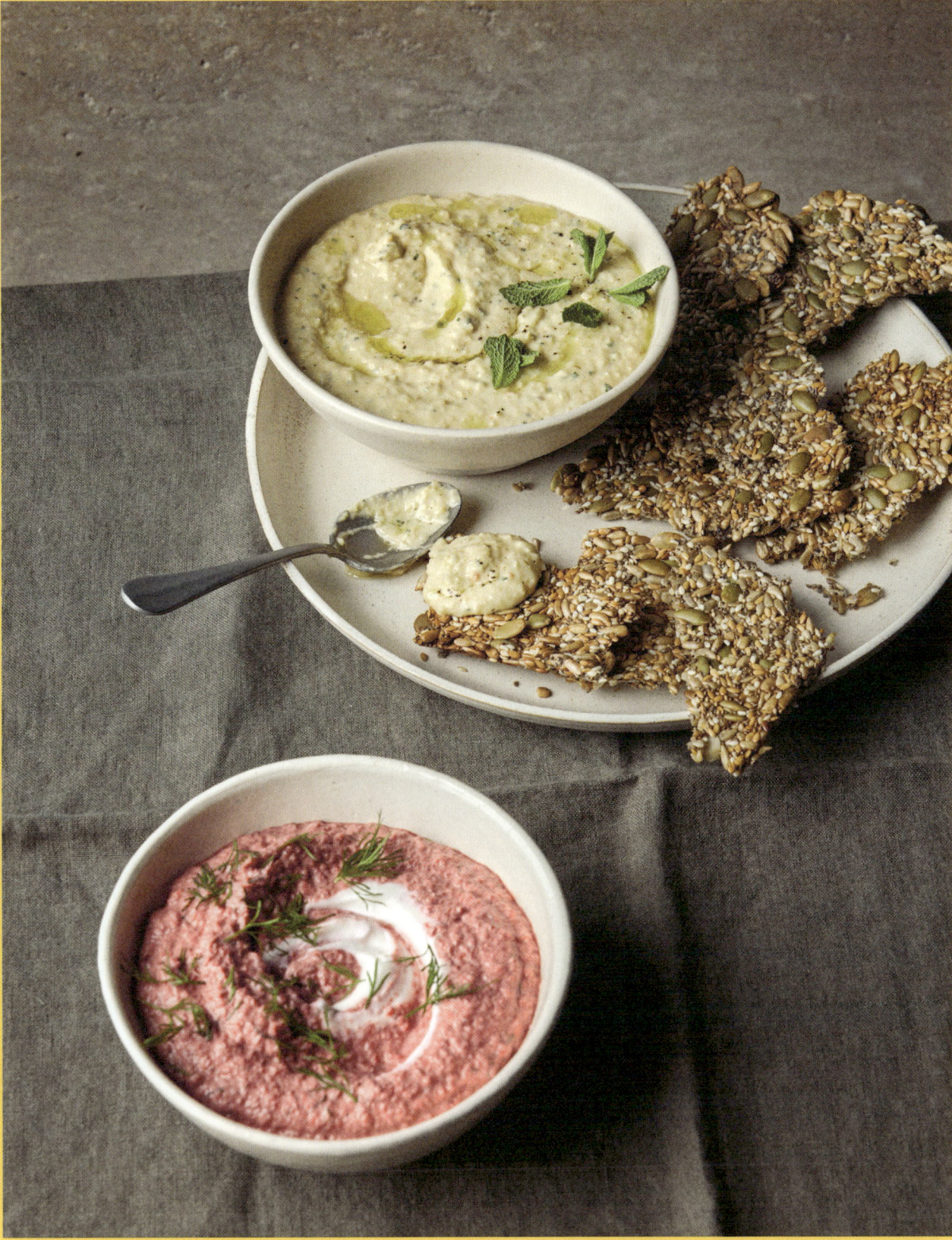

Chilli and mint hummus

● **Makes** 400g (14oz)　　● **Prep** 10 mins　　● **Cook** 8 mins

½ tsp cumin seeds

1 mild red chilli, pierced with the tip of a knife

1 garlic clove, chopped

Juice of 1 large lemon

50g (2¾ tbsp/1¾oz) tahini

100g (scant ½ cup/3½oz) olive oil

1 × 400g (14oz) can chickpeas, drained and rinsed (save the aquafaba for another use—page 207)

Small handful of mint leaves

Sea salt and freshly ground black pepper

Store-bought hummus is incredibly convenient, but did you know it's super easy to make at home and much more cost-effective? This delicious dip is perfect for loading into flatbreads (page 179), dolloping on salads, or used as a dip for carrots and cucumber (or the chips over on page 176). Stored in an airtight container in the fridge, this will keep for 5 days. Pictured on page 173.

1. Set a small frying pan (skillet) over a medium heat and, when hot, toast the cumin seeds for 1 minute, then immediately transfer the toasted seeds to a blender or food processor.

2. Return the pan to the heat, add the chilli, and dry fry 6–8 minutes, occasionally pushing it against the base of the pan with the back of a spoon, until charred all over and tender. Place in a small bowl and cover with cling film (plastic wrap) for 10 minutes. When cool enough to handle, remove and discard the skin, stem, and seeds.

3. Meanwhile, add the garlic, lemon juice, tahini, olive oil, ½ teaspoon salt, and 2 tablespoons of water to the blender and blitz until smooth.

4. Add half the chilli to the blender, along with the chickpeas and mint, and blitz again until smooth, adding more water as needed. Taste, and if you think you'd like a bit more heat, add the rest of the chilli and blitz again.

5. Check the seasoning, adding salt and pepper to taste, then scoop into a serving bowl.

Nutritional info per portion

Fibre 8.2g
Protein 23g
Plant Points 7.25

Beetroot, dill, and yogurt dip

- **Makes** 400g (14oz)
- **Prep** 5 mins
- **Cook** 0 mins

Another dip with plenty of protein that will brighten up any plate; it's great served with the seedy crackers (right). If you'd like to make this vegan, simply use a mix of soy yogurt (for added protein) and coconut yogurt (for added flavor). Stored in an airtight container in the fridge, this will keep for 5 days. Pictured on page 173.

250g (9oz) cooked vac-paced or canned beetroot (beets), halved

1 small garlic clove, chopped

1 tbsp apple cider vinegar

2 tbsp olive oil

40g (2¼ tbsp/1½oz) tahini

125g (generous ½ cup/4½oz) Greek yogurt or coconut yogurt

Handful of dill, finely chopped

Sea salt and freshly ground black pepper

1. Place the beetroot, garlic, vinegar, olive oil, and ½ teaspoon of salt in a blender or food processor and blitz until smooth.

2. Transfer to a serving bowl and stir in the tahini, yogurt, and dill. Taste and add salt and pepper if needed.

Nutritional info per 100g

Fibre 42g
Protein 5.4g
Plant Points 3

Seedy crackers

- **Makes** about 260g (9oz)
- **Prep** 20 mins
- **Cook** 35 mins

Avoid store-bought crackers, which tend to contain palm oil and plenty of unneeded extra ingredients, and make these omega-3-rich crackers instead. Stored in an airtight container at room temperature, these will keep for 2 weeks. Pictured on page 173.

40g (5 tbsp/1½oz) chia seeds

75g (½ cup/2¾oz) pumpkin seeds

100g (¾ cup/3½oz) sunflower seeds

40g (5 tbsp/1½oz) linseeds (flaxseeds)

25g (3 tbsp/1oz) sesame seeds

Sea salt

1. Preheat the oven to 160°C/140°C fan/325°F and line a baking sheet with baking paper (parchment paper).

2. Place the chia seeds and ¼ teaspoon salt in a bowl, then stir in 160ml (⅔ cup/5½fl oz) water. Set aside for 15 minutes.

3. Once the chia seeds have absorbed the water, stir in the rest of the ingredients. Spread the mixture onto the baking sheet as thinly and smoothly as possible.

4. Bake for 35–40 minutes until firm and crisp to the touch. Allow to cool completely on the baking sheet, then break into pieces to serve.

Nutritional info per 100g

Fibre 8.3g
Protein 13g
Plant Points 5

Tortilla chips with butter bean and onion dip

Serves 4–6   **Prep** 10 mins   **Cook** 15 mins

4–6 large wholemeal (whole wheat) wraps (see Note)

Olive oil, for drizzling and brushing

1 tsp hot paprika

Sea salt and freshly ground black pepper

For the dip

Bunch of spring (green) onions, trimmed

125g (½ cup/4½oz) olive oil

1 garlic clove, chopped

Zest and juice of 1 small lemon

2 × 400g (14oz) can butter (lima) beans, drained and rinsed

Replacing your favourite snack with your own homemade chips and dip is a no-brainer—the best part is that you don't need to worry about any added salt, sugars, and preservatives. Butter beans are vastly underrated: they are cheap, creamy, versatile, and an amazing source of protein. I also sometimes add a couple of tablespoons of tahini when adding the butter beans to the blender, to add a velvety texture and boost the protein levels even further. This dip freezes well and you can keep the chips in an airtight container for up to 3 days to maintain their crispness.

1. Preheat your oven on a hot grill (broiler) setting.

2. Add the spring onions to a baking sheet, drizzle with a little oil, and place under the grill for 6–8 minutes, turning them over halfway. Watch them closely—once they are charred all over, remove from the oven and set aside.

3. Adjust the oven setting and preheat to 200°C/180°C fan/400°F. Line a couple of baking sheets with baking paper (parchment paper).

4. Brush the wraps on both sides with olive oil, then cut them into triangles. Spread them out on the lined baking sheets in an even layer (they can overlap a little) and bake for 6–8 minutes until pale golden and firm to the touch. Transfer to wire racks, sprinkle with a little salt, and leave to cool (they will crisp up more as they cool).

5. Roughly chop the charred spring onions and add them to a blender or food processor along with the oil, garlic, lemon zest and juice, and 1 teaspoon of salt. Blitz until finely chopped, then add the butter beans and blitz again until smooth. Taste and add salt and pepper if needed, then transfer to a serving bowl.

6. Add the paprika to a small pan along with 2 tablespoons of olive oil. Set it over a low heat and gently warm for 10–15 seconds—just long enough to let the flavors infuse.

7. Drizzle the paprika oil over the dip, then serve with the tortilla chips on the side for dipping.

Note You can also make the chips in your air fryer! Heat the air fryer to 180°C/350°F and air fry the chips for 3–5 minutes, tossing them halfway. Depending on the size of your air fryer, you may need to cook them in batches. Do check the label of the wraps to ensure the ingredients list contains just flour, water, olive oil, and salt.

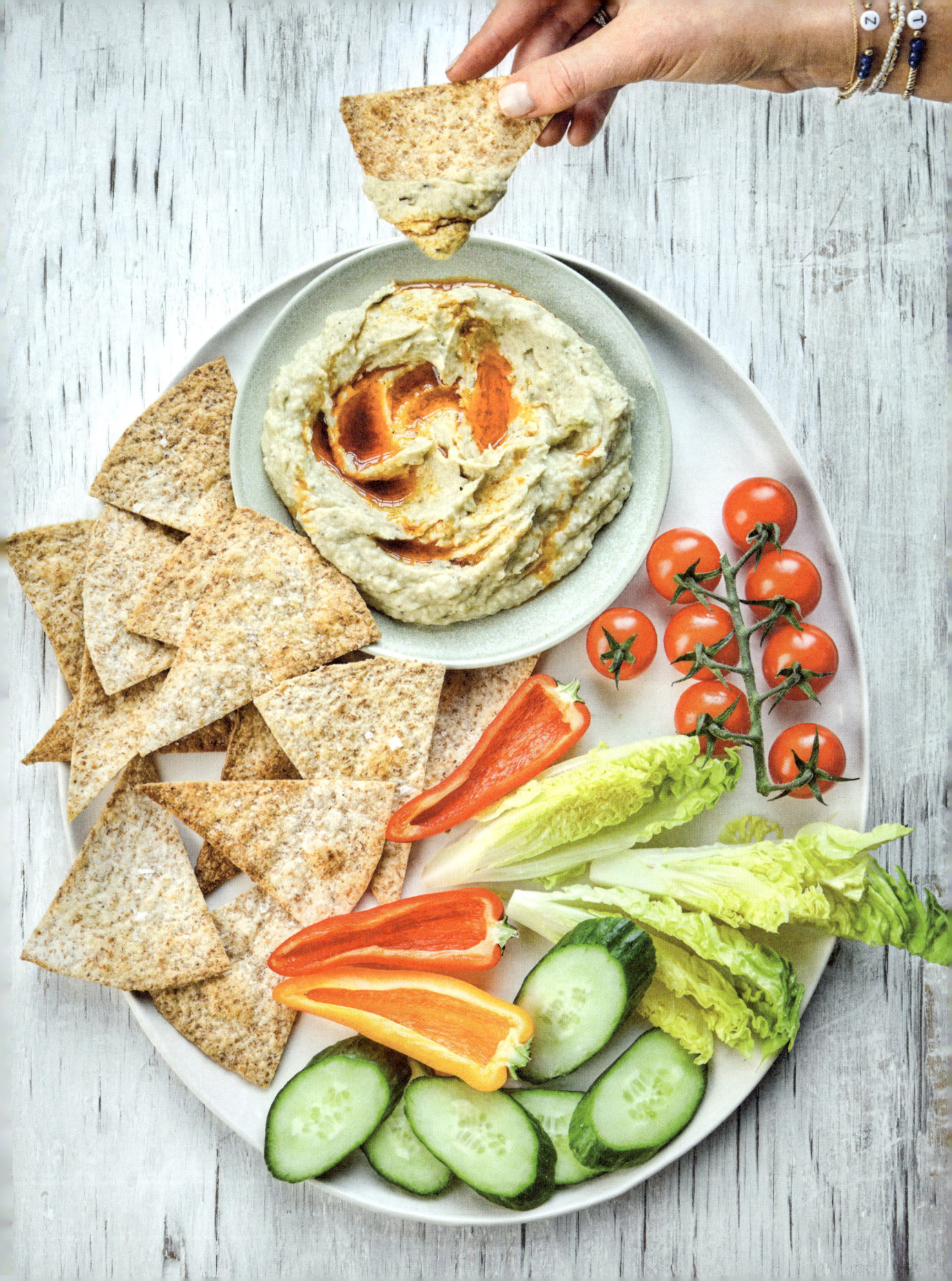

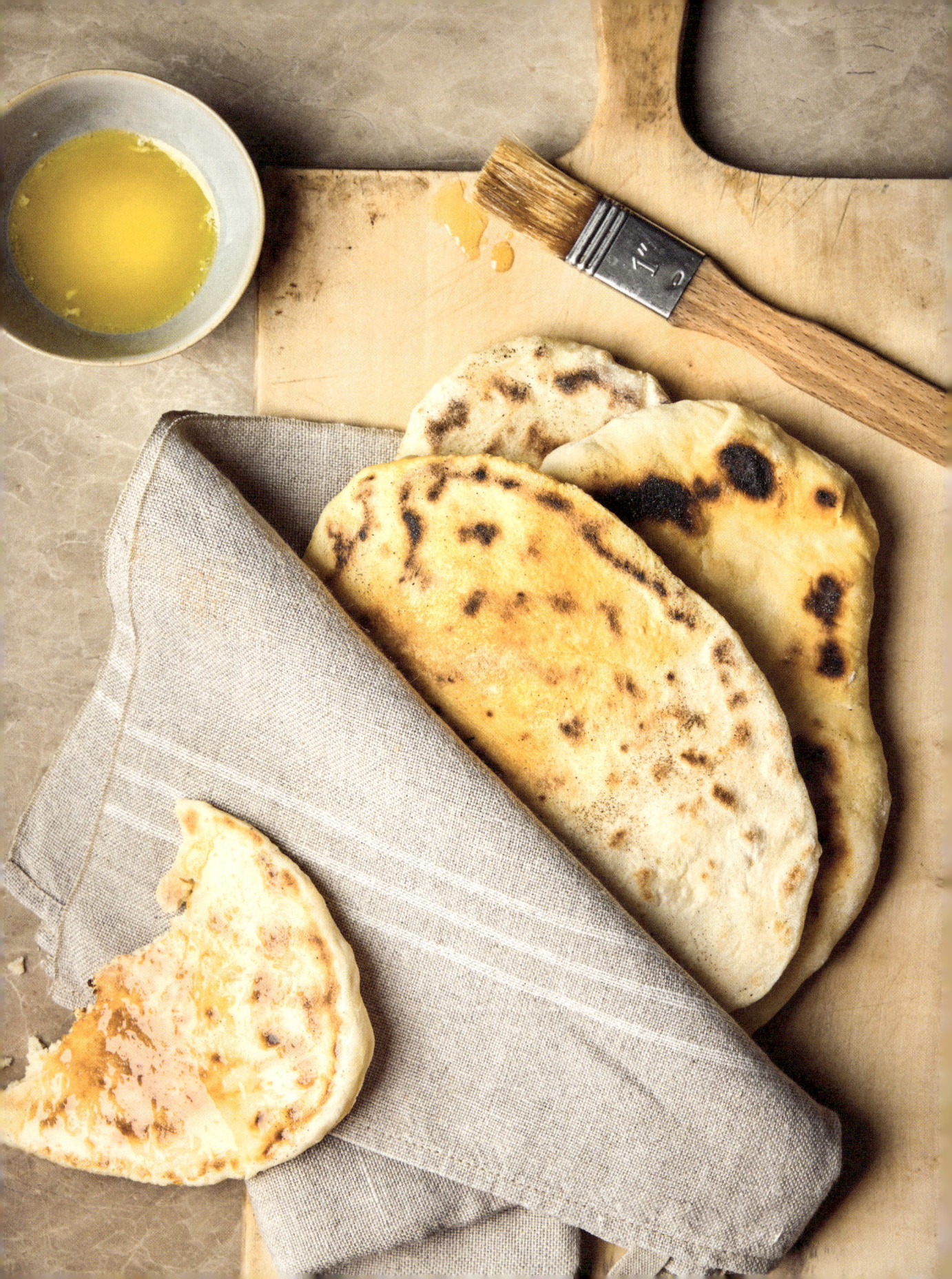

Easy yogurt flatbreads

Nutritional info per portion

Fibre 3.1g
Protein 13g
Plant Points 1.25

Makes 6   **Prep** 10 mins   **Cook** 10 mins

400g (3 cups/14oz) white spelt or wholemeal (whole wheat) flour, plus extra to dust

1 tbsp baking powder

1 tsp sea salt

1 tsp olive oil, plus extra for frying if needed

200g (1 cup/7oz) skyr, Greek yogurt or coconut yogurt

These flatbreads are such a useful recipe to have up your sleeve, and you can use whatever flour you have to hand. Each type of yogurt and flour has different hydration levels, so this recipe is just a guide—if you find the dough is too dry, add splashes of water until it comes together; if you find it's too wet, simply add more flour. Once you've got the hang of the basic recipe, feel free to experiment by adding some of the optional extras to the dough. The flatbreads are also delicious brushed with a little melted butter as they come out of the pan.

1. Combine the flour, baking powder, and salt in a bowl, then stir in the olive oil and yogurt (add any additional extras now too). Mix with your hands until the dough comes together, then tip onto a flour-dusted surface and knead for a couple of minutes until you have a smooth dough. Divide the dough into 6 equal balls, cover with a clean kitchen towel, and allow to rest for at least 10 minutes.

2. Meanwhile, set a griddle pan or non-stick frying pan (skillet) over a high heat.

3. Roll each dough ball into a flatbread shape about 20cm (8 inches) long and 2mm (⅛ inch) thick. If your pan isn't non-stick or you want a slightly crisp finish to your flatbreads, brush both sides of the flatbreads with a little olive oil.

4. When the pan is searingly hot, add a flatbread to the pan and cook for 60–90 seconds until char marks appear, then flip it over and cook the other side until nicely charred too. Wrap the flatbread in a kitchen towel while you cook the rest.

Optional extras

· Freshly ground black pepper
· Grated garlic
· Nigella seeds
· Cumin seeds
· Chopped coriander (cilantro) leaves
· Sliced spring (green) onion
· Desiccated (dried shredded) coconut

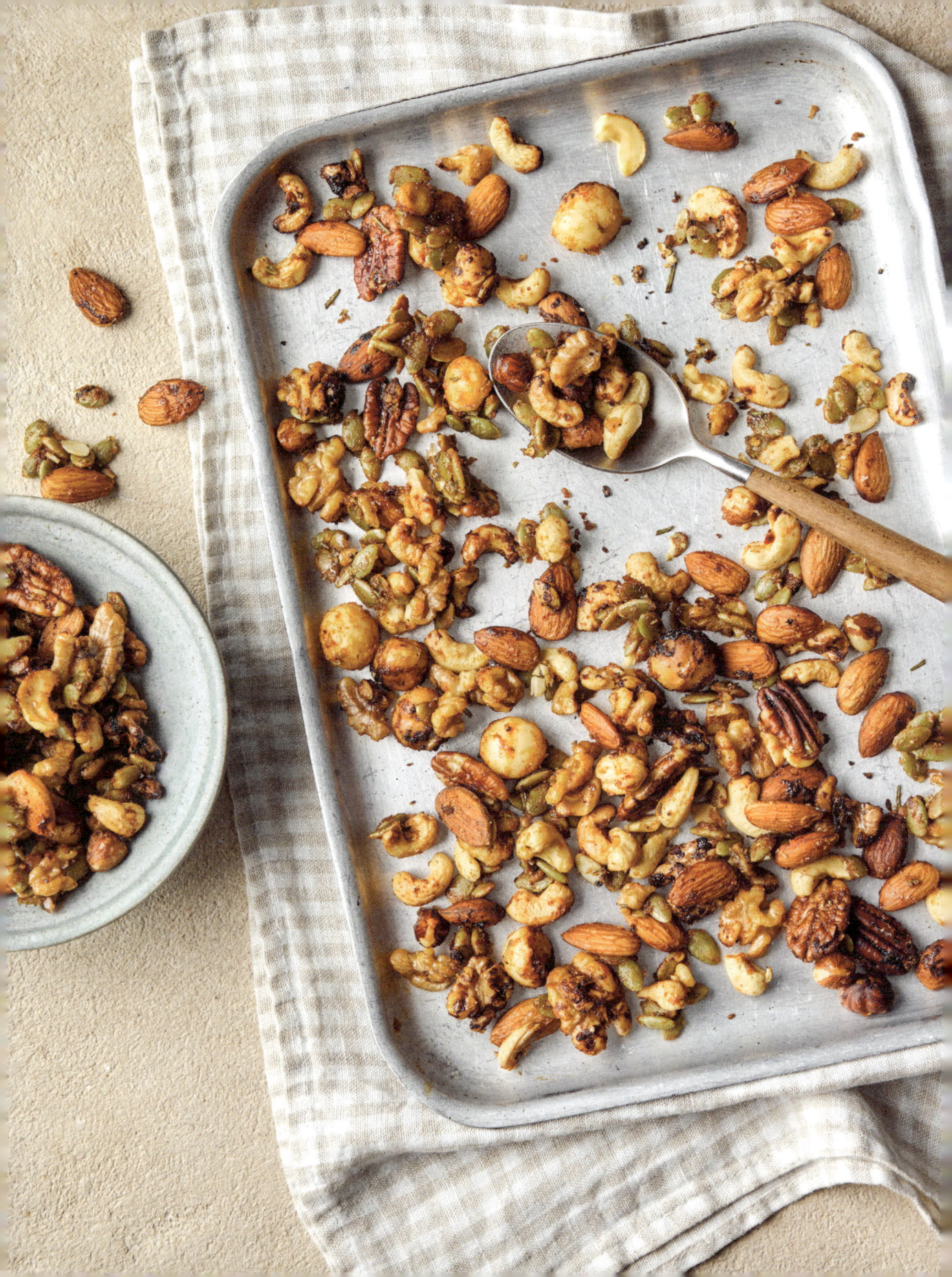

Miso-roasted nuts

Nutritional info per portion

Fibre 6.8g
Protein 14g
Plant Points 8.25

Makes about 500g (18oz)

Prep 2 mins

Cook 15 mins

2 tbsp brown or white miso

3 tbsp maple syrup

3 tbsp olive oil

1 tbsp chopped rosemary

1 tsp sweet paprika

½ tsp dried chilli (red pepper) flakes (optional)

500g (18oz) nuts (I use a mix of cashews, walnuts, pecans, hazelnuts, macadamia nuts, and skin-on almonds)

100g (¾ cup/3½oz) pumpkin seeds

Sea salt and freshly ground black pepper

The miso gives these nuts a moreish sweet and savory flavor—you'll be amazed at how delicious they are! They are perfect for snacking on, but I also love adding them to salads or roasted veggie suppers for an extra crunch and boost of healthy fat. Stored in an airtight container at room temperature, these will keep for 2 weeks.

1. Preheat the oven to 170°C/150°C fan/350°F and line a baking sheet with baking paper (parchment paper).

2. Place everything except the nuts and seeds in a bowl with ½ teaspoon each of salt and pepper and mix well. Add the nuts and seeds and stir so everything is nicely coated, then spread out in a single layer on the baking sheet.

3. Roast for 13–17 minutes, stirring occasionally, until the nuts turn golden brown. Allow to cool fully on the tray, then serve or store.

Note You can also make these in your air fryer! Heat the air fryer to 150°C/350°F and air fry for 10 minutes, tossing halfway.

For those of you with a sweet tooth, I see you! There's always room for dessert, and that's perfectly fine most of the time, especially when enjoying homemade treats. However, consistently purchasing UPF chocolate bars, cakes, and other sweet items can quickly push your daily sugar intake over the limit, without offering much in terms of nutritional value (just a lot of extra additives!).

With many confectionery items around the world still containing questionable additives, it's reassuring to know that you can make something healthier at home with ingredients you trust. By adding veggies and fruits to your sweet treats, you can also boost your fibre intake, reduce the amount of refined sugar they contain, and even add a boost of protein.

Something sweet

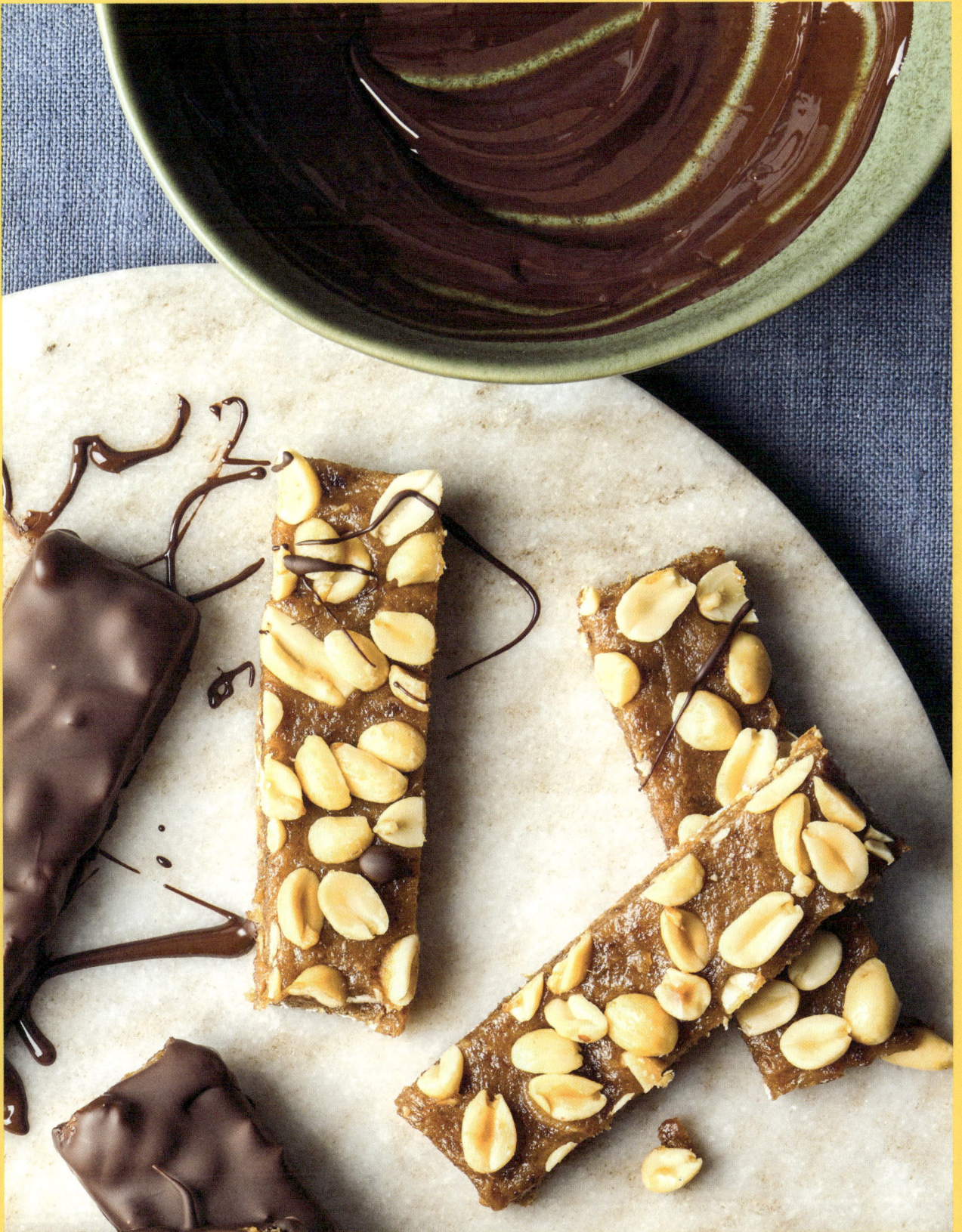

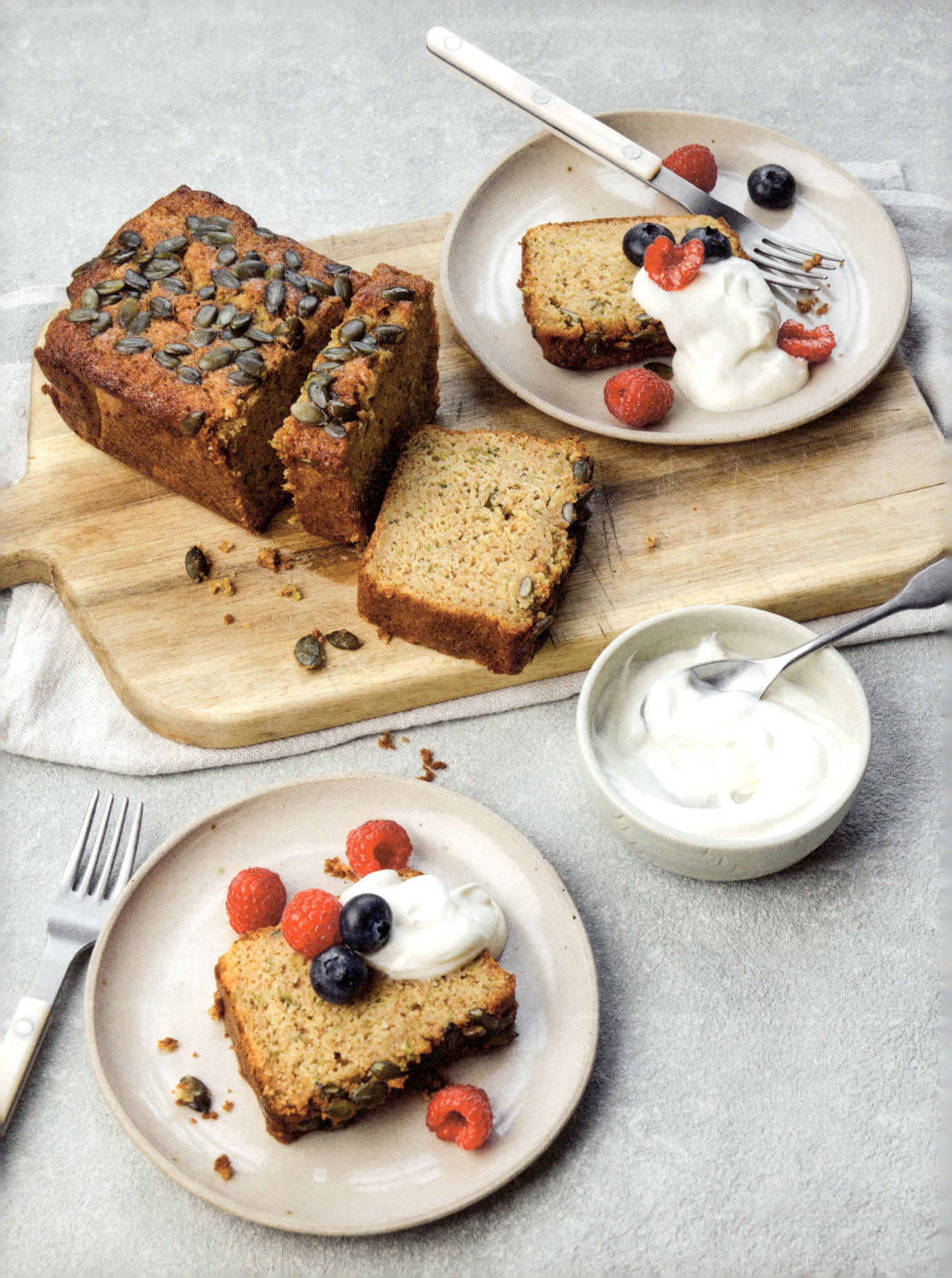

Courgette, miso, and olive oil cake

Nutritional info per 100g

Fibre 2.8g
Protein 10g
Plant Points 4.25

Makes 1 loaf (serves 6–8)

Prep 10 mins

Cook 40 mins

350g (12½oz) courgettes (zucchini)

150g (¾ cup/5½oz) light brown sugar

3 tbsp white miso

3 eggs

Zest of 2 lemons

90g (⅓ cup/3¼oz) olive oil, plus extra for greasing

175g (1¼ cups/6¼oz) spelt flour (wholemeal/whole wheat or white)

2 tsp baking powder

40g (5 tbsp/1¾oz) pumpkin seeds

Greek yogurt or skyr, to serve (optional)

Miso is a fermented ingredient, which is not only beneficial for your gut, but also adds a wonderful umami flavor to this cake. If you'd like to make this vegan, substitute the eggs for 3 tablespoons of aquafaba—just be sure to whisk it until fluffy before using. Stored in an airtight container at room temperature, this will keep for 5 days.

1. Preheat the oven to 180°C/160°C fan/350°F. Grease and line the base and sides of a 450g (1lb) loaf pan with olive oil and baking paper (parchment paper).

2. Coarsely grate (shred) the courgette straight onto a clean kitchen towel, pull up the sides and wring out any excess moisture over the sink, squeezing out as much liquid as possible. Set aside.

3. Add the sugar, miso, eggs, and lemon zest to a large mixing bowl. Whisk to combine, then slowly pour in the oil, whisking constantly until it just comes together. Sift in the flour and baking powder and fold to combine. Finally, gently stir through the courgette. Transfer the mixture to the lined loaf pan, smooth the top with a spatula, then sprinkle with the pumpkin seeds.

4. Bake in the middle of the oven for 40–50 minutes until a skewer inserted into the centre comes out clean. Allow to cool in the pan for 10 minutes, then turn out onto a wire rack to cool completely. Serve in slices with a dollop of yogurt, if you like.

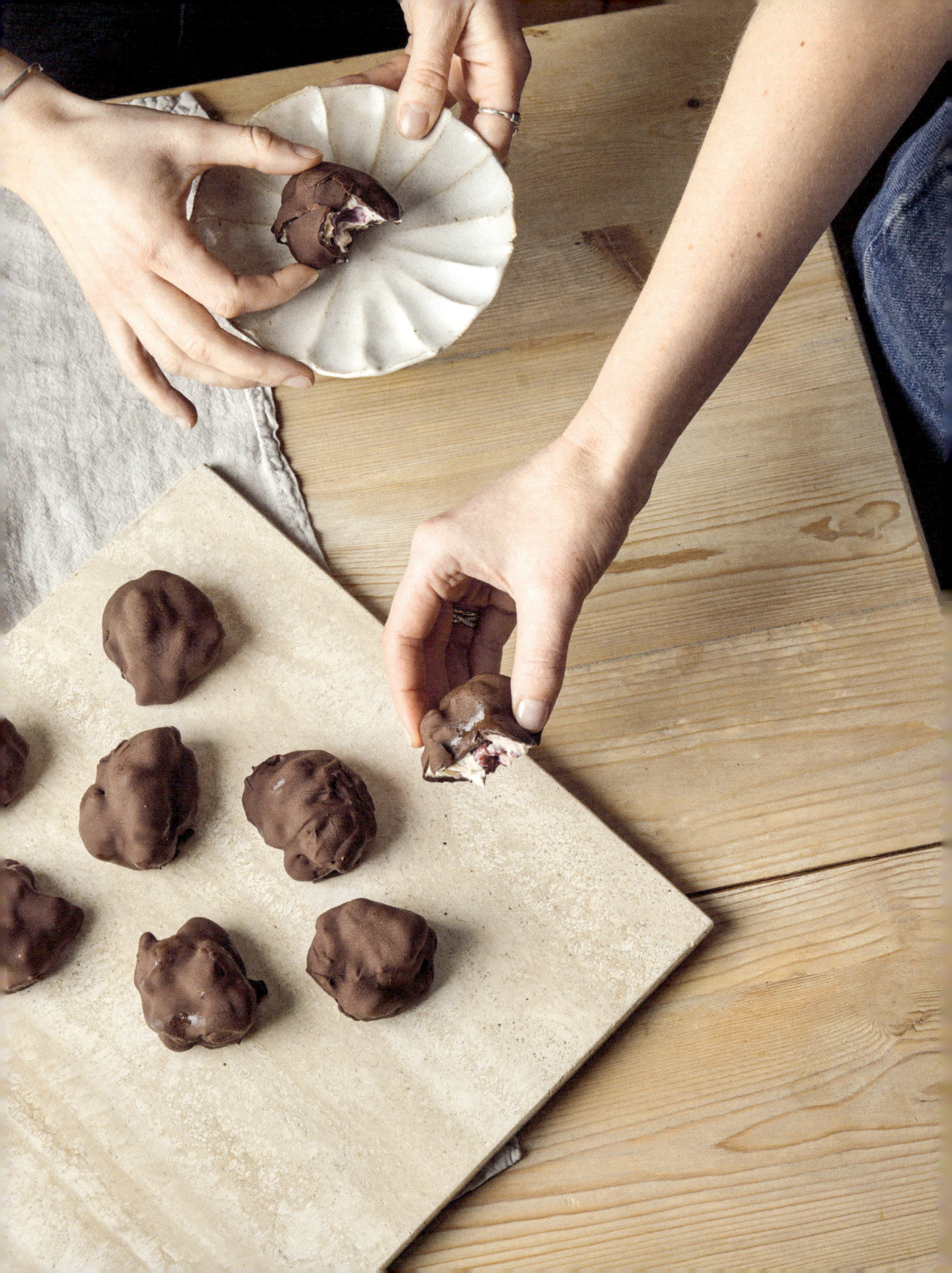

Frozen berry yogurt clusters

Makes 12

Prep 20 mins (plus freezing)

Cook 5 mins

175g (generous ¾ cup/ 6¼oz) Greek yogurt

2½ tbsp nut butter, such as peanut, cashew, or almond

½ tsp vanilla extract

125g (4½oz) frozen berries (I use a mix of blackberries, blueberries, and raspberries)

185g (6½oz) dark chocolate (at least 72% cocoa solids), broken into small pieces

1½ tsp coconut oil, plus extra for greasing

Ideal for hot summer days, these protein-rich and incredibly delicious bites are the perfect way to use up the frozen berries lurking in your freezer. You can use fresh berries if you prefer, and they're also lovely with some chopped banana added. These should be stored in the freezer and will keep for up to 1 month.

1. Line a baking sheet with baking paper (parchment paper) and grease the paper with a little coconut oil.

2. Add the yogurt, nut butter, and vanilla to a bowl and stir to completely combine, then fold in the berries.

3. Dollop heaped tablespoons of the mixture onto the lined baking sheet (you should have about 12), shaping them into little mounds. Place in the freezer for at least 2 hours until frozen solid.

4. Add the chocolate and coconut oil to a heatproof bowl set over a pan of barely simmering water and heat until just melted, stirring to combine. Alternatively, heat in a microwave on the lowest setting in 30-second blasts, stirring between each, until just melted. If you have a cooking thermometer, the chocolate is ready when it reads 45–50°C (113–122°F).

5. Remove the clusters from the freezer and reserve the lined baking sheet. Working quickly, toss the frozen berry clusters one at a time in the melted chocolate, using two forks to turn and fully coat them. Lift out of the bowl with one of the forks, allowing the excess chocolate to drip back into the bowl, then transfer them back to the lined sheet.

6. Once all the clusters are coated in chocolate, return the baking sheet to the freezer for at least 15 minutes until the chocolate is set. Store in an airtight container in the freezer and serve frozen.

Coconut rice pudding with mango

● **Serves** 4　　● **Prep** 2 mins　　● **Cook** 30 mins

150g (¾ cup/5½oz) pudding (short grain) rice

1 × 400g (14oz) can coconut milk

350ml (1½ cups/12½fl oz) almond milk

3 tbsp light brown sugar or coconut sugar, plus an extra 1 tsp

½ tsp ground cinnamon, plus extra to serve

A few gratings of nutmeg

2 tbsp pumpkin seeds

2 tbsp sunflower seeds

2 tbsp white and/or black sesame seeds

4 tbsp desiccated (dried shredded) coconut

1 ripe mango, peeled, de-stoned, and sliced

Sea salt

Creamy, comforting, and nourishing, this is quite a loose rice pudding, so simply use less milk if you prefer it thicker (although remember that it'll also thicken as it cools). Use whatever seeds you have to hand—I've used pumpkin, sunflower, and sesame seeds here, but linseeds (flaxseeds) and chia seeds would also be great. If you've got any leftover seed mix, use it to top your morning porridge.

1. Place the rice, coconut milk, almond milk, 3 tablespoons of sugar, the spices, and a pinch of salt in a heavy-bottomed saucepan set over a low–medium heat and bring to a simmer. Cook, stirring often, for 25–30 minutes until the rice has plumped-up and is tender.

2. Meanwhile, place a small frying pan (skillet) over a low–medium heat and add the pumpkin seeds. Cook, stirring, for 2–3 minutes until they begin to color and pop, then add the sunflower seeds, sesame seeds, and coconut. Cook for a further 3–4 minutes, stirring constantly, until everything is golden and toasted. Take off the heat, then stir in the 1 teaspoon of sugar and a pinch of salt.

3. Serve the rice pudding warm or chilled, topped with the fresh mango, a sprinkle of the coconutty toasted seeds, and an extra pinch of cinnamon.

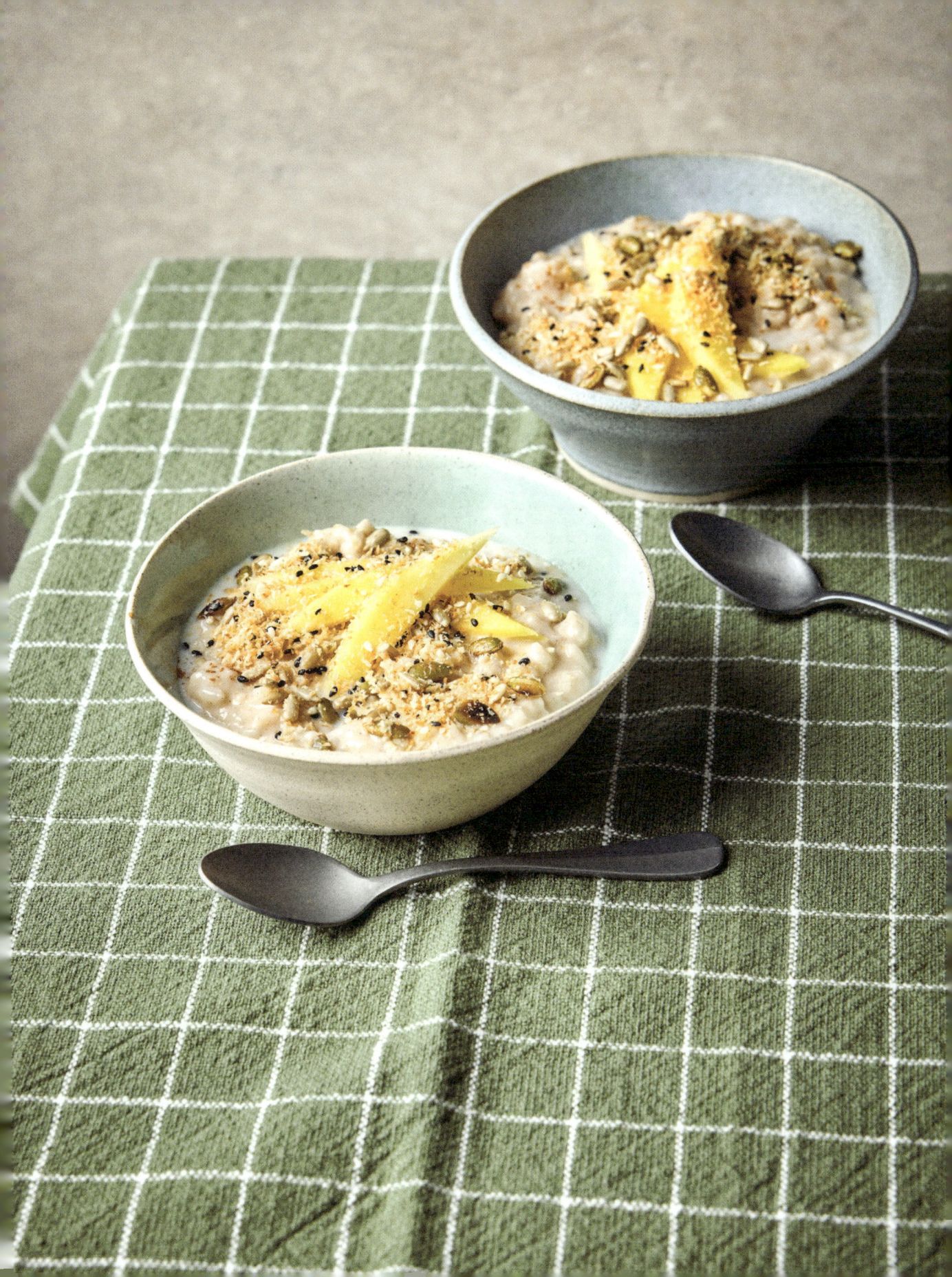

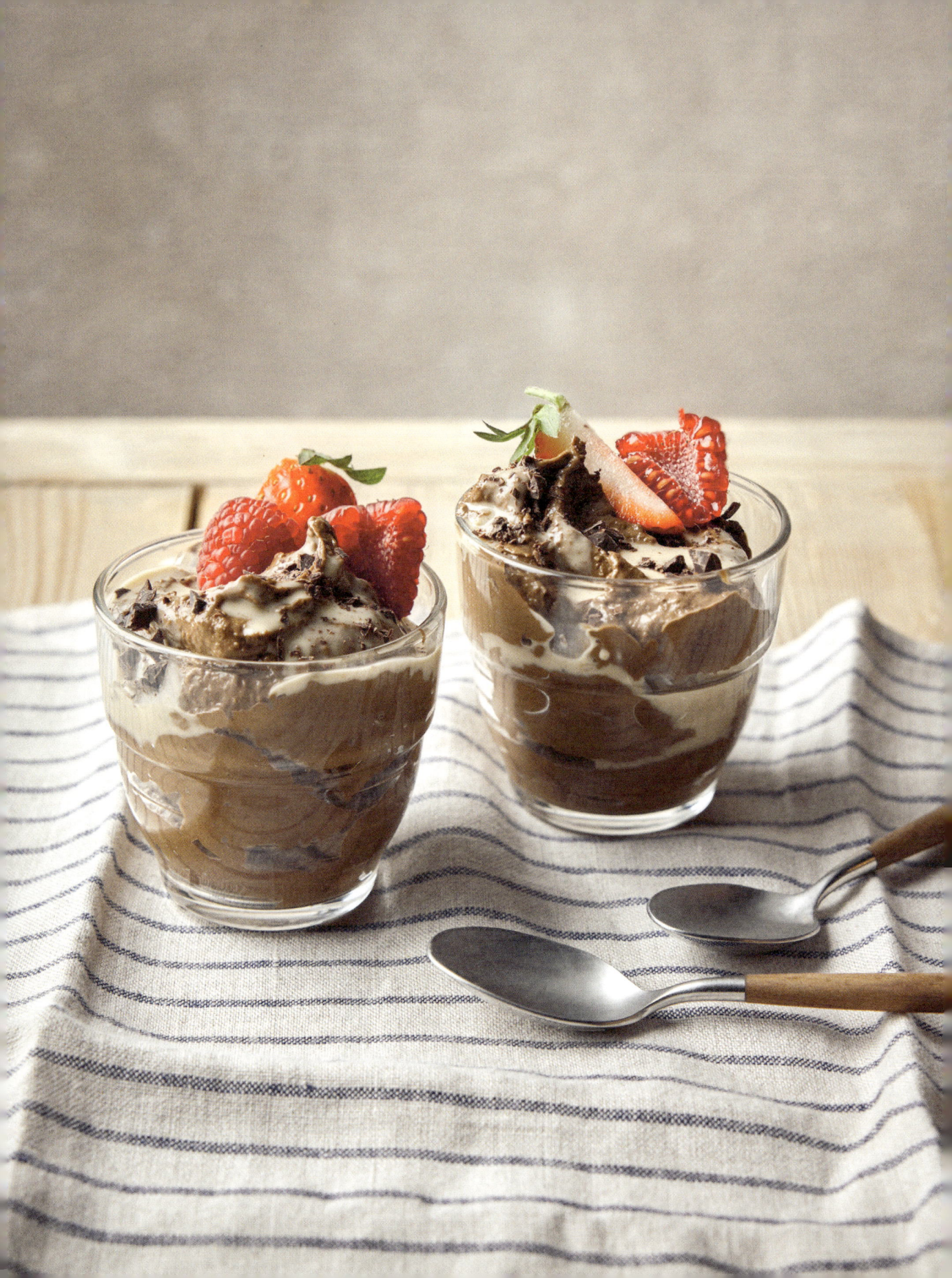

Avocado chocolate mousse

Makes 4   **Prep** 10 mins   **Cook** 0 mins

2 ripe avocados, peeled and de-stoned

1 small ripe banana

3 tbsp nut butter, such as peanut, cashew, or almond

2½ tbsp maple syrup or honey

2½ tbsp unsweetened cocoa powder

10g (⅓oz) dark chocolate (at least 72% cocoa solids), finely chopped (optional)

Fresh berries, to serve

Sea salt

Who would've thought an indulgent chocolate mousse could actually be good for you? Packed with protein and healthy fats, this tasty dessert could almost double up as breakfast. It's also great if you're having people over for dinner and want to get ahead on prep—simply make these the day before and store in the fridge until ready to serve.

1. Add the avocados, banana, 2 tablespoons of the nut butter, 2 tablespoons of the maple syrup, the cocoa powder, and a pinch of salt to a blender or food processor and blitz until smooth. Divide the mixture between 4 glasses or small serving bowls.

2. Whisk together the remaining tablespoon of nut butter and ½ tablespoon of maple syrup in a small bowl until completely combined, then very slowly whisk in ½–1 tablespoon water until you have a smooth, runny sauce.

3. Drizzle some sauce over each mousse, then sprinkle with chopped chocolate (if using) and a little sea salt. Decorate with a few berries, if you like, then serve immediately or chill in the fridge for up to 1 week.

Ice pops (2 ways)

Making homemade ice pops is such a great thing to do with little ones, and ensures they're treated to a little nutrition too. You'll need a 6-hole ice lolly (ice pop) mold for this recipe.

Makes 6

Prep 5 mins (plus freezing)

Cook 0 mins

Berry banana

250g (9oz) frozen mixed berries

1 ripe banana

250g (1 cup/9oz) Greek yogurt or coconut yogurt

2½ tbsp maple syrup or honey

½ tsp vanilla extract (optional)

1. Place everything in a blender or food processor, then blitz until whipped up and smooth.

2. Divide the mixture evenly between the molds and place in the freezer for at least 4 hours until frozen.

3. Dip the mold in hot water to loosen before serving.

Mango and lime

350g (12½oz) ripe mango chunks

Zest and juice of 1 lime

250ml (1 cup/9fl oz) fresh orange juice

2½ tbsp maple syrup or honey (optional)

1. Place the mango, lime zest and juice, and the orange juice in a blender or food processor, then blitz until whipped up and smooth. Taste for sweetness (if the mango wasn't fully ripe it may not be that sweet) and add the maple syrup or honey if needed and blitz again to combine.

2. Divide the mixture evenly between the molds and place in the freezer for at least 4 hours until frozen.

3. Dip the mold in hot water to loosen before serving.

Nutritional info per 100g

Fibre 1.3g
Protein 4.6g
Plant Points 4–6

Nutritional info per 100g

Fibre 14g
Protein 0.7g
Plant Points 3

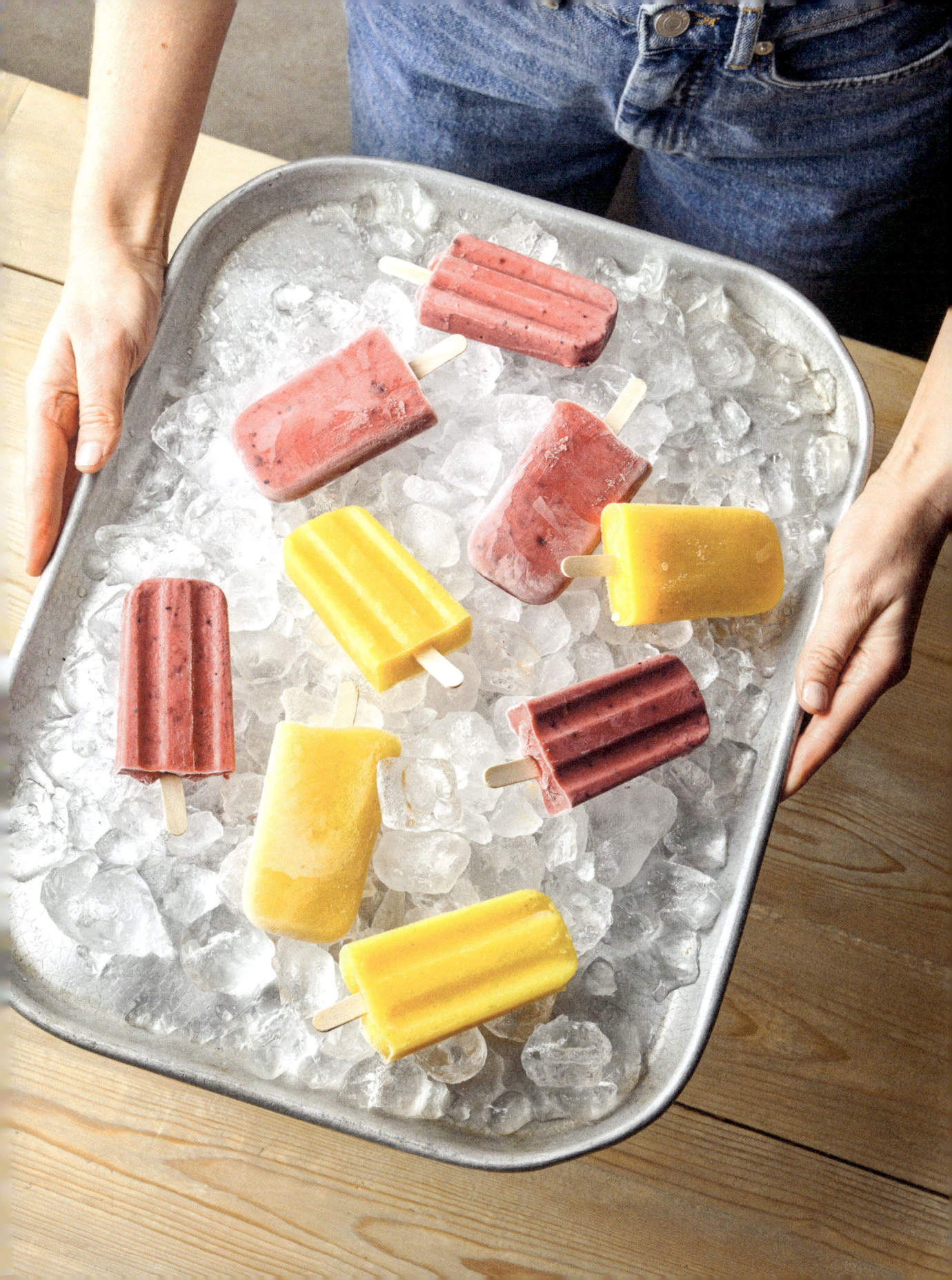

Chocolate, peanut, and date bars

Nutritional info per bar

Fibre 3.3g
Protein 5g
Plant Points 5

Makes about 15 bars

Prep 20 mins (plus freezing)

Cook 5 mins

75g (2¾oz) jumbo or rolled (old fashioned) oats

300g (10½oz) pitted Medjool dates

4 tbsp smooth peanut butter

1½ tsp vanilla extract

¼ tsp sea salt

80g (2¾oz) unsalted roasted peanuts

175g (6¼oz) dark chocolate (at least 72% cocoa solids), broken into small pieces

2 tsp coconut oil

Sticky, nutty, and chocolatey, these are the ultimate pick me up. You can slice these into smaller bars if you like, but if doing so, be aware that you may need a little more chocolate to coat all of them. In the summer, I love to eat these straight out of the freezer sprinkled with a tiny pinch of flaky salt!

1. Line a 20cm (8 inch) square cake pan with baking paper (parchment paper), with plenty of overhang. Place the oats in a blender or food processor and blitz to a fine flour, then tip into a bowl and set aside.

2. Place the dates in the blender or food processor (no need to clean it) with the peanut butter, vanilla, and salt. Roughly blitz, then slowly add 75ml (5 tbsp/2½fl oz) water until you have a smooth, thick paste. Be sure to scrape down the sides occasionally. Remove 300g (10½oz) of the date mix to a bowl and set aside.

3. Add the oat flour back to the blender or food processor containing the remaining date mix and pulse a few times until nicely combined. Tip the mixture into the base of the lined pan and use wet fingertips to spread it into a smooth layer that fills the tin.

4. Spread the reserved date mixture on top, smoothing it with a spatula. Evenly sprinkle over the nuts, pushing them in a little. Place in the freezer for at least 6 hours or ideally overnight until frozen and firm.

5. Lift the frozen slab out of the pan and slice into 15 bars. Line a baking sheet with baking paper (parchment paper).

6. Add the chocolate and coconut oil to a heatproof bowl set over a pan of barely simmering water and heat until just melted, stirring to combine. Alternatively, heat in a microwave on the lowest setting in 30-second blasts, stirring between each, until just melted. If you have a cooking thermometer, the chocolate is ready when it reads 45–50°C (113–122°F).

7. Working one at a time, submerge the bars in the melted chocolate, using two forks to turn them. Lift out of the bowl using the forks, allowing the excess chocolate to drip back into the bowl, then transfer them to the lined sheet. Once all the bars are coated in chocolate, return the sheet to the freezer or fridge for at least 15 minutes until the chocolate is set. Store in an airtight container in the fridge for up to 2 weeks or freezer for up to 4 weeks, but I assure you they won't last long!

Note If you can't find roasted peanuts, simply use unroasted peanuts and roast them in the oven at 180°C/160°C fan/350°F for 8–12 minutes until golden. Then use in the recipe as specified.

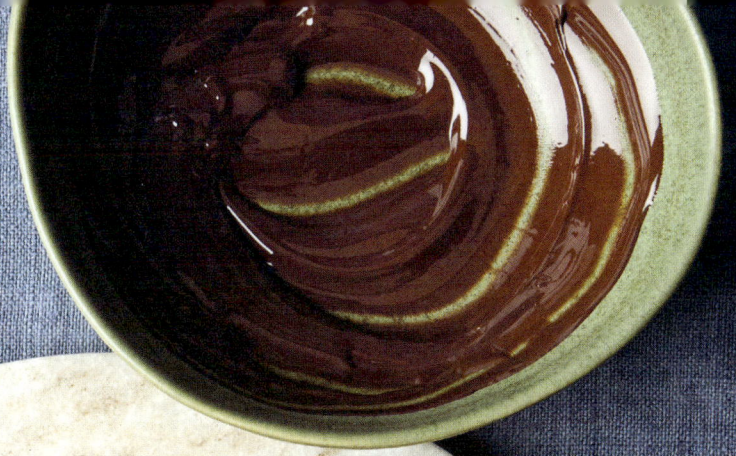

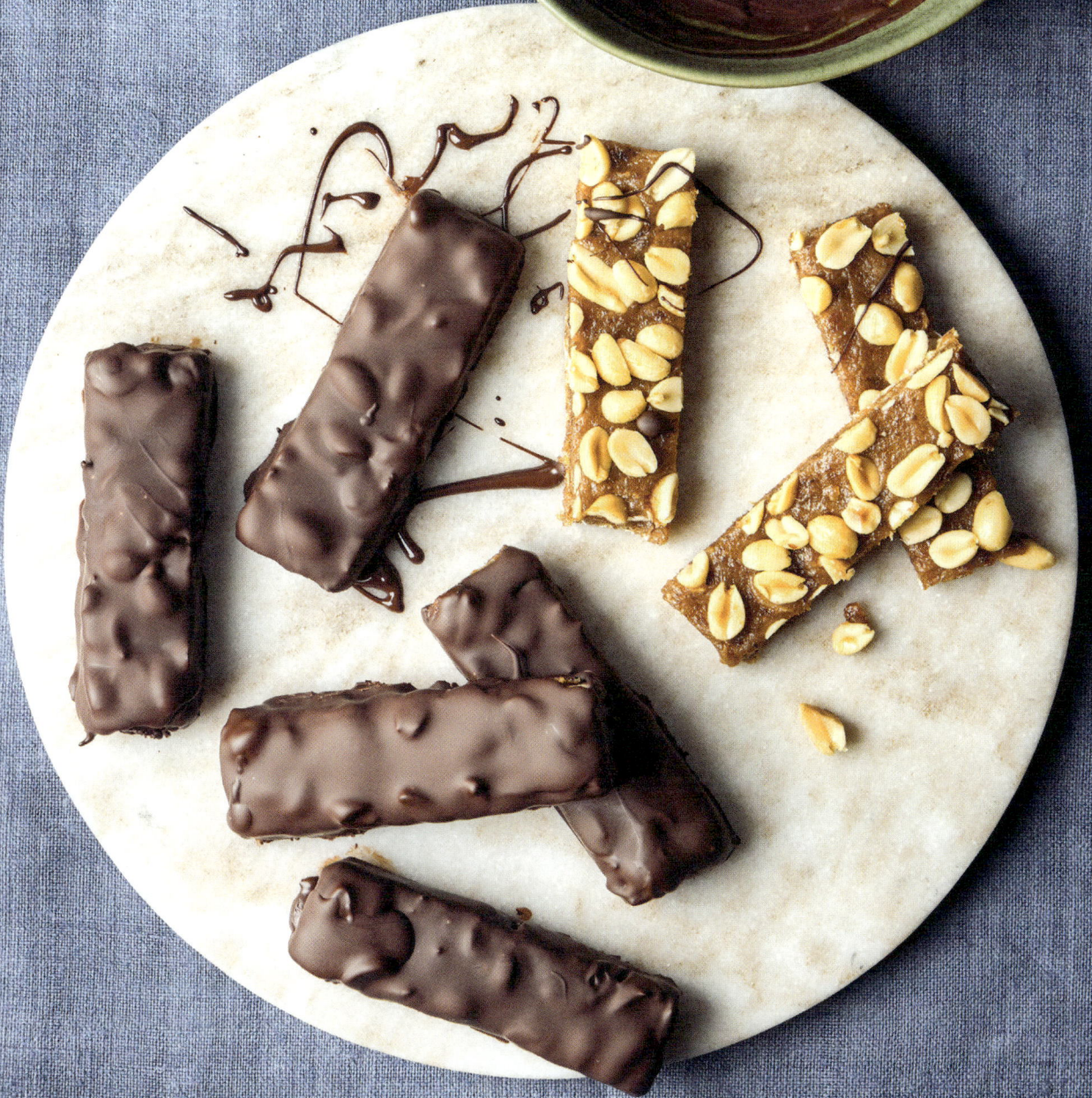

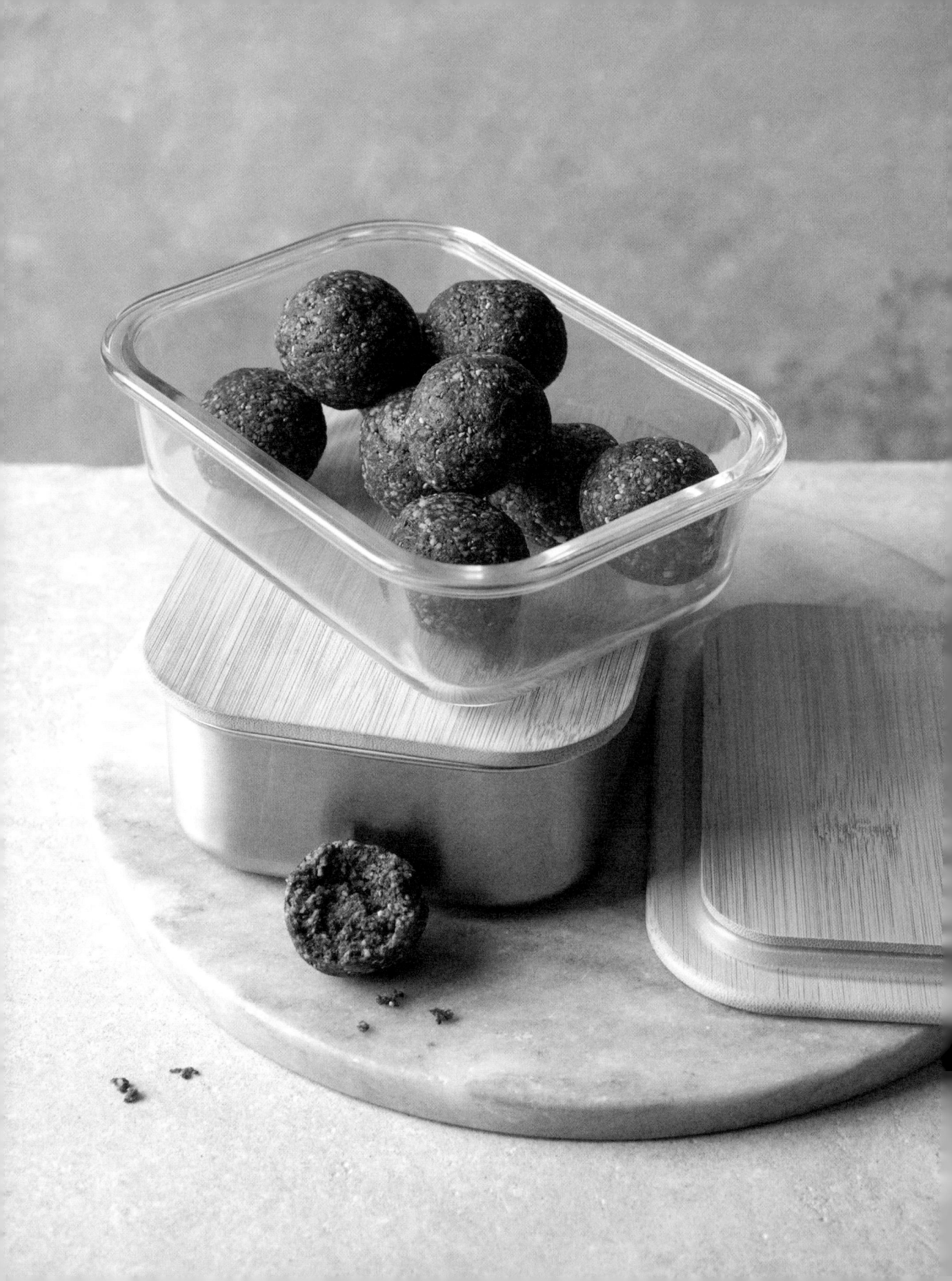

Coconut, date, and orange energy balls

Nutritional info per ball

Fibre 11g
Protein 10g
Plant Points 7

Makes 10

Prep 10 mins
(plus chilling)

Cook 0 mins

75g (2¾oz) skin-on or blanched almonds

25g (1oz) walnuts or hazelnuts

120g (4oz) pitted Medjool dates

1 tbsp chia seeds

50g (¾ cup/1¾oz) desiccated (dried shredded) coconut

2 tbsp unsweetened cocoa powder

1 tbsp coconut oil

Zest of ½ orange

½ teaspoon of sea salt

These little balls are packed with healthy fats and protein to give you a boost. Ideal before or after a workout or as an on-the-go snack for both adults and kids, it's always worth having a batch of these to hand.

1. Place all the nuts in a food processor and blitz until finely ground. Add the dates to the processor and keep blitzing for 1–2 minutes until the dates are puréed and the mixture is just beginning to clump.

2. Add all the remaining ingredients to the food processor and blitz until everything is just combined.

3. With damp hands, roll the mixture into 30g (1oz) balls (you should have about 10 balls). Place the balls on a plate or tray in the fridge for at least 1 hour to firm up before enjoying. Stored in an airtight container in the fridge, they'll keep for 2 weeks.

Fruit roll-ups

**Nutritional info
per ⅙ of a tray**

Fibre 12g
Protein 1.8g
Plant Points 2

Makes 1 tray

Prep 5 mins

Cook at least
12 hours

1 tsp flavorless oil

200g (7oz) cooking apples,
(such as Granny Smith,
Gala or Jonagold) peeled,
cored, and cut into large
chunks

400g (14oz) fresh or frozen
strawberries, hulled

**This twist on classic jelly candies is actually very simple to whip up. You can
replace the strawberries with any berries or fruit you like, depending on preference,
the season, or what you need to use up (although be sure not to replace the apples
as they help the rolls set). Although these have a long oven time, they're very
hands-off—I tend to prep them in the evening before I go to bed, then leave them
in the oven overnight.**

1. Preheat the oven to 50°C/120°F (do not use the fan setting). Line your largest
   baking sheet with baking paper (parchment paper), then rub the paper with the oil.

2. Place all the fruit in a large saucepan, cover with a lid and cook over a medium heat
   for 10–15 minutes until the apple is completely soft and tender and the berries have
   collapsed. Use an electric hand-held blender to blitz until completely smooth, then
   pass through a sieve (strainer) into a bowl, using a spoon to push it through.

3. Pour the sieved purée onto the lined baking sheet and use a spatula to evenly
   smooth it out to about 5mm (¼ inch) thick. Place in the oven for about 12 hours
   until it feels firm but flexible and not tacky.

4. Cut it into strips with scissors, then peel off the paper and roll them up. Stored in an
   airtight container at room temperature, they will keep for up to 2 weeks.

Alternative fruits

- Mango
- Blackberries
- Raspberries
- Blueberries
- Plum
- Pineapple
- Pear

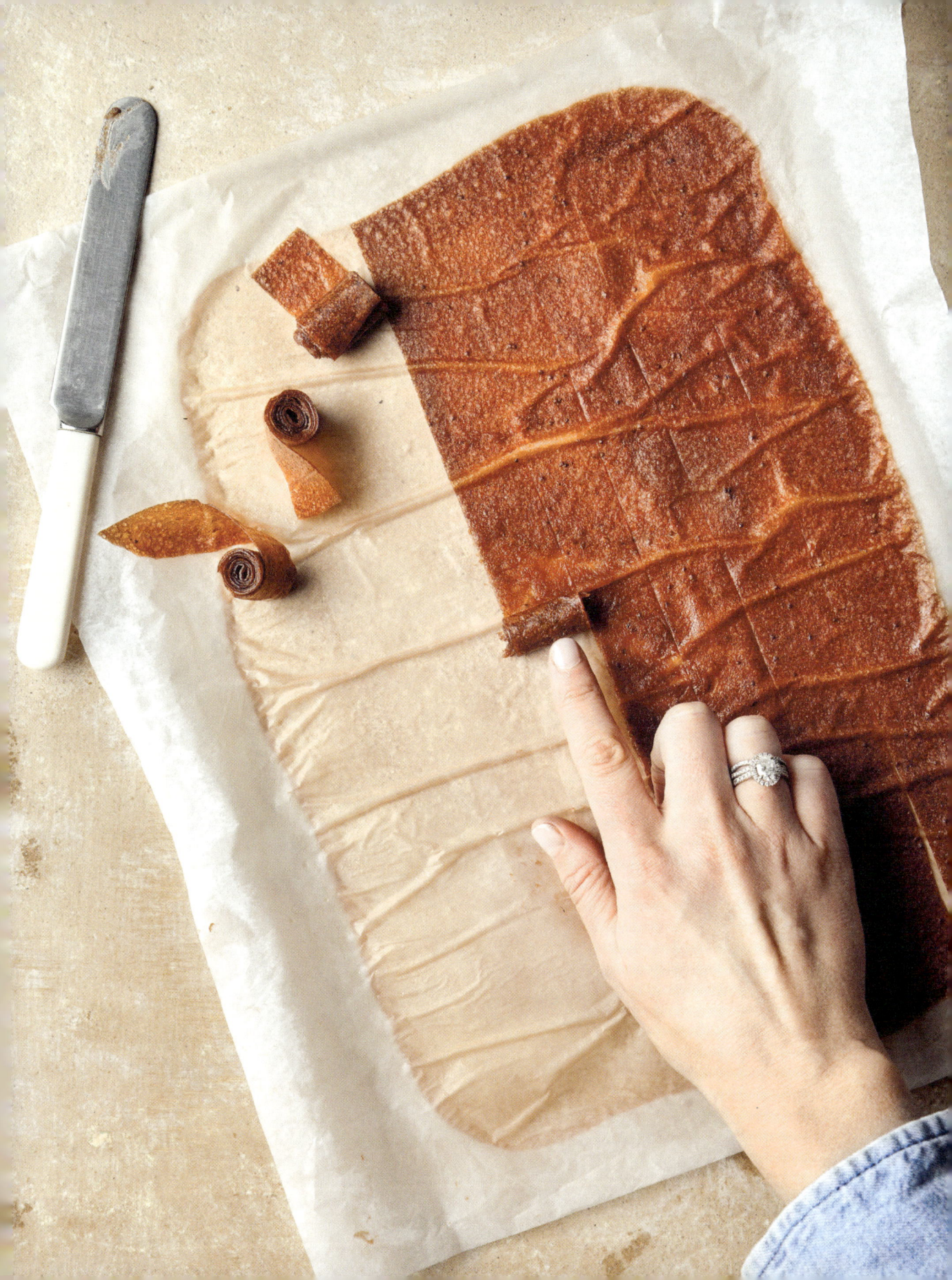

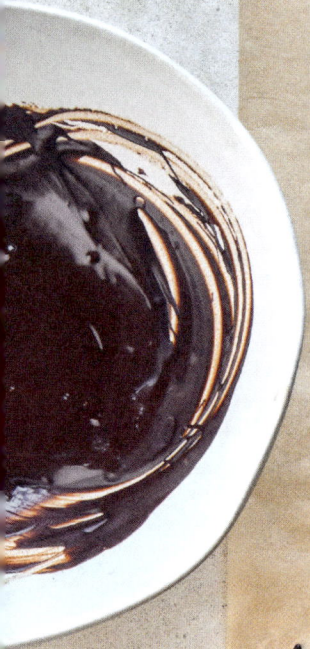

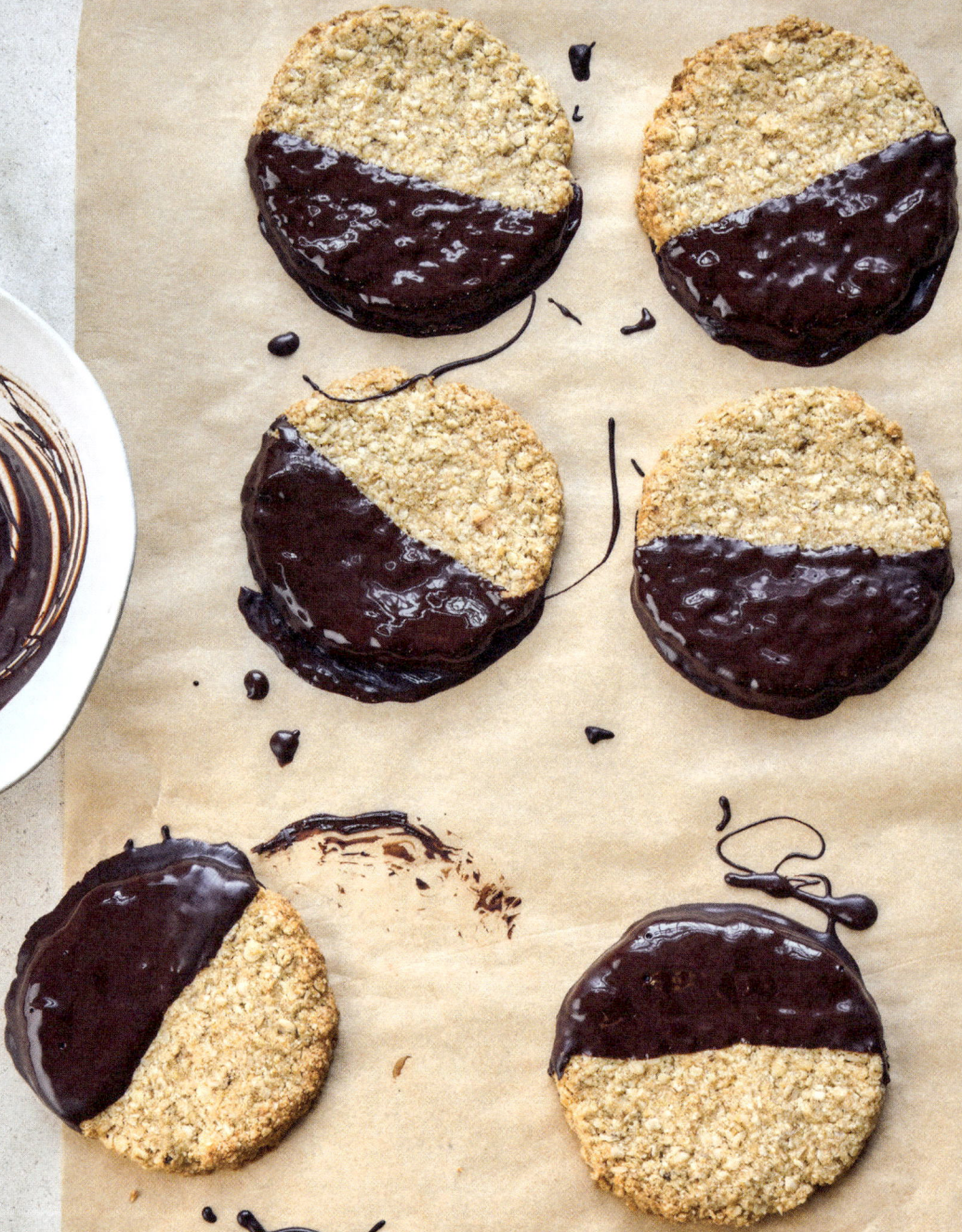

Dark chocolate and oat cookies

Nutritional info per cookie

Fibre 2.3g
Protein 4.1g
Plant Points 3

Makes about 14   **Prep** 15 mins   **Cook** 20 mins

200g (7oz) rolled (old fashioned) oats

75g (¾ cup/2¾oz) ground almonds

½ tsp sea salt

120g (½ cup/4oz) coconut oil

120ml (½ cup/4fl oz) maple syrup

100g (3½oz) dark chocolate (at least 72% cocoa solids), broken into small pieces

Who doesn't love a biscuit with a cup of tea? It may come across as very British, but I am convinced that biscuits and cookies have become ingrained in our food love language, no matter where you are in the world. These lower-UPF cookies use chocolate that has at least 75% cocoa solids, which adds to your plant points for gut health alongside the oats, antioxidants, minerals, and flavanols. Most chocolate you buy will have additives included (it's hard to avoid this) but chocolate is an incredible food if you keep the cocoa percentage high, plus the higher the percentage, the less added sugar there is.

1. Preheat the oven to 180°C/160°C fan/350°F and line a large baking sheet with baking paper (parchment paper).

2. Place 60g (2oz) of the oats in a blender or food processor and blitz to a fine powder. Tip this into a large bowl along with the remaining oats, the ground almonds, the and salt.

3. In a small saucepan set over a low heat, gently melt the coconut oil, then allow it to cool slightly. Stir in the maple syrup, then pour the wet mixture over the dry ingredients and mix to completely combine.

4. Divide the mixture into about 14 equal balls, rolling them between your hands to shape them. Place them on the lined baking sheet, then gently press each ball down with the base of a glass to create cookie shapes.

5. Bake for 15–18 minutes until firm to the touch and lightly golden on the edges. Allow the cookies to cool slightly on the sheet before transferring to a wire rack to cool completely (do not discard the lined baking sheet).

6. Add the chocolate to a heatproof bowl set over a pan of barely simmering water and heat until just melted. Alternatively, heat in a microwave on the lowest setting in 30-second blasts, stirring between each, until just melted. If you have a cooking thermometer, the chocolate is ready when it reads 45–50°C (113–122°F).

7. Dip the cooled cookies halfway into the melted chocolate. Place them back on the lined baking sheet and place in the fridge or somewhere cool for 10–15 minutes, until the chocolate is firm to the touch. These will keep for up to 5 days in an airtight container at room temperature or the fridge.

Most of us don't think twice about adding condiments to our food when we're out and about. But if you check the ingredients, you'll often find they're packed with additives, salt, sugar, and fat—things that help preserve flavor and shelf life. In this section, I'll show you that it's entirely possible to make these condiments at home without compromising on taste. In fact, they're not only better for your taste buds but also for your health.

Sauces and essentials

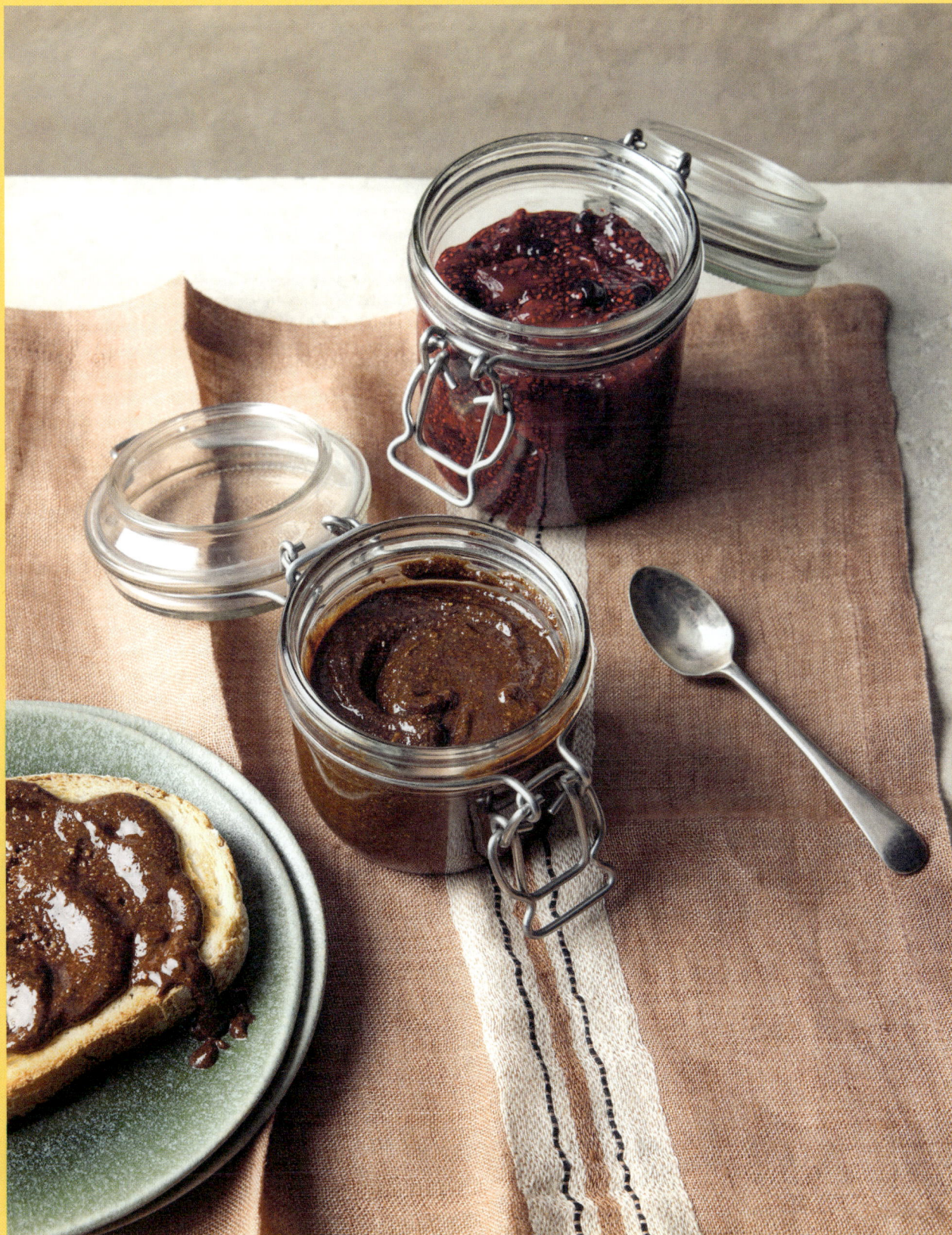

Chia and berry jam

Nutritional info per 100g

Fibre 8.2g
Protein 3.6g
Plant Points 2

Makes 1 large jar about 650g (23oz)

Prep 2 mins

Cook 10 mins

500g (18oz) frozen berries, such a raspberries, blueberries, strawberries, or blackcurrants

6–8 tbsp honey, date syrup, or maple syrup, plus extra to taste

5 tbsp chia seeds

I make this every month with my children because it's so easy, nutritious, and far superior health-wise to store-bought jam (jelly). It contains omega-3 from chia seeds, and the frozen berries, with their delicious, dark colors, provide polyphenols and anthocyanins, which support brain health. Pictured on page 203.

1. Add the berries, the honey or syrup and 4 tablespoons of water to a medium saucepan and place over a low heat. Cook for 5–8 minutes, stirring occasionally, until the berries have broken down.

2. At this stage, depending on how textured you like your jam, you can either leave the berries whole, crush them with a potato masher, or blitz them into a smooth purée with an electric hand-held blender. Add more honey or syrup, to taste, if needed.

3. Stir in the chia seeds, then transfer to a sterilized jar. Allow to cool, then store in the fridge for up to 5 days.

Nutty chocolate spread

Nutritional info per 100g

Fibre 9g
Protein 13g
Plant Points 2

Makes 300g (10½oz)

Prep 10 mins

Cook 0 mins

250g (9oz) blanched roasted hazelnuts

20g (2¼ tbsp/¾oz) unsweetened cocoa powder

60g (5 tbsp/2oz) dark brown sugar

¼ tsp sea salt

Everyone loves chocolate spread, but did you know that it's super simple to make at home with just a blender and a handful of ingredients? This never lasts long in our house, so while you have the chance, slather it on soda bread (page 97) or serve it with sliced apple for dipping as a mid-afternoon snack. Pictured on page 203.

1. Place the nuts in a high-speed blender or food processor and blitz until they turn into a smooth butter. The mixture will clump and then loosen again and you'll need to scrape down the sides a few times to get it to blend properly. If you feel the blender or processor overheating, stop, let it cool, then continue blitzing.

2. Once you have a smooth, fairly wet nut butter, add the rest of the ingredients and continue to blitz for another 2–3 minutes to allow the sugar to dissolve.

3. Transfer the nutty chocolate spread to a sterilized jar and store at room temperature for up to 2 weeks.

Note If you can only find skin-on, unroasted hazelnuts, simply roast them for 8–10 minutes at 180°C (350°F). As soon as they come out of the oven, rub them between a kitchen towel to remove the skins.

Spiced tomato ketchup

Nutritional info per 100g

Fibre 1.4g
Protein 0.9g
Plant Points 4.25

Makes 1 large jar about 525g (18½oz)

Prep 5 mins

Cook 1 hour

2 tbsp olive oil, cold-pressed rapeseed oil, or avocado oil

1 onion, chopped

1 tbsp chopped fresh ginger

2 garlic cloves, chopped

½ tsp ground cumin

½ tsp ground cinnamon

¼ tsp ground allspice

¼ tsp sweet paprika

⅛ tsp ground cloves

4 tbsp apple cider vinegar

4 tbsp dark brown sugar

2 × 400g (14oz) cans chopped tomatoes

Sea salt and freshly ground black pepper

This is very satisfying to make, and tastes less sweet than its store-bought counterpart. Dollop it onto fridge-raid omelette muffins (page 105) or take a leaf out of my kids' book and use as a dip for fish sticks (page 168). Pictured on page 209.

1. Drizzle the oil into a large deep saucepan set over a medium heat. When the oil is hot, add the onion and a pinch of salt and cook for 10 minutes until soft.

2. Add the ginger and garlic and cook for a further 2–3 minutes until fragrant, then add all the spices and stir them into the onions for 30 seconds.

3. Next add the vinegar, sugar, tomatoes, 1 teaspoon of salt, and a good grinding of pepper and bring to a simmer. Reduce the heat to low, and leave to cook for 45 minutes, stirring often to make sure it isn't catching, until thickened and reduced.

4. Use an electric hand-held blender (or regular blender) to blitz the ketchup until completely smooth, then pass it through a sieve (strainer) set over a bowl, using a spoon to push it through. Check and adjust the seasoning, if needed.

5. Transfer to a sterilized glass jar or bottle, allow to cool, then store in the fridge for up to 3 weeks.

Aquafaba mayonnaise

Nutritional info per 100g

Fibre 0g
Protein 0.5g
Plant Points 0.75

Makes 400g (14oz)

Prep 5 mins

Cook 0 mins

100ml (⅓ cup/3½fl oz) aquafaba (see intro)

1 small garlic clove, chopped

2 tsp Dijon mustard

2 tbsp apple cider vinegar, white wine vinegar or lemon juice

150g (⅔ cup/5½oz) mild olive oil

150g (⅔ cup/5½oz) sunflower oil

Sea salt and freshly ground black pepper

Aquafaba is the liquid that canned or jarred pulses are cooked in, and it can act as a great substitute for eggs. Chickpea and white bean aquafaba in particular have a very neutral flavor, so are ideal for making mayonnaise. Save the liquid from the can when making hummus (page 174), so you can whip up this simple mayo. Pictured on page 209.

1. Place the aquafaba, garlic, mustard, 1 teaspoon salt, and the vinegar or lemon juice in a jug (pitcher) and blitz with an electric hand-held blender (or regular blender) on the highest setting for about 15 seconds until completely blended and frothy.

2. Combine both the oils in a separate small jug, then very slowly drizzle them into the aquafaba mixture with the blender still running. If using, move the hand-held blender up and down constantly to get as much air into the mixture as possible. You'll soon find the mayonnaise begins to thicken. Once all the oil has been incorporated, taste the mayonnaise and add some black pepper and a little extra vinegar or salt if needed.

3. Store in an airtight container in the fridge for up to 1 week.

Note If you want to jazz up your mayo, try stirring in a little smoked paprika or chilli powder, or some chopped herbs, capers, or anchovies.

Tartare sauce

Nutritional info per 100g

Fibre 0.8g
Protein 6g
Plant Points 3

Serves 4   **Prep** 5 mins   **Cook** 0 mins

2 spring (green) onions or 2 small shallots, finely chopped

1½ tbsp capers in brine, plus 4 tbsp brine from the jar

Small handful of dill or parsley leaves, finely chopped

150g (½ cup/5½oz) Greek yogurt

50g (3½ tbsp/1¾oz) aquafaba mayonnaise (page 207), or 3½ tbsp Greek yogurt mixed with 1 tbsp olive oil)

Sea salt and freshly ground black pepper

This sauce is perfect with most fish, like my seeded wholemeal fishcakes (page 156) or fish sticks, chips, and peas (page 168) and is also ideal for topping jacket (baked) potatoes.

1. Combine all the ingredients in a small bowl and mix well, then season to taste with salt and pepper. It should be quite punchy and acidic, so add a little more caper brine if you feel it needs it.

2. Store in an airtight container in the fridge for up to 1 week.

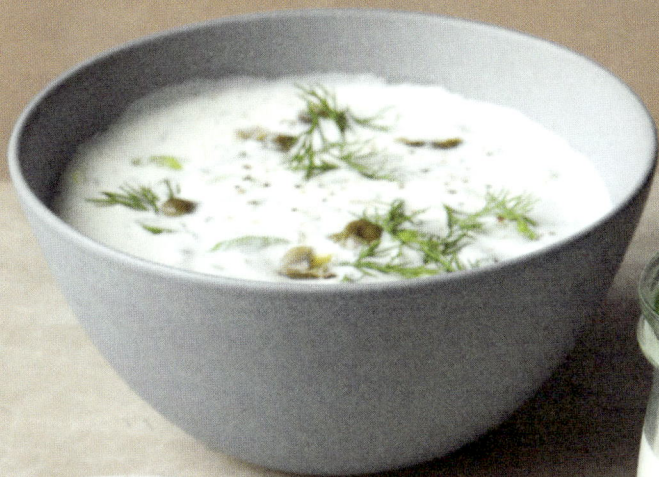

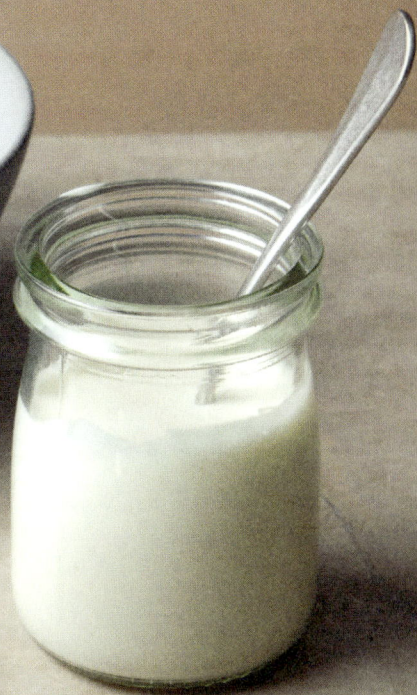

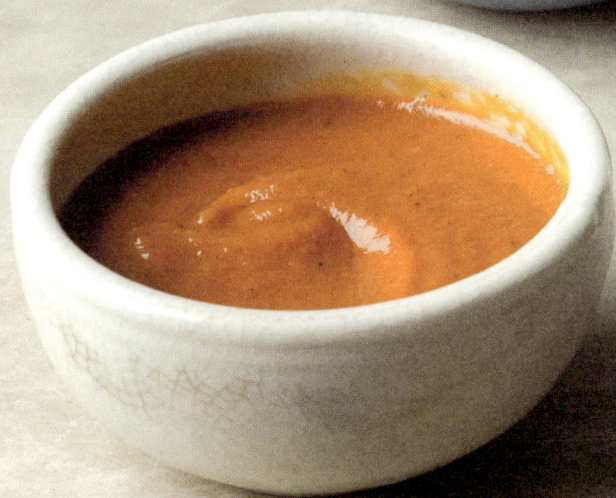

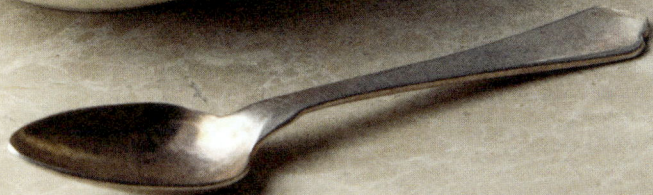

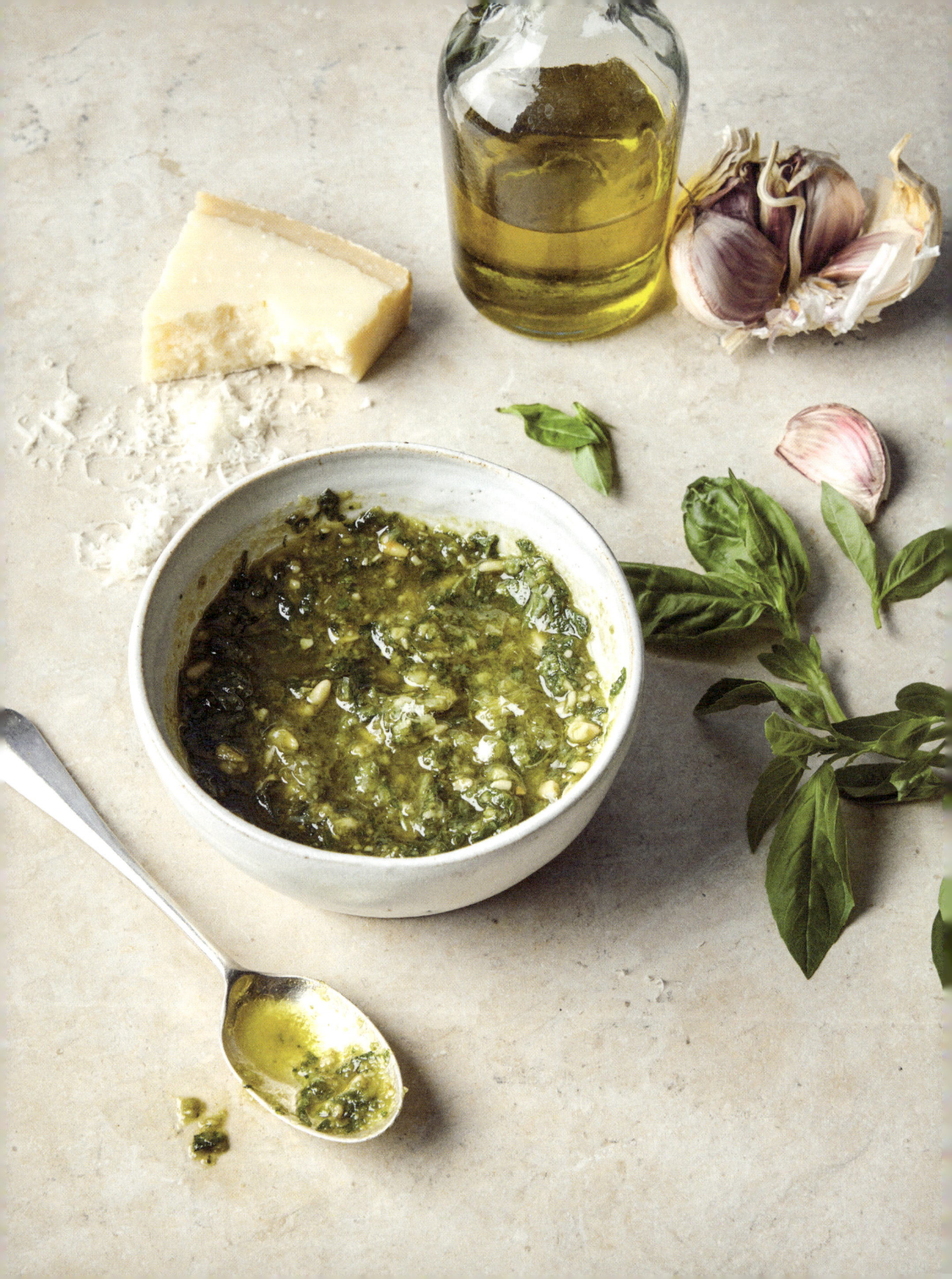

Green pesto

Makes 300g (10½oz)

Prep 10 mins

Cook 0 mins

60g (2oz) pine nuts

1 small garlic clove, chopped

75g (2¾oz) basil leaves

50g (1¾oz) Parmesan (or veggie/vegan alternative), finely grated

125g (½ cup/4oz) extra-virgin olive oil, plus extra if needed

Sea salt

Once you've got the hang of making basic pesto, you can try recreating it with almost any nut or seed and a range of different herby or peppery leaves (see below for a few different ideas). If you plan to store the pesto in the fridge instead of using it immediately, drizzle the top with olive oil to help preserve the vibrant color. This recipe makes enough to toss with pasta for about 4–6 people.

1. Place the nuts, garlic and ¼ teaspoon of salt in a small food processor (or a pestle and mortar) and blitz (or pound) until you have very small chunks.

2. Add the basil and pulse (or pound) until finely chopped, then add the Parmesan and olive oil and blitz until you have a bright green paste. Season to taste with more salt, if needed.

3. Stir straight into hot pasta or store in the fridge for up to 5 days (see intro), or in the freezer for up to 1 month.

Note Add leftover cooked peas or greens to the blender when making pesto as an easy way to get some extra vegetables into your diet.

Alternative nuts or seeds

- Roasted hazelnuts
- Walnuts
- Almonds
- Macadamia nuts
- Pumpkin seeds

Alternative leaves

- Rocket (arugula)
- Parsley
- Wild garlic
- Spinach

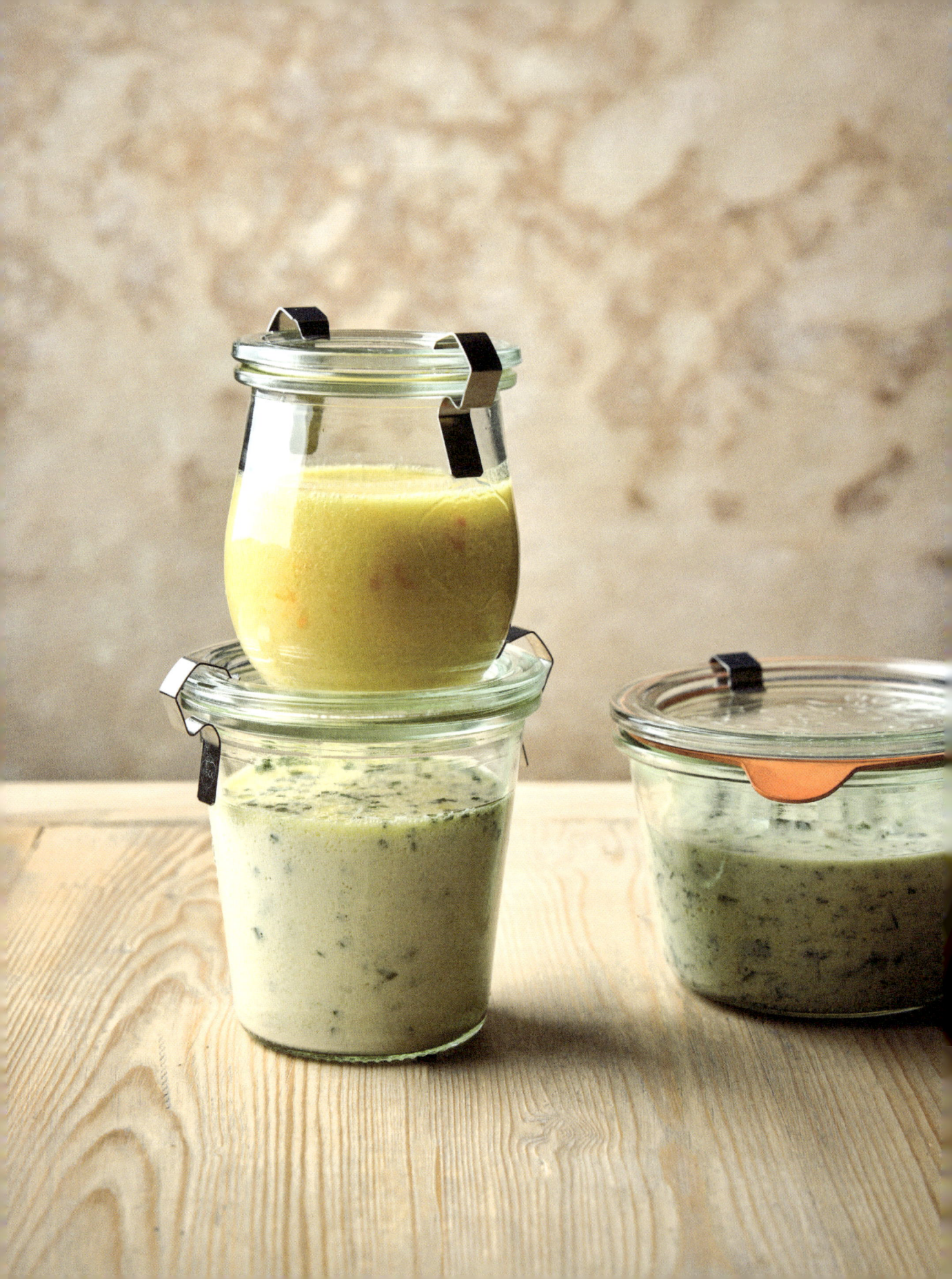

Dressing (3 ways)

These three dressings will elevate your salads to new heights! Try tossing them with leaves, grains, seeds, and roasted veggies for a flavor-packed lunch.

Makes 250g (9 oz)   **Prep** 5 mins   **Cook** 0 mins

Sour cream and sauerkraut

1 small garlic clove, grated

6 tbsp sour cream or Greek yogurt

1 heaped tbsp Dijon mustard

1 tsp maple syrup (optional)

125ml (½ cup/4fl oz) sauerkraut brine or 2 tbsp white wine vinegar

6 tbsp extra-virgin olive oil

1 heaped tbsp chopped chives

Sea salt and freshly ground black pepper

1. Stir all the ingredients together in a small bowl and season to taste.

2. Store in an airtight container in the fridge for up to 5 days.

Green Goddess

½ small garlic clove, grated

1½ tbsp capers in brine, plus 1 tbsp brine from the jar

Small handful of parsley leaves

Small handful of dill leaves

Small handful of mint leaves

Zest and juice of 1 small lemon

8 tbsp Greek yogurt

5 tbsp extra-virgin olive oil

½ shallot, finely chopped

Sea salt and freshly ground black pepper

1. Place everything except the shallot and seasoning in a blender or food processor and blitz until smooth.

2. Stir in the shallot and season to taste with salt and pepper.

3. Store in an airtight container in the fridge for up to 5 days.

Ginger and miso

2½ tbsp white miso

1 tsp grated fresh ginger

Juice of 1 lemon

Zest and juice of 1 orange

200g (scant 1 cup/7oz) extra-virgin olive oil

Sea salt and freshly ground black pepper

1. Whisk all the ingredients together in a small bowl until emulsified, then season to taste with salt and pepper.

2. Store in an airtight container in the fridge for up to 5 days.

Nutritional info per 100g

Fibre 0g
Protein 1.6g
Plant Point 1

Nutritional info per 100g

Fibre 1.2g
Protein 5g
Plant Points 3.75

Nutritional info per 100g

Fibre 1.2g
Protein 1.4g
Plant Points 2.75

Soup and salad sprinkles

Use these crunchy and crispy sprinkles to top your favourite salads and soups to add texture and an extra punch of nutrition.

Makes 220g (8oz)　　**Prep** 2 mins　　**Cook** 35 mins

Roast butter beans and chickpeas

1 × 400g (14oz) can of butter (lima) beans, drained and rinsed
1 × 400g (14oz) can of chickpeas, drained and rinsed
3 tbsp olive oil, cold-pressed rapeseed oil, or avocado oil
1½ tsp sweet paprika
½ tsp sea salt

1. Preheat the oven to 180°C/160°C fan/350°F and line a baking tray with baking paper (parchment paper).

2. Use paper towels to roughly dry the pulses, then transfer them to a medium bowl and add the oil, paprika, and salt. Toss to combine, then spread over the baking tray in a single layer—the more space they have, the crisper they'll get.

3. Roast for 30–35 minutes until everything is golden. The cooking time will vary, so keep checking them until they're done. Set aside—they'll crisp more as they cool.

4. Use within a few hours for ultimate crispiness, though they do reheat well in the oven. Store in an airtight container at room temperature for up to 1 week.

Nutritional info per 100g

Fibre 7.3g
Protein 21g
Plant Points 3

Tamari seeds

100g (generous ¾ cup/3½oz) pumpkin seeds
100g (¾ cup/3½oz) sunflower seeds
20g (2½ tbsp/¾oz) sesame seeds
4 tbsp tamari or soy sauce

1. Place a large frying pan (skillet) over a medium heat. When hot, add the pumpkin seeds. Toast, occasionally shaking the pan until they start to pop and the majority have darkened, then add the sunflower and sesame seeds and toast for a further 2–3 minutes until they've got a bit of color too.

2. Turn off the heat and immediately add the tamari or soy sauce. Stir to make sure all the seeds are coated, then leave to cool in the pan. Store in an airtight container at room temperature for up to 2 weeks.

Note You can cook these using your air fryer too! Heat the air fryer to 180°C/350°F and air fry for 10–12 minutes, tossing occasionally.

Nutritional info per 100g

Fibre 5.1g
Protein 7.1g
Plant Points 2.5

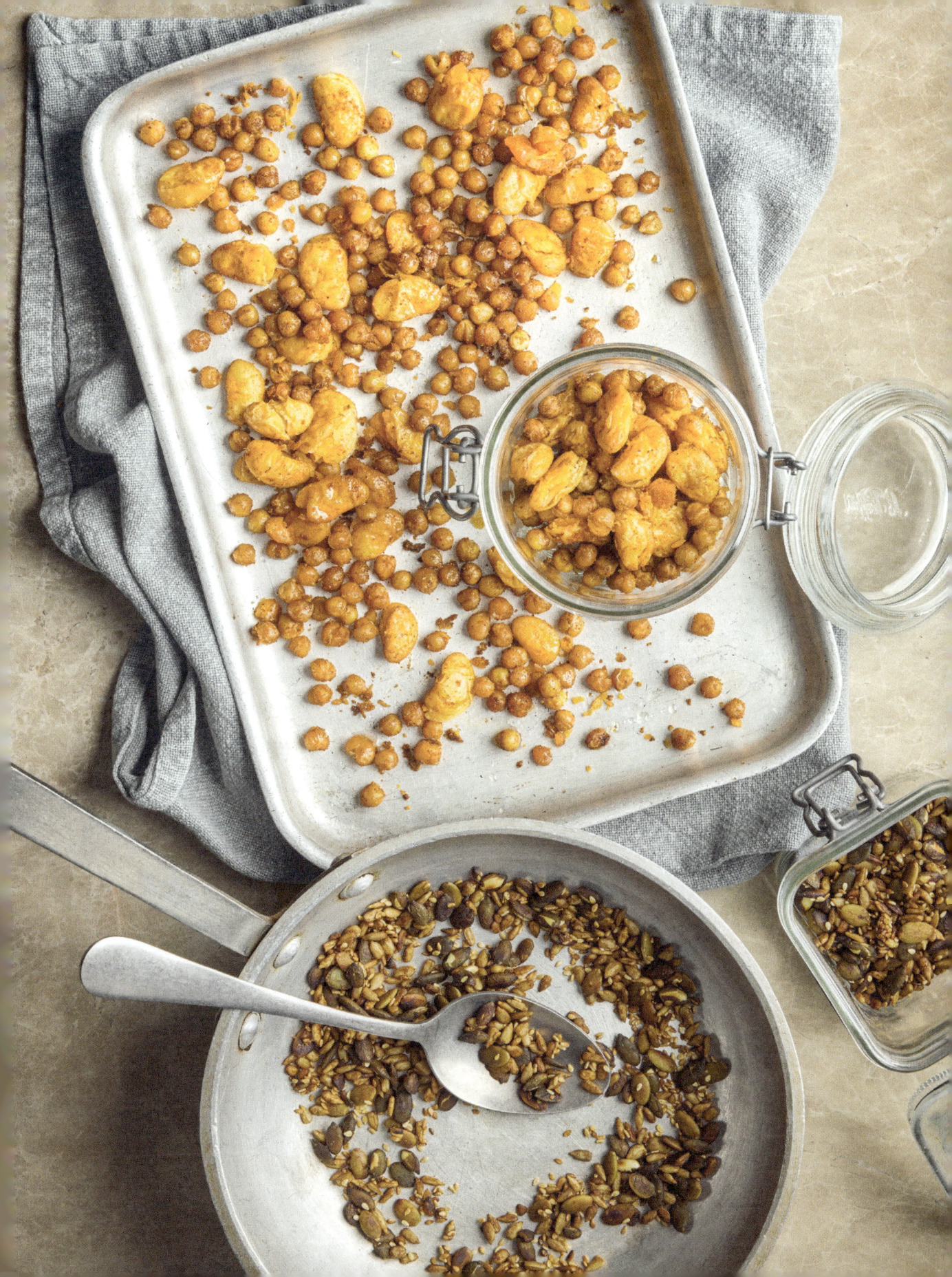

Recipe notes

- When possible, always use **organic** ingredients to reduce pesticide exposure (the difference between organic and non-organic is marginal when it comes to the availability of nutrients, though).

- Use **locally sourced** produce when possible.

- Avoid products containing **palm oil**.

- Opt for **unwaxed fruits**.

- **Fish** should be MSC certified. Always try new varieties; the oceans are already over-farmed.

- **Meat** should be free-range and sustainably sourced.

- **Eggs** should be free-range. Try to research the farm they travel from for welfare standards

- Use **natural sweeteners** like honey, maple syrup, or mashed fruit instead of artificial sweeteners. Reduce reliance on ultra-processed syrups and sweeteners where possible.

- Where possible, choose **dark chocolate** with more than 72% cocoa solids with minimal added ingredients.

- I mostly use sea **salt** flakes when cooking, but these measurements are not interchangeable with fine salt. If using fine salt, halve the amount stated in the recipe.

- Reduce the amount of food you buy in **plastic** and make active switches when you see produce available that is either recyclable or not packaged at all.

- Always use food in date and check the full ingredients list for salt, sugar, and saturated fat levels.

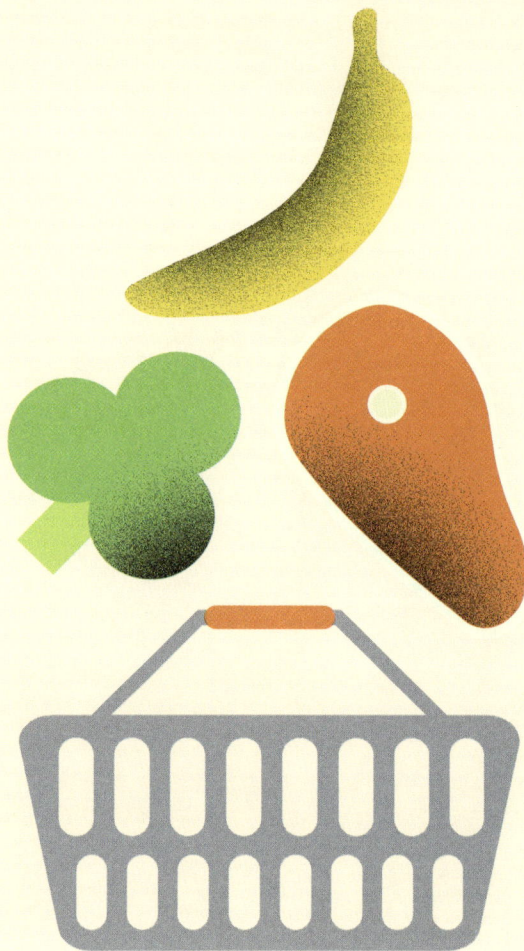

Resources and bibliography

Books

Every Body Should Know This by Federica Amati

Ravenous: How to get ourselves and our planet into shape by Henry Dimbleby

Spoon Fed by Tim Spector

The 30 Plan by Catherine Rabess

The Science of Nutrition by Rhiannon Lambert

The Science of Plant-Based Nutrition by Rhiannon Lambert

Ultra-processed People by Chris van Tulleken

Unprocess Your Life by Rob Hobson

Well Fed by James Collier

Why Calories Don't Count by Giles Yeo

Podcasts

A Thorough Examination with Drs Chris and Xand van Tulleken

Food for Thought with Rhiannon Lambert

The Proof with Simon Hill

The Wellness Scoop with Ella Mills and Rhiannon Lambert

ZOE Science and Nutrition with Jonathan Wolf

Websites

BDA, www.bda.uk.com

Dietitians Australia, www.dietitiansaustralia.org.au

Dietitians of Canada, www.dietitians.ca

Eat Right, www.eatright.org

Food Facts, www.foodfacts.org

International Agency for Research on Cancer, www.iarc.who.int/news-events

Pub Med, pubmed.ncbi.nlm.nih.gov/30744710/

Rhitrition, www.rhitrition.com

The Soil Association, www.soilassociation.org/causes-campaigns/ultra-processed-foods

The World Healt,h Organization www.who.int

World Obesity, www.worldobesity.org/resources/journals

ZOE, zoe.com/learn

Find all scientific references for the information provided in this book here:

www.dk.com/uk/information/the-unprocessed-plate/

The publisher would like to thank the following for their kind permission to reproduce their data:

16 MDPI: Data of infographic: Rauber, F.; Da Costa Louzada, M.L.; Steele, E.M.; Millett, C.; Monteiro, C.A.; Levy, R.B. Ultra-Processed Food Consumption and Chronic Non-Communicable Diseases-Related Dietary Nutrient Profile in the UK (2008–2014). Nutrients 2018, 10, 587. https://doi.org/10.3390/nu10050587. **18-19 Cambridge University Press:** © The Author(s), 2023. Published by Cambridge University Press on behalf of The Nutrition Society / Data From: Dicken SJ, Qamar S, Batterham RL. Who consumes ultra-processed food? A systematic review of sociodemographic determinants of ultra-processed food consumption from nationally representative samples. Nutrition Research Reviews. 2024;37(2):416-456. doi:10.1017/S0954422423000240. **22 Nutritics, 2024:** Data From:Nutritics. (2024). Libro (v.09) [Mobile application software]. Dublin. Retrieved from https://www.nutritics.com. **24 Nutritics, 2024:** Nutritics. (2024). Libro (v.09) [Mobile application software]. Dublin. Retrieved from https://www.nutritics.com. **25 Food & Nutrition Research 2013:** Ravn A.-M., Gregersen N. T., Christensen R., Rasmussen L. G., Hels O., Belza A., Raben A., Larsen T. M., Toubro S., & Astrup A. (2013). Thermic effect of a meal and appetite in adults: an individual participant data meta-analysis of meal-test trials. Food & Nutrition Research. https://doi.org/10.3402/fnr.v57i0.19676. **59 Our World in Data | https://ourworldindata.org/:** Data From:Poore, J., & Nemecek, T. (2018). Reducing foods environmental impacts through producers and consumers. Science. – processed by Our World in Data. "Greenhouse gas emissions per kilogram [dataset]. Poore, J., & Nemecek, T. (2018). Reducing foods environmental impacts through producers and consumers. Science. [original data].

Index

A

added sugars 40–41, 48
addiction, UPFs and 22–23
additives 14, 26–33, 36, 65
    in baby formula 49
    effect on gut health 54, 55
    in processed meat 38
adult consumption of UPFs 16, 17, 45
air fryers 76
allergens 62, 63
almonds: chicken, date, and almond
    pilaf 166
anticaking agents 28, 47
antioxidants 29, 31, 44, 49, 53, 69, 73, 84
apples: apple, tahini, and cinnamon
    overnight oats 93
    fruit roll-ups 198
appliances 75, 76
aquafaba mayonnaise 207
ascorbic acid 65
aspartame 26, 41, 65
Atwater, Wilbur Olin 25
avocado: avocado chocolate mousse 191
    grapefruit salsa 140
    rainbow rice bowl 117
    the ultimate pasta salad 114

B

babies 44, 49, 52
baked beans 37
    baked beans with speedy hash
browns 102
balanced plates 70–71
bananas: berry banana ice pops 192
    wholesome banana muffins 100
basil: green pesto 211
beans 37, 46
    baked beans with speedy hash
    browns 102
    smoky tomato, pepper, and bean
    soup 121
    see also individual types of bean
beets: baked ricotta, beet, and walnut
traybake 139
    beetroot, dill, and yogurt dip 175
    rainbow rice bowl 117
berries: berry banana ice lollies 192
    berry blast overnight oats 92
    chia and berry jam 204
    frozen berry yogurt clusters 187
best by dates 63
beta carotene 65
black beans: shrimp tacos 140
the brain 22, 23, 54

bread 12, 13, 29, 36, 44, 73, 78
    cottage cheese bread 110
    easy yogurt flatbreads 179
    soda bread 97
breakfast 35, 74
broccoli: baked ricotta, beet, and walnut
    traybake 139
    super green soup 122
butter, spreadable 36
butterbeans: eggplant, tomato, and
    butterbean stew 158
    butterbean and onion dip 176
    roast butterbeans and chickpeas 214

C

Caesar salad, chicken 110
cake 35
    carrot and yogurt breakfast loaf 107
    courgette, miso, and olive oil cake 185
calories 24–25
cancer 36, 56–57
candy 37, 40, 79
capers: tartare sauce 208
carbohydrates 40, 44
    balanced plates 70, 71
    complex carbs 25, 42
    refined carbs 22, 23
    starchy carbs 51
    what to buy 73
carboxymethyl cellulose (CMC) 32
carcinogen classifications 56, 57
cardiovascular disease 41, 48, 54
carotenes 51
carrageenans 32
carrot and yogurt breakfast loaf 107
celery root: super green soup 122
celluloses 32
cereals 35, 40, 48, 64, 78
cheese: eggplant, tomato, and butterbean
    stew with baked feta 158
    salad bag pasta 147
    spanakopita pie 155
chermoula 161
chia and berry jam 204
chicken 40, 45
    chicken Caesar salad 110
    chicken, date, and almond pilaf 166
    chicken, pumpkin, and chickpea
    traybake 161
    sweet potato and chicken curry 136
chickpeas: chicken, pumpkin, and
chickpea traybake 161
    chili and mint hummus 174

    roast butter beans and chickpeas 214
children 44, 48, 49, 50–51, 65
chili and mint hummus 174
chocolate 22, 23, 79, 80
    avocado chocolate mousse 191
    chocolate and coffee overnight
    oats 93
    chocolate, peanut, and date bars 194
    dark chocolate and oat cookies 201
    frozen berry yogurt clusters 187
    nutty chocolate spread 205
Clément, Nicolas 24
climate change 58
coconut, date, and orange energy
    balls 197
coconut milk: coconut rice pudding with
    mango 188
    sweet potato and chicken curry 136
    triple protein dhal 152
coffee: chocolate and coffee overnight
    oats 93
convenience meals 35
collagen 46–47
colorings 27, 28, 29, 50, 54
cookies 37, 79
    dark chocolate and oat 201
cooking from scratch 74–77
cost of food 19, 42
cottage cheese: cottage cheese
    bread 110
    green fritters with whipped herby
cottage cheese 126
    spanakopita pie 155
crackers, seedy 175
creatine 46
Crohn's disease 32
cucumber raita 152
culture 19, 45
curry: eight veg curry 143
    sweet potato and chicken curry 136

D

dairy 51, 58, 73
dal, triple protein 152
dates: chicken, date, and almond pilaf 166
    chocolate, peanut, and date bars 194
    coconut, date, and orange energy
    balls 197
diabetes 37, 38, 43, 50, 65
diglycerides 32
dips: beet, dill, and yogurt dip 175
    butterbean and onion dip 176
    chilli and mint hummus 174
disordered eating 20

dopamine 22, 23
drinks 36, 40, 74, 79, 87

E

E-numbers 27, 32, 33
eggplant, tomato, and butterbean stew
    158
eggs: fridge-raid omelet muffins 105
    quinoa Niçoise salad 112
emulsifiers 12, 29, 32–33, 47, 49, 54, 65
endometriosis 52
energy balls, coconut, date, and
    orange 197
energy drinks 36
environment, effect of UPFs on 58–59
equipment 76–77
expiration dates 62

F

fast food 42–43
fats 25
    balanced plates 70, 71
    health halos 67, 73
    saturated fat 22, 23, 35, 45
    unsaturated fats 45, 67, 73
fennel: baked ricotta, beet, and walnut
    traybake 139
fertility, effect of UPFs on 52–53
fiber 17, 25, 51, 54, 55, 67
filo (phyllo) pastry: spanakopita pie 155
fish 36, 39, 84
    fish sticks, fries, and peas 168
    quinoa Niçoise salad 112
    seeded wholemeal fishcakes 156
flatbreads, easy yogurt 179
flavorings 12, 28, 29, 47, 65
folate 44, 65
folic acid 26, 44, 53, 65
food: building healthy relationships with
    20–21
    food addiction 22–23
    food matrix 17
    food poisoning 30
    food waste 58, 62, 84
    storage of 31
formula milk 44, 49
fortifiers 27
freezers 84–85
fridge-raid omelette muffins 105
fries 45
    fish sticks, fries, and peas 168
fritters, green 126
frozen berry yogurt clusters 187
fructose 40, 41
fruit 32, 42, 43, 55
    fruit-based snacks 36
    fruit roll-ups 198
    seasonal eating 68–69

spelt and oat pancakes 98
    what to buy 72
fruit juice 79

G

galactose 40
ginger and miso dressing 213
glucose 40, 41
glycerol 27, 65
granola 35
    seedy granola 95
grapefruit salsa 140
gravy 81
green beans: quinoa Niçoise salad 112
green fritters 126
green goddess dressing 213
green pesto 211
green sauce 139
greenhouse gases 58, 59
guar gum 26, 32
gut health 32, 37, 41, 42, 54–55

H

ham 38, 40
hash browns, speedy 102
hazelnuts: nutty chocolate spread 205
health claims, nutritional 66
health halos 66, 67
healthy eating, cost of 19
healthy relationships with food 20–21
heart disease 38, 39
herbs 54, 70, 81
    chermoula 161
    green goddess dressing 213
home cooking 74–77, 86
honey 80
hummus 35
    chilli and mint hummus 174
hydration 74, 87
hyperactivity 48

I

ice cream 33, 79
ice pops 192
immune function 54
infertility 52–53
ingredients: food labels 63, 64, 65
    processed culinary ingredients 12
    storing 82–83
    UPF-free 72–73, 80–81
insulin resistance 52, 56, 65
International Agency for Research on
Cancer (IARC) 56, 57

J

jams (jelly) 80
    chia and berry jam 204

K

ketchup 36, 81
    spiced tomato ketchup 206
kimchi: rainbow rice bowl 117

L

labels, food 62–67, 73
larb, tofu 131
lasagna, veggie-loaded 151
leaky gut 55
lecithin 32, 65
leeks: super green soup 122
leftovers 74, 84
legumes 45, 54
lemon: pork ragu with milk, lemon, and
sage 133
lentils: baked ricotta, beetroot, and walnut
traybake 139
    triple protein dal 152
    veggie-loaded lasagna 151
lettuce: chicken Caesar salad 110
    tofu larb 131
lime: mango and lime ice pops 192
low-density lipoprotein (LDL)
    cholesterol 35, 38
low-income households 18–19
lunch 50, 86

M

male fertility 52, 53
maltodextrin 65
mango: coconut rice pudding with
mango 188
    mango and lime ice pops 192
margarine 36
marketing 42
mayonnaise 36, 81
    aquafaba mayonnaise 207
meal planning 72, 74, 75, 86
meat 56, 58, 59
    plant-based meat 38
    processed meat 16, 36, 38, 44, 54,
    55, 65, 79
microplastics 59
microwaves 76
milk: pork ragu with milk, lemon, and
sage 133
milks, plant-based 35, 44
miso 80
    courgette, miso, and olive oil cake 185
    creamy miso and peanut butter
ramen 144
    ginger and miso dressing 213

miso-roasted nuts 181
monoglycerides 32
monosodium glutamate (MSG) 35, 65
Monteiro, Carlos 12
mousse, avocado chocolate 191
muffins 35
    fridge-raid omelette muffins 105
    wholesome banana muffins 100
mushrooms: roast mushrooms with
  polenta and salsa verde 165
    veggie-loaded lasagna 151

N

"natural" foods 34
Niçoise salad, quinoa 112
nitrates 36, 65
noodles 35
    creamy miso and peanut butter ramen
    144
    tahini noodle salad 125
NOVA classification 12, 23, 167
nut butters 80
nutrition: how our bodies metabolize 25
    nutritional health claims 66
nuts 17, 54
    miso-roasted nuts 181
    nutty chocolate spread 205
    seedy granola 95

O

oats 35
    cottage cheese bread 110
    dark chocolate and oat cookies 201
    overnight oats 92–93
    seedy granola 95
    spelt and oat pancakes 98
obesity 41, 48, 56
    and increase in UPF consumption 12,
    19, 35, 36, 42, 52
olive oil 73
    courgette, miso, and olive oil cake 185
omega-3 fatty acids 39, 51, 53, 67, 73, 84
omelette muffins, fridge-raid 105
on-the-go items 86
oranges: coconut, date, and orange
  energy balls 197
ovens 76
overeating 22, 23
overnight oats 92–93
oxidative stress 56, 59, 69

P

packaging 58, 59
palm oil 58
pancakes, spelt and oat 98
pasta: pork ragu with milk, lemon, and
  sage 133
    salad bag pasta 147

the ultimate pasta salad 114
    veggie-heavy pasta bake 163
    veggie-loaded lasagna 151
pasta sauces 36
pasteurization 14, 29
peanut butter: chocolate, peanut, and
  date bars 194
    creamy miso and peanut butter
ramen 144
    wholesome banana muffins 100
peas: fish sticks, fries, and peas 168
    green fritters with whipped herby
cottage cheese 126
    pearl spelt and pea risotto 134
    super green soup 122
    triple protein dhal 152
pectin 65
peppers: smoky tomato, pepper, and bean
  soup 121
    sweet and sour sticky tofu 171
pesto, green 211
pie, spanakopita 155
pilaf, chicken, date, and almond 166
pine nuts: green pesto 211
pineapple: sweet and sour sticky tofu 171
plant-based diets 38, 54, 55, 58, 73
plant-based milks 35, 44
plastics 58, 59
polenta: roast mushrooms with polenta
  and salsa verde 165
polycystic ovary syndrome (PCOS) 54
polysorbate 80 (P80) 32
popcorn 46
pops, ice 192
pork ragu with milk, lemon, and sage 133
portion control 70, 84
potatoes: seeded wholemeal
  fishcakes 156
    speedy hash browns 102
preservatives 29, 30–31, 43, 47, 65
privilege 18–19, 45
processed foods: additives 26, 33
    definition of 12–15
protein 44, 51, 84, 86
    balanced plates 70, 71
    content in UPFs 25
    health halos 67
    protein bars 36, 66
    protein powder 46, 47
    sources of 38–39
    what to buy 73
pumpkin: chicken, pumpkin, and chickpea
traybake 161

Q

quality ingredients 73
quinine yellow 65
quinoa Niçoise salad 112

R

ragu: pork ragu with milk, lemon, and sage
  133
rainbow rice bowl 117
raita, cucumber 152
ramen, creamy miso and peanut butter 144
rice: chicken, date, and almond pilaf 166
    coconut rice pudding with mango 188
    rainbow rice bowl 117
ricotta: baked ricotta, beet, and walnut
  traybake 139
risotto, pearl spelt and pea 134

S

salad dressings 87, 213
salad sprinkles 214
salads: chicken Caesar salad 110
    quinoa Niçoise salad 112
    salad bag pasta 147
    tahini noodle salad 125
    the ultimate pasta salad 114
salmon 22, 41
salsa, grapefruit 140
salsa verde 165
salt 25, 30, 31, 45, 67
sauces 44, 75, 79, 81
    see also individual sauces
sauerkraut: sour cream and sauerkraut
  dressing 213
sausages 36, 38
school lunches 50
scientific words 64
seafood 59
seasonal eating 68–69, 72
seeds 54
    overnight oats 92–93
    seeded wholemeal fishcakes 156
    seedy crackers 175
    seedy granola 95
    tamari seeds 214
selenium 39, 57
sell by dates 62
sensory properties of food 26
shelf-life 17, 26, 27, 32
shopping: average UPF content 34
    UPF-free 72–73
shrimp tacos with grapefruit salsa 140
slow cookers 76
smoky tomato, pepper, and bean soup 121
snacks 36, 48, 78, 87
soda bread 97
sodium benzoate (E211) 65
sodium nitrate (E251) 65

sorbitol 43
soup 35
    smoky tomato, pepper, and bean
soup 121
    soup sprinkles 214
    super green soup 122
sour cream and sauerkraut dressing 213
soy 58, 73
soy lecithin 49
soy sauce 81
spanakopita pie 155
Spector, Tim 6–7, 17
spelt: pearl spelt and pea risotto 134
    spelt and oat pancakes 98
spices 54, 70, 81
spinach: salad bag pasta 147
    spanakopita pie 155
    super green soup 122
spoilage 30, 31
spreads 79, 80
    nutty chocolate spread 205
spring onions: butterbean and onion
    dip 176
sprinkles, soup and salad 214
stabilizers 15, 29, 38
stevia 41
stew, aubergine, tomato, and
    butterbean 158
stock 81
store cupboards: ingredients 75, 80–81
    reorganizing 82–83
stovetops 76
strawberries: fruit roll-ups 198
    strawberries and cream overnight
        oats 92
sucrose 40
sugar 23, 40–42, 67
    content in UPFs 25, 35, 48
    free sugars 40–41, 45
super green soup 122
supplements 46–47
swaps 44, 78–79, 87
sweet and sour sticky tofu 171
sweet potatoes: fish fingers, chips, and
    peas 168
    sweet potato and chicken curry 136
sweeteners 27, 29, 40–41, 47, 54, 65
sweets 37, 79

T
tacos, shrimp 140
tahini: apple, tahini, and cinnamon
    overnight oats 93
    tahini noodle salad 125
tamari seeds 214
tartare sauce 208
thermic effect of food (TEF) 25
thickeners 29, 47, 65
toddlers 48
tofu: sweet and sour sticky tofu 171
    tofu larb 131
tomatoes: eggplant, tomato, and
    butterbean stew 158
    baked beans with speedy hash
browns 102
    quinoa Niçoise salad 112
    smoky tomato, pepper, and bean
soup 121
    spiced tomato ketchup 206
    the ultimate pasta salad 114
    veg-loaded lasagne 151
tortillas: shrimp tacos 140
    tortilla chips 176
trans-fats 45
traybakes: baked ricotta, beetroot, and
    walnut traybake 139
    chicken, pumpkin, and chickpea
traybake 161
tuna: quinoa Niçoise salad 112

U
ultra-processed foods (UPFs):
    addictiveness of 22–23
        additives 14, 26–33, 34, 38, 49, 54,
            55, 65
        adult consumption 15, 17, 45
        avoiding when out and about 86–87
        babies and children 48–51
        calories 24–25
        categorizing 16–17
        common everyday UPFs 34–35
        definition of 12–15
        easy swaps 78–79
        effect on fertility 52–53
        effect on gut health 54–55
        fast food 42–43
        impact on the environment 58–59
        link to cancer 56–57
        link to privilege 18–19
        most eaten UPFs 16
        occasional consumption of 44
        supplements 46–47
        who eats the most 18–19
    use by dates 62

V
vegetables 44, 45, 51, 54
    balanced plates 70, 71
    eight veg curry 143
    fridge-raid omelette muffins 105
    seasonal eating 68–69
    veggie-heavy pasta bake 163
    veggie-loaded lasagna 151
    what to buy 72
vitamins 67
    B vitamins 28, 51, 53
    vitamin A 51, 65
    vitamin C 51, 65, 69, 84
    vitamin D 51, 53, 84

W
walnuts: baked ricotta, beet, and walnut
    traybake 139
water 30, 59, 87
watercress: salad bag pasta 147
wheat flour, fortified 28
wholegrains 44, 45, 54, 73, 87
women and fertility 52–53
World Health Organisation (WHO) 28, 41,
    45, 50, 65
wraps 87

X
xantham gum 32

Y
yogurt 35, 40, 48, 64, 79
    beetroot, dill, and yogurt dip 175
    carrot and yogurt breakfast loaf 107
    cucumber raita 152
    easy yogurt flatbreads 179
    frozen berry yogurt clusters 187
    green goddess dressing 213
    tartare sauce 208

Z
zinc 51, 57
zucchini, miso, and olive oil cake 185

About the Author

Rhiannon Lambert is celebrated as one of the UK's leading practitioners in the complex field of nutritional science. Her stellar academic achievements, practical expertise as a nutritionist, authorship, and work as a podcast host have cemented her reputation as a trusted voice in the industry. Her philosophy is refreshingly simple: to empower individuals with evidence-based knowledge, enabling them to embrace a healthy lifestyle through the food they love and the lives they lead.

In 2016, Rhiannon founded **Rhitrition**, her private clinic on London's Harley Street. Rooted in scientific evidence, the clinic stands in sharp contrast to the sea of pseudoscience often promoted by fad diets. She has worked with both individuals and globally recognized brands – including Deliveroo, Wagamama, Samsung, Alpro, Yeo Valley, and Tesco – helping them transform how they think about and approach nutrition.

Registered with the Association for Nutrition, Rhiannon obtained a first-class degree in Nutrition and Health and a Master's degree in Obesity, Risks, and Prevention. She holds additional diplomas in sports nutrition and pre- and post-natal nutrition. She is a Master Practitioner in Eating Disorders, accredited by The British Psychological Society, and a Level 3 Personal Trainer. These qualifications reflect her comprehensive and multidisciplinary approach to health and nutrition.

A prolific author, Rhiannon has penned five books, two of which – *The Science of Plant-Based Nutrition* (2024) and *The Science of Nutrition* (2021) – achieved Sunday Times Bestseller status.

In 2018, Rhiannon launched her highly acclaimed podcast, *Food for Thought*. Offering practical, evidence-based advice for healthier living, the podcast has garnered enduring popularity with over 10 million downloads since its inception. Since 2025 Rhiannon has also co-hosted the hugely popular podcast *The Wellness Scoop* with Deliciously Ella founder, Ella Mills. Consistently ranked among the top nutrition podcasts, both shows have become a go-to resource for listeners seeking clarity amidst the noise of modern health trends. Her influence extends to Instagram, where her community of more than 450,000 followers engages with her relatable, science-backed content.

Expanding her mission, Rhiannon re-launched **Rhitrition+** in 2023, an innovative web-based supplement brand designed to cut through the misinformation that often clouds the supplement industry. Focused on products like Vegan Multivitamins, Vitamin D sprays for adults and children, and Pregnancy Multivitamins, the brand is a testament to Rhiannon's commitment to creating science-backed solutions for optimal health.

Among her many roles, Rhiannon cherishes her life as a wife and as a mother to two young boys, Zachary and Theodore, and her Cat Aurora. Balancing her personal and professional life, she remains dedicated to creating a brighter, healthier future for both people and the planet. Her work continues to inspire individuals and communities to make informed, sustainable choices in their journey towards better health.

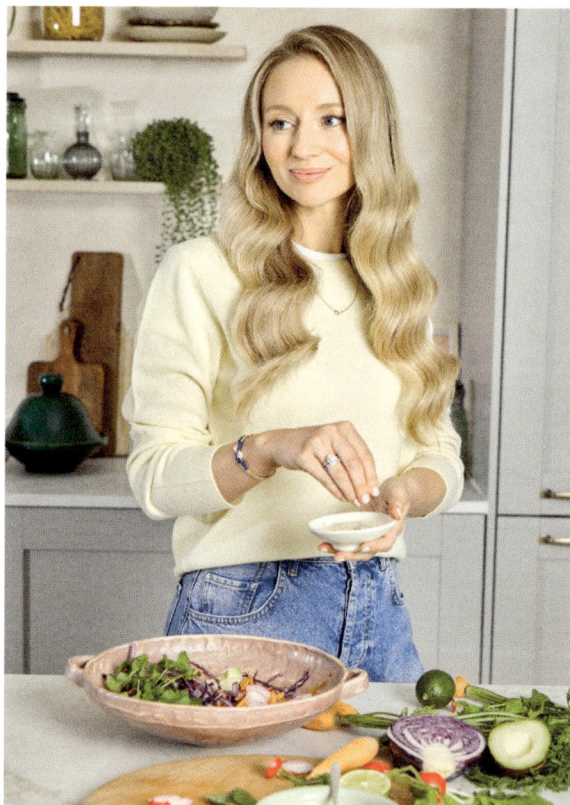

Acknowledgments

This book is dedicated to everyone who feels confused or overwhelmed by the conflicting nutrition messaging surrounding ultra-processed foods. It is the result of a collective mission, made possible by the incredible contributions of so many remarkable individuals.

To the exceptional team at DK, including Izzy, Cara, Harriet, Georgia, Clare, Tania, Holly, Charlie, and everyone working behind the scenes – thank you for your unwavering support in bringing this mission to life. Your dedication to empowering others through education is inspiring, and I am deeply grateful for all your hard work.

Thank you to Pam Lyddon, for her incredible enthusiastic, unwavering supportive work; Victoria Simmonds, the most amazing stylist, for assisting with the shoot days for this book; and to Melissa Oldridge my wonderful MUA, ensuring that even with no sleep I look awake when capturing all of the hard work that has gone into this book. Thank you also to Secret Spa, especially Claire L and Claire P, who have been there for me for the past ten years (I always appreciate the glow up!).

My heartfelt thanks also go to my fantastic Rhitrition team. Bryony Landricombe, your unwavering loyalty and support mean the world. Aoibhínn Connolly, your creative genius, passion, and drive have been instrumental in shaping this book. Maya Tu and Kitty Costelloe, your enthusiasm for our shared mission have been invaluable, and Ana Lopez, for your wonderful support over the past few years. The amazing Rhitrition clinic team, with a special thank you to Catherine Rabess RD for reviewing this book, her knowledge and expertise have given the book's gut health science the ultimate edge. A special mention must go to my right-hand woman, Abi Robertson – this book truly wouldn't have been possible without you, from the late nights working on text to the last-minute studies cropping up, I appreciate your help and support so much. Watching you all immerse yourselves in the latest scientific research with such genuine enthusiasm has been a joy to witness.

This has been one of the most challenging periods of my adult life, navigating motherhood and work in uncertain times. Balancing the demands of family life and business ownership has not been easy, but I feel incredibly fortunate to be surrounded by such an exceptional team who have supported me every step of the way.

Finally, to my family – thank you for your endless love and understanding. To my two little boys, Zachary and Theodore, you are my constant inspiration and the driving force behind my desire to make a positive contribution to the world.

Publisher's acknowledgments

DK would like to thank Georgia Levy for the recipe development, Sarah Epton for proofreading, and Vanessa Bird for indexing. DK would also like to thank Noor Ali for her design assistance, Dr. Ginger Hultin for her consultant work, and Harriet Webster and the team at Studio Noel for all their work on this project.

DK [RED] | Penguin Random House

Editorial Director Cara Armstrong
Project Editor Izzy Holton
Senior Designer Tania Gomes
Editorial Assistant Athena Stacy
Sales and Jackets Coordinator Emily Cannings
Senior Production Editor Tony Phipps
Senior Production Controller Stephanie McConnell
Art Director Maxine Pedliham
Publisher Stephanie Jackson

Editorial Harriet Webster
Designer Studio Noel
Photographer Claire Winfield
Recipe Developer Georgia Levy
Food Styling Holly Cowgill, Georgia Levy
Prop Styling Charlie Phillips
Food Styling Assistants Lu Cottle, Georgia Rudd
US Consultant Dr. Ginger Hultin DCN RDN CSO

First American Edition, 2025
Published in the United States by DK RED, an imprint of DK Publishing, a division of Penguin Random House LLC
1745 Broadway, 20th Floor, New York, NY 10019

Text copyright © Rhitrition Limited 2025

Rhiannon Lambert has asserted her right to be identified as the author of this work.

Copyright © 2025 Dorling Kindersley Limited
25 26 27 28 29 10 9 8 7 6 5 4 3 2 1
001-350622-Jun/2025

A catalog record for this book is available from the Library of Congress.
ISBN 979-8-2171-2646-0

DK books are available at special discounts when purchased in bulk for sales promotions, premiums, fund-raising, or educational use. For details, contact: DK Publishing Special Markets, 1745 Broadway, 20th Floor, New York, NY 10019
SpecialSales@dk.com

Printed and bound in Slovakia

www.dk.com

Disclaimer

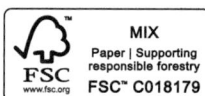

FSC MIX
Paper | Supporting responsible forestry
FSC™ C018179
www.fsc.org

This book was made with Forest Stewardship Council™ certified paper – one small step in DK's commitment to a sustainable future.

Learn more at www.dk.com/uk/information/sustainability